I bel[illegible]g to:-

=Judith A. Kirk=

MIDWIFERY

MIDWIFERY

Maureen A. Hickman
BA, SRN, SCM, MTD
Senior Midwifery Teacher
Somerset District School of Midwifery

SECOND EDITION

BLACKWELL SCIENTIFIC PUBLICATIONS
OXFORD LONDON EDINBURGH
BOSTON PALO ALTO MELBOURNE

Editorial offices:
Osney Mead, Oxford, OX2 0EL
8 John Street, London, WC1N 2ES
23 Ainslie Place, Edinburgh, EH3 6AJ
52 Beacon Street, Boston
Massachusetts 02108, USA
667 Lytton Street, Palo Alto
California 94301, USA
107 Barry Street, Carlton
Victoria 3053, Australia

First published 1978 as *Introduction to Midwifery*
Revised reprint 1980
Reprinted 1981
Second Edition 1985

Printed in Great Britain
by the University Press,
Cambridge

DISTRIBUTORS
USA
Blackwell Mosby Book Distributors
11830 Westline Industrial Drive
St Louis, Missouri 63141
Canada
Blackwell Mosby Book Distributors
120 Melford Drive, Scarborough
Ontario M1B 2X4
Australia
Blackwell Scientific Publications
(Australia) Pty Ltd
107 Barry Street, Carlton
Victoria 3053

British Library
Cataloguing in Publication Data

Hickman, Maureen A.
Midwifery.—2nd ed.
1. Obstetrics
I. Title
II. Hickman, Maureen A.
Introduction to midwifery
618.2 RG524

ISBN 0-632-01375-3

Contents

Preface, vii

Introduction
Basic terminology, 1
Prefixes used in obstetrics, 2
Abbreviations, 3
Definitions, 5
Pre-conception care, 7

Section I Normal Pregnancy, Labour and Puerperium
1 Menstrual Cycle, 13
2 Normal Pregnancy, 17
3 Anatomy and Physiology, 57
4 Management of Labour, 144
5 Management of the Puerperium, 163

Section II Abnormal Pregnancy, Labour and Puerperium
6 Abnormal Pregnancy, 171
7 Medical Disorders Associated with Pregnancy, 211
8 Abnormal Labour, 237
9 Abnormal Puerperium, 295

Section III The Fetus and Neonate
10 The Fetus, 309
11 The Neonate, 331
12 Neonatal Complications, 343

Section IV Associated Subjects
13 Sociological Aspects in Relation to Childbearing, 401
Classification of social class, 409
The National Health Service, 410
The social services, 426
The voluntary organisations, 442
Acts of Parliament, 443
Vital statistics, 444
14 Psychological Aspects in Relation to Childbearing, 458
Psychological aspects of pregnancy, labour and the postnatal period, 458

15 An Introduction to Genetics, 466
Genetics, 466
16 Medico-Legal Aspects in Relation to Childbearing, 478

Section V The Midwifery Profession
17 The History of Midwifery, 487
18 The Practice of Midwifery, 495
19 The Midwife, 502

Index, 505

Preface

The aim of this book is to provide student midwives with a comprehensive textbook arranged in a logical sequence. The book has five sections: the first section covers normal aspects of pregnancy, labour and the puerperium and the second the abnormalities that may occur. Section three relates to the fetus and neonate; section four deals with subjects associated with childbearing and section five with the midwifery profession.

I am grateful to the publishers for allowing me to extend the book, which has given me the opportunity to develop the existing material and introduce new subjects. As a result, it has been decided to change the title as being more appropriate to the extended content which includes chapters on sociological, psychological and medico-legal aspects associated with childbearing and an introduction to genetics.

I am indebted to many people for their constructive criticism and suggestions. I am especially grateful to Ruth White for her patience and skill in typing the manuscript.

Maureen Hickman

Introduction

Students coming to midwifery for the first time are faced with a host of new terms, which, whilst not exclusive to the subject, may not have been encountered before. I have incorporated the following lists of definitions, prefixes and abbreviations at the beginning of this book to remind the reader that it is important to understand the language of a subject in order to appreciate its meaning.

Basic terminology

This list is intended to deal only with very general terms. An explanation of the many other terms used will be given as they present in the text.

Gestation. Pregnancy.
Trimester. Three months.
Gravid. Pregnant.
Gravida (pl. ae). A term applied to a woman who is pregnant.
Primigravida (pl. ae). A woman who is pregnant for the first time.
Multigravida (pl. ae). Pregnant not for the first time.
Parous. Having borne one or more than one viable child.
Nullipara. A woman who has never borne a child.
Primipara (adj. ous). A woman who has borne one viable child.
Multipara (adj. ous). A woman who has borne more than one viable child.
Grand multipara. A woman who has borne five or more viable children.
Natal. Birth.
Antenatal. Before birth.
Prenatal. Before birth.
Postnatal. After birth.
Parturition. The birth process.
Antepartum. Before birth.
Intrapartum. During labour.
Postpartum. After birth.
Embryo. A term used to describe the fetus during its developmental phase.
Fetus. An unborn child.
Perinatal. Around birth.
Neonatal. Newborn.
Neonate. The baby during first month of life.

Infant. A child during the first year of life.
Cephalic. Pertaining to the head.
Vertex. That part of the fetal head between the anterior and posterior fontanelles and the two parietal eminences.
Zygote. Fertilised ovum produced by fusion of ovum and spermatozoon.

Prefixes used in obstetrics

An understanding of many words used in obstetric practice can be achieved if you learn the meaning of a few basic prefixes. Set out below are prefixes, their meaning and an example of their use in obstetric practice.

Ante (*before*). Antenatal; period before birth.
Auto (*self*). Autolysis; self-digestion.
Bi(s) (*having two, twice*). Bimanual examination; using two hands. Binovular (twins); from two ova.
Dys (*difficult*). Dystocia; abnormal uterine action.
Endo (*within, lining*). Endometrium; lining of the uterus.
Eu (*well*). Eutocia; normal uterine action.
Ex (*out of, without*). Extrauterine pregnancy; pregnancy outside the uterus.
Haem (*blood*). Haematoma; a collection of blood.
Hetero (*different*). Heterozygote (ous); an individual who has inherited contrasting members of a pair, or series, of genes.
Homo (*same*). Homozygote(ous); an individual who has inherited similar members of a pair, or series, of genes.
Hydro (*to do with water*). Hydrocephaly; a condition resulting from the accumulation of cerebrospinal fluid within the skull.
Hyper (*over, above*). Hypertonic uterine action; excessive uterine contractions.
Hypo (*under, below*). Hypotonic uterine action; weak uterine contractions.
Inter (*between*). Intertuberous; a pelvic diameter measured between the ischial tuberosities.
Intra (*within*). Intrapartum; during labour.
Mal (*bad*). Malpresentation; abnormal presentation.
Mega (*great*). Megaloblast; a primitive red blood cell.
Micro (*small*). Microcephaly; a small head.
Mono (*one, single*). Monozygotic; arising from one zygote.
Neo (*new*). Neonatal; newborn, baby within one month of birth.
Oligo (*little, less than normal*). Oligohydramnios; a deficiency in the amount of amniotic fluid.
Para (*alongside*). Parametrium; pelvic connective tissue at the side of the uterus.
Peri (*round about*). Perinatal mortality; stillbirths and deaths in the first week of life.

Poly (*much, many*). Polyhydramnios; excessive amount of amniotic fluid.
Post (*after*). Postpartum; after birth.
Pre (*before*). Prenatal; before birth.
Retro (*behind, backwards*). Retroplacental; behind placenta. Retroverted (uterus); the uterus that is tilted backwards.
Tri (*three*). Trimester; a period of three months.
Ultra (*lying beyond*). Ultrasound; beyond range of human hearing.
Uni (*one*). Uniovular (twins); from one ovum.

Abbreviations

The use of abbreviations leads to confusion and sometimes error. This list is included, not to encourage their use, but to help the newcomer to unravel the confusion their usage may create.

AF; artificially fed.
AFP; Alpha–fetoprotein.
AN, ANC; antenatal, antenatal clinic.
APH; antepartum haemorrhage.
ARM; artificial rupture of membranes.
BBA; born before arrival.
BF; breast fed.
Br; breech.
C; Celcius.
cm; centimetre.
CMB; Central Midwives Board.
CTG; cardiotocgraph.
Cx; cervix.
DTA; deep transverse arrest.
DVT; deep vein thrombosis.
ECV; external cephalic version.
EDD(C); expected date of delivery/confinement.
Eng; engaged.
F; Fahrenheit.
FBS; fetal blood sampling.
FD; forceps delivery.
FH(H); fetal heart (heard).
FSH; follicle stimulating hormone.
g; gram.
GTT; glucose tolerance test.
Hb; haemoglobin.
HCG; human chorionic gonadotrophin.
HDN; haemolytic disease of the newborn.

HPL; human placental lactogen.
HVS; high vaginal swab.
IPPV; intermittent positive pressure ventilation.
IU(C)D; intrauterine (contraceptive) device or death.
IUGR; intrauterine growth retardation.
K; menarche.
kg; kilogram.
LBW; low birth weight (baby).
LFD; light-for-dates (baby).
LH; luteinising hormone.
LMP; last menstrual period.
LMA (L) (P); left mentoanterior (lateral) (posterior) (position).
LOA (L) (P); left occipitoanterior (lateral) (posterior) (position).
LSA (L) (P); left sacroanterior (lateral) (posterior) (position).
L/S; lecithin sphingomyelin ratio.
LSCS; lower segment caesarean section.
LTH; luteotrophic hormone.
m; metre.
ml; millilitre.
MV; mentovertical (diameter).
ND; normal delivery.
NND; neonatal death.
OA; occipitoanterior position.
OF; occipitofrontal (diameter).
OFS; obstetric flying squad (the emergency obstetric unit).
OP; occipitoposterior position.
P_{CO_2}; symbol for carbon dioxide pressure.
P_{O_2}; symbol for oxygen pressure.
PE; pre-eclampsia or pulmonary embolism.
pH; a symbol used to denote the hydrogen ion concentration, and hence the degree of acidity or alkalinity of a solution.
PN (C); postnatal (clinic).
PNM (R); perinatal mortality (rate).
POP; persistent occipitoposterior (position).
PPH; postpartum haemorrhage.
PV; *per vaginum.*
RCM; Royal College of Midwives.
RDS; respiratory distress syndrome.
Rh; Rhesus.
RMA (L) (P); right mentoanterior or (lateral) (posterior).
ROA (L) (P); right occipitoanterior (lateral) (posterior).
RSA (L) (P); right sacroanterior (lateral) (posterior).
SB; stillbirth.

SCBU; Special Care Baby Unit.
SFD; small-for-dates (fetus).
SOB; suboccipitobregmatic (diameter).
SOF; suboccipitofrontal (diameter).
SMB; submentobregmatic (diameter).
STD; sexually transmitted disease(s).
SVD; spontaneous vaginal delivery.
TOL; trial of labour.
UKCC; United Kingdom Central Council.
VE; vaginal examination or vacuum extraction.
VD; venereal disease(s).
Vx; vertex.

Definitions

Included under this heading are definitions of words used that it would be inappropriate to define as part of the text. But an understanding of them may lead the student to a better knowledge of the subject as a whole.
Other more important words are defined as used, and are included in the index for reference.

Adnexa. Appendages; Adnexa uteri—ovaries and Fallopian tubes.
Agglutinin. A substance in the blood causing agglutination.
Aldosterone. A hormone secreted by the adrenal cortex.
Anabolism. Constructive metabolism; building up of body tissue.
Antibody. A protein appearing in the blood and body fluids in response to the stimulus of an antigen.
Antigen. Any substance which when introduced into the blood or tissues is capable of stimulating formation of antibody.
Asynclitism. Engagement of the fetal head with the sagittal suture anterior or posterior to the transverse diameter of the pelvic brim.
Atelectasis. The condition of incomplete expansion of the lungs.
Atresia. Absence or closure of a natural passage, e.g. anus or oesophagus.
Bacteraemia. The presence of bacteria in the bloodstream.
Bacteriuria. The presence of bacteria in the urine.
Bilirubin. A pigment found in bile; a breakdown product of haemoglobin.
Biology. The science dealing with the phenomena of life.
Catabolism. Destructive metabolism; breaking down of body tissue.
Caucasian. Person of European origin.
Congenital. Pertaining to a trait or quality present at birth.
Cytology. The science of the structure of cells.
Diastole. The moment in the heart cycle when the heart is in a state of relaxation. It occurs after atrial and ventricular systole.

Enzyme. A complex protein formed in the living cell, but able to act independently of the cell.
Endogenous. Growing from within.
Exogenous. Growing from outside.
Fibrin. An insoluble protein resulting from the interaction of fibrinogen with thrombin during the clotting of blood.
Gammaglobulin. The fraction of the blood globulin containing immune bodies.
Genotype. Classification of an individual according to the genes he has inherited.
Globin. A type of protein present in tissues.
Haemolysis. Destruction of red blood cells.
Heredity. The characteristics received by an individual at the fusion of ovum and spermatozoon.
Heterozygous. An individual who has inherited contrasting members of a pair, or series of genes.
Homozygous. An individual who has inherited similar members of a pair, or series of genes.
Hormone. A substance having a definite chemical composition, secreted in the cells of a gland and discharged directly into the bloodstream.
Hydraemia. Excess of water in the blood.
Hyperchromia. Abnormal increase in the colour of the cell due to an increase in the haemoglobin of the red blood cells.
Hypochromia. Decrease in the colour of the cell due to a decrease in the haemoglobin in the normal content of haemoglobin in the red blood cells.
Hyperplasia. An abnormal increase in the number of normal cells in a tissue.
Hypertrophy. Increase in size of an organ or structure.
Iatrogenic. Induced by effects of treatment.
Idiopathic. A disease of unknown origin.
Immune. Protected against a particular disease, either naturally, or by means of immunisation.
Immunoglobulin. See Gammaglobulin.
Isoimmunisation. Immunisation by an antigen.
Isotonic. Having the same tone or tension.
Isometric. Having equal length.
Lysis. Chemical destruction of cells.
Molecule. A unit particle of a substance.
Morbidity. The condition of suffering from a disease.
Mutation. A change in a gene or chromosome capable of producing a modification which can be inherited.
Necrosis. Death of tissue.
Non-Caucasian. Person of non-European origin.
Occult. Concealed, hidden.
Odema. An excessive accumulation of fluid in the tissue spaces.

Osmosis. The passage of a solvent through a semi-permeable membrane separating solutions of different concentrations.
Physiology. The science of function in living organisms.
Plasma. The fluid part of the blood in which the cellular elements are suspended.
Promontory. A process jutting out from a part of the body.
Racemose. Resembling a bunch of grapes.
Ratio. A numerical expression of the quantitative relationship between different factors or elements.
Reticulocyte. An immature blood cell.
Systole. The moment in the heart cycle when both ventricles are in a state of contraction and blood is injected into the pulmonary artery and aorta.
Thrombin. An enzyme which converts fibrinogen to fibrin, causing clotting of blood.
Vaccination. Inoculation with a vaccine.
Vasa. Vessels.

Preconception care

The idea that a woman (and her husband) should seek advice before conception is based on the knowledge that many of the abnormalities present in the baby at birth or revealed in the months and years after birth, are the result of damage caused early in pregnancy, including at the time of conception. This knowledge is not new, but the improvement in the standard and uptake of antenatal care, and other factors (see p. 449) have resulted in reduction of the stillbirth and infant mortality rates and this has brought morbidity into sharper focus.

In addition to the obvious congenital malformations many children suffer from hyperactivity and learning difficulties. Factors that are known to cause congenital defects are implicated in only 30–35% of cases; the remaining 65–70% are of unknown causes. Figures such as this raise many questions most of which remain unanswered. It seems likely that birth malformations have multifactorial causation with some factors more important than others. It is only by reducing the risk factors that it should, in time, be possible to identify the primary cause(s) in all cases.

It is probable that nutritional imbalance at the stage of organogenesis is one of the unknown factors. Recent research has shown that the incidence of neural tube defects in a group of women at high risk was 0.6% where they were given a multivitamin supplement compared with 5% in a control group of women not given the supplement. The supplement was taken at least twenty-eight days before conception and at least until the second missed period. The supplement included Vitamins A, C and D with vitamins from the B group, folic acid, iron, calcium and phosphate, and therefore leaves unanswered the question which of these is or are important? Hibberd and Smithells in 1965 reported a link between folate deficiency and neural tube deficiency, thus giving an indication for future research.

It seems inevitable that when the benefits of antenatal care in the second and third trimesters of pregnancy had reached a plateau, the attention should move to the first trimester, and from there eventually to the pre-pregnant/pre-conception state. Foresight—The Association for the Promotion of Pre-Conceptual Care, is responsible for much of the awareness within the professions and among prospective parents, for the need for this new approach to care. But who are the professions who should be involved? Certainly general practitioners, but why not midwives and obstetricians?

Major stages in development of the embryo will have already taken place before most women seek professional advice, and therefore much of the future pattern of development of the individual will already have been decided. For example, the neural tube normally closes approximately twenty-five days after conception. Therefore, damage to this structure may already have been caused before most women would consider seeking confirmation of the pregnancy.

Many of the routine investigations and tests performed at booking are used to exclude/detect abnormality, but as such must be considered as only secondary to prevention, especially as they are not without hazard. For example, the recent introduction of routine/selective screening of women for raised serum alphafetoprotein may need to be followed by amniocentesis to confirm/exclude neurotubal abnormality; a procedure that is not without risk to the fetus (see p. 474), which may be normal. Also, if abortion is recommended, this procedure is not without hazard to the woman (see p. 176), particularly as it is usually performed beyond the time of optimal safety.

The need to reduce further the risks to the fetus has focused attention on the pre-pregnancy state. Much of the advice given to the woman early in pregnancy is also appropriate in preparation for pregnancy, and in most cases is more timely when given before conception.

1 Contraception. The introduction of effective methods of contraception had made it possible for pregnancies to be planned and therefore pre-conception care a realistic idea. But as so often happens the very method that assists can also have disadvantages; for example, oral contraceptives affect absorption by the body of essential minerals, therefore advice on alternative methods of contraception may be indicated for a period of time before conception. A barrier method used in conjunction with a spermicidal lubricant is a good alternative choice (see p. 419).

2 Diet. The refining of foods leads to the removal of nutrients that are essential for health, therefore dietary advice should stress the importance of whole foods as well as fresh fruit and vegetables. Experimental evidence has shown that deficiencies in both water and fat soluble vitamins can have an adverse effect upon the fetus.

3 Alcohol readily crosses the placenta and circulates in the fetal blood in the same concentrations as in the expectant mother's blood. Maternal alcohol consumption is now recognised as potentially harmful to the fetus (see p. 41).

4 Smoking. The adverse effects of smoking on the fetus are well recognised; carbon monoxide interferes with the uptake of oxygen and therefore oxygenation of the fetus and thus with its growth. The nicotine content of tobacco causes vasoconstriction of maternal and fetal blood vessels resulting in decreased uteroplacental blood flow contributing to fetal growth retardation.

Smoking also depresses the appetite and therefore has an adverse effect on dietary intake. In men, smoking lowers testosterone levels and effects spermatogenesis resulting in an increase in chromosomal aberrations.

5 Drugs. When considering the harmful effects of drugs on the conceptus and developing embryo, there are several situations that need to be given consideration. The one that has received most publicity is taking drugs to relieve nausea and vomiting in the early weeks of pregnancy. But in addition to this the intermittent use of medication must be discussed as well as routine use of drugs in the treatment of a chronic illness. The woman should be advised not to take any drug unless it is specifically prescribed for her, and to discuss her plans for pregnancy with her general practitioner so that he is fully aware of the situation.

6 Pre-existing disease. Where a woman (or her husband) has a disease or a family history of disease, medical advice should be sought, so that the risks can be discussed. In the case of prescribed drugs a review of the treatment should be made to take an account of the planned pregnancy. It may not be appropriate to change the treatment and therefore any risks should be discussed, or if there are no risks reassurance can be given.

7 Rubella. The harmful effects of the rubella virus on the embryo and developing fetus are well recognised (see p. 372). It is, therefore, an important aspect of pre-conception care to test the woman for immunity and to give the rubella vaccine if indicated. The importance of not conceiving until at least eight weeks after vaccination must be stressed and suitable methods of contraception discussed.

8 Dental care. It would be appropriate for the woman to have a dental check and treatment prior to pregnancy so that X-rays that are often used to assist in locating dental caries, are not used in pregnancy, and septic foci, which undermine the health and are a potential hazard, are treated.

9 Environmental factors are becoming increasingly important as we are made more aware of the potentially harmful substances in the atmosphere. To advise a woman to take exercise in the fresh air presupposes the air is unpolluted, but comparisons of blood lead concentrations of people living in urban and rural areas showed a significant difference.

10 Emotional security. A happy, secure, loving environment is surely every woman's right when she is carrying and caring for a baby. Teaching the

partner to fulfil his role in meeting the woman's needs is another important aspect of pre-natal care. Enlisting his cooperation may be crucial in persuading the woman to take a particular course of action.

Indications are that it is important to give attention to the general health and nutritional status of prospective parents before a child is conceived as well as the expectant mother during pregnancy. As more is learned of the factors which have the potential to harm the ovum and sperm, before conception and the embryo and fetus before birth, pre-conception advice will become more specific.

SECTION I

NORMAL PREGNANCY, LABOUR AND PUERPERIUM

Chapter 1
Menstrual Cycle

It is important to have an understanding of the menstrual cycle before learning about pregnancy, for it is an interruption in this cycle, manifested by amenorrhoea, that leads most women to suspect that they are pregnant, and to consult their doctor.

The menstrual cycle involves (Fig. 1.1):

1 The cerebral cortex which controls the hypothalamus by producing the gonadotrophin releasing factor.

2 The hypothalamus which is concerned with the rhythmical control of the ovarian-menstrual cycle. It produces follicle stimulating and luteinising hormone releasing factors which act on the anterior lobe of the pituitary gland.

3 The anterior lobe of the pituitary gland produces follicle stimulating hormone which causes ripening of the Graafian follicles, and luteinising hormone which, combined with follicle stimulating hormone causes ovulation and subsequently maintains the corpus luteum.

4 The ovaries secrete oestrogens from the Graafian follicle and oestrogens and progesterone from the corpus luteum. These ovarian hormones bring about changes in the endometrium and myometrium.

5 The uterus. Menstrual, proliferative and secretory changes occur in the endometrium and contraction of the myometrium takes place.

The menstrual cycle is closely associated with the ovarian cycle, and the physiological purpose of the ovarian-menstrual cycle is ovulation which takes place fourteen days prior to menstruation. Menstruation is the physiological bleeding from the endometrium at regular intervals from puberty to the menopause. The menstrual cycle extends from the first day of menstruation to the day prior to commencement of the next menstrual flow. The average cycle lasts for twenty-eight days and is divided into three phases as follows:

1 Menstrual phase. The endometrium is shed down to its basal layer. It degenerates due to spasm of the arteries and deprivation of blood flow. Necrosis occurs and the lining is expelled by contraction of the myometrium under the influence of oestrogens. It lasts for about five days during which time 50–100 ml of blood are lost.

2 Proliferative phase. Regeneration of the tubular glands and stroma of the endometrium occurs from the basal layer, and is under the influence of oestrogens from the developing Graafian follicle. It lasts for about ten days.

In a prolonged or short cycle it is the proliferative phase that is extended or shortened, not the secretory phase.

3 Secretory phase. The tubular glands become tortuous and produce secretions under the influence of oestrogens and progesterone from the corpus luteum. This phase lasts for fourteen days.

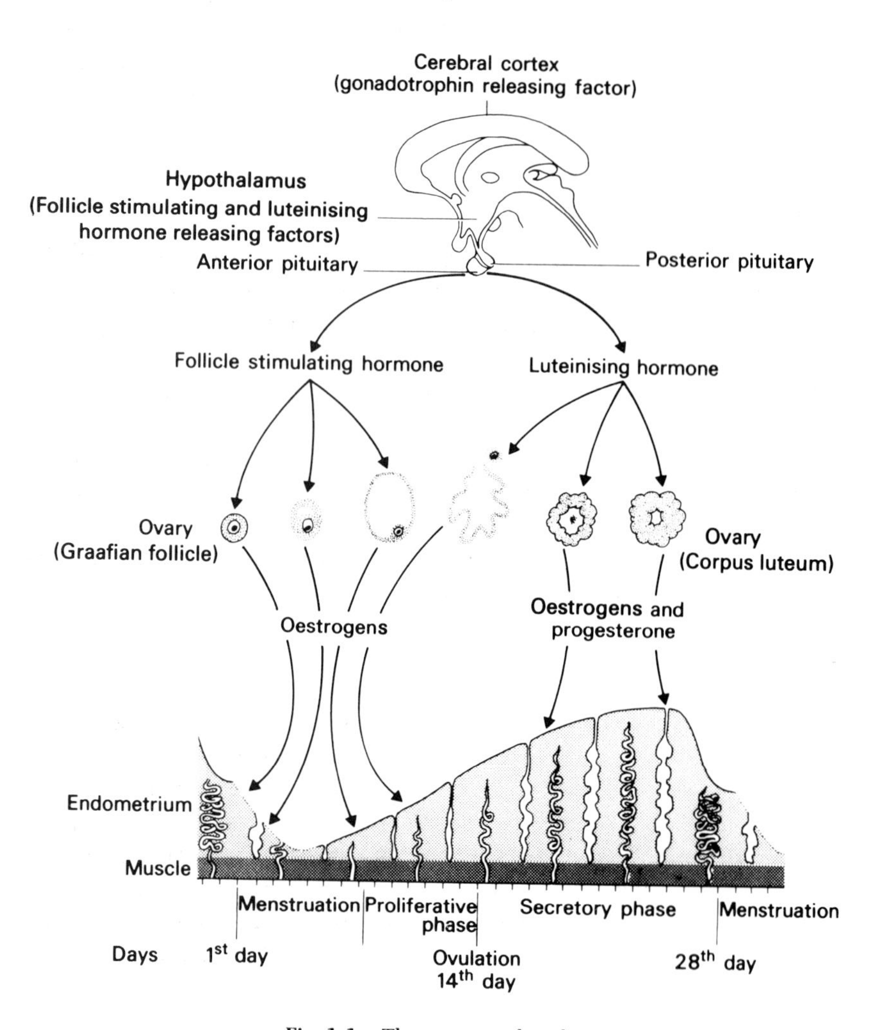

Fig. 1.1 The menstrual cycle.

Ovulation and fertilisation

Maturation of the ovum

Prior to ovulation the ovum undergoes maturation. Division of the ovum occurs and the chromosomes in the cell nucleus are reduced from forty-six to twenty-three. The two resultant cells, which are unequal in size, are the ovum which resembles the original ovum in size and the first polar body which is very small (see p. 467).

Ovulation

The ovum surrounded by the discus proligerus (see p. 84) is expelled into the peritoneal cavity and received into the fimbrial end of the Fallopian tube.

The empty follicle collapses, bleeding occurs into the cavity and the granulosa cells proliferate. The structure, known as the corpus luteum, produces oestrogens and progesterone which bring about the secretory changes in the endometrium.

The fact that ovulation has taken place is indicated by a rise in the basal temperature. If ovulation is followed by fertilisation this rise of temperature persists into pregnancy. If fertilisation does not take place, the corpus luteum degenerates to become the corpus albicans, progesterone levels fall and menstruation occurs fourteen days after ovulation.

Fertilisation

This usually occurs in the ampulla of the Fallopian tube within twenty-four hours of ovulation. Following fertilisation the second maturation division takes place, the second polar body is extruded, and the female pronucleus is formed. The resultant cell, the zygote, undergoes division producing two cells of equal size. Cell division continues until the structure comprises a mass of equal-sized cells called the morula. It is important to note that the morula is the same size as the original ovum and, therefore, is able to pass along the Fallopian tube. Fluid develops between the cells, and the structure is now known as a blastocyst.

While these changes are taking place the ovum is passing along the Fallopian tube towards the uterine cavity. The passage through the tube is effected as a result of movement of the cilia and peristaltic contractions.

The blastocyst enters the uterine cavity about six days after ovulation or five days after fertilisation.

Before the blastocyst is ready to embed in the endometrium, the cells undergo a process of rearrangement. A capsule of cells develops and is known as the trophoblast, and the remaining cells form a clump at one end of the blastocyst known as the inner cell mass. The cells of the trophoblast produce a hormone—human chorionic gonadotrophin.

This hormone maintains the corpus luteum until the placenta takes over the production of oestrogens and progesterone. It suppresses the production of follicle stimulating and luteinising hormones by the anterior lobe of the pituitary gland, and forms the basis of immunological tests of pregnancy (see p. 20).

The blastocyst embeds in the endometrium eight days after ovulation and seven days after fertilisation. Thus, with the levels of oestrogens and progesterone maintained, amenorrhoea, one of the earliest signs of pregnancy occurs.

It is perhaps interesting to note at this stage the effects of oral contraceptives on the ovarian-menstrual cycle. They prevent the anterior lobe of the pituitary gland producing follicle stimulating hormone, thus suppressing ovulation; there is rapid regeneration and then atrophy of the endometrium; and the cervical mucus remains thick and hostile to spermatozoa. A more detailed description of these changes is included later (see pp. 417–18).

Chapter 2
Normal Pregnancy

Signs and symptoms of pregnancy

Pregnancy results in changes not only in the genital tract but in the woman's body as a whole.

These physiological changes, due mainly to hormonal, circulatory and metabolic factors, are responsible for the signs and symptoms by which pregnancy is recognised and the minor disturbances about which women seek reassurance.

The signs and symptoms of pregnancy and their causes can be considered in many ways but it is perhaps more practical to relate them to the period of pregnancy at which they present.

Early pregnancy (first trimester)

AMENORRHOEA

This may be physiological when it occurs as the result of pregnancy (see p. 16) or the menopause, or pathological. If pathological it may be due to:

1 a severe debilitating disease, e.g. anorexia nervosa;
2 endocrine disorders such as hypothyroidism or adrenogenital syndrome;
3 emotional stress.

NAUSEA AND VOMITING

Morning sickness is present in about half of all pregnancies, usually appearing about the sixth to eighth week. Characteristically, the woman vomits a small quantity of fluid on rising in the morning and for the rest of the day is not sick. Sometimes the vomiting is more frequent, occurring two or three times during the day. Sometimes only nausea is complained of. This vomiting produces no ill effects; the woman does not feel ill, nor lose weight and only rarely does ketosis present. Very occasionally the vomiting is so pronounced that it becomes pathological. It is then termed hyperemesis gravidarum (see p. 188).

BREAST CHANGES (Fig. 2.1)

The earliest symptom is a feeling of fullness, the breasts are also tense and tender and a tingling sensation is noted. This is apparent at about four weeks. The breasts become nodular by about the sixth week, due to increased

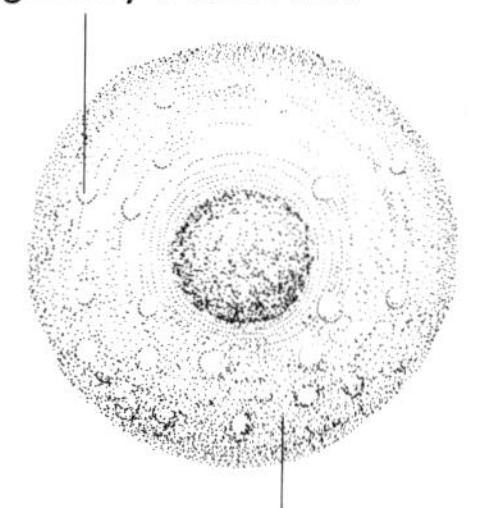

Fig. 2.1 Early breast changes.

vascularity possibly as a result of progesterone. By the eighth week of pregnancy the superficial veins become more prominent and a venous network becomes apparent. By the twelfth week the nipples are more prominent and there is a fullness of the areola.

In a primigravida, the pink colour of the areola changes to brown and is most marked in brunettes. This is referred to as the primary areola and is accompanied by enlargement of the sebaceous glands situated in the deeper layers of the skin. These are known as Montgomery's tubercles. They appear as fifteen to twenty raised spots paler than the surrounding areola and secrete sebum to lubricate the nipple. These signs are more marked in the primigravida as many of them persist following pregnancy and, therefore, the changes are less obvious in subsequent pregnancies.

FREQUENCY OF MICTURITION

The bladder is indented by the growing anteverted uterus and cannot therefore contain a normal amount of urine, resulting in the necessity for frequent emptying of the bladder. This is aggravated by an increased fluid intake and blood supply, and stretching of the urethral sphincter allowing small amounts of urine to escape into the urethra. This makes the woman feel she wants to pass urine.

THE VAGINA

Due to the increased vascularity the vagina is observed to be a violet colour. This is known as Jacquemier's sign. There is also an increase in the vaginal secretions.

THE CERVIX

Softening can be detected round the internal os as early as the sixth week. The cervix is seen to have the same purple discolouration as the vagina.

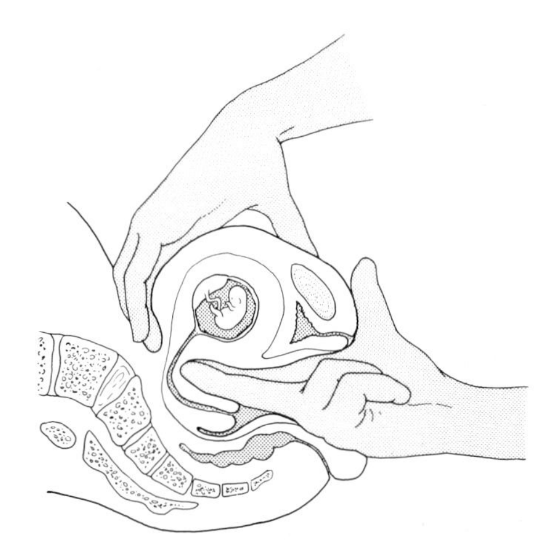

Fig. 2.2 Hegar's sign.

HEGAR'S SIGN (Fig. 2.2)

This sign is present from the sixth to the tenth week. It is dependent on the enlargement and softening of the uterus and cervix, caused by pregnancy, and the fact that in the early stages the developing embryo does not completely fill the uterine cavity (see p. 88).

On bimanual examination, the body of the uterus is found to be soft, cystic and enlarged, while at the junction of the cervix and body an empty area is felt so that the fingers on the abdomen and the fingers in the anterior fornix come into close contact.

Pulsation of the uterine arteries, Osiander's sign, can be detected by digital examination of the lateral fornices.

PIGMENTATION

This is a manifestation of hormonal activity and is due to an increase in the melanin stimulating hormone from the pituitary gland. In addition to the pigmentation of the breasts already mentioned, deposits of pigment also occur in other places, especially on the face, abdomen and vulva. On the face, a mask-like area of pigmentation covering the forehead and upper part of the cheeks is seen. This is known as the chloasma. On the abdomen the linea nigra may be noted. It extends from the symphysis pubis to the umbilicus, and when well marked encircles the umbilicus and extends upwards towards the xiphisternum.

ULTRASONOGRAPHY

Pregnancy can be visualised at five weeks and the fetal heart seen to beat seven to eight weeks after the last menstrual period.

PREGNANCY TESTS

Laboratory tests for pregnancy depend on the presence of human chorionic gonadotrophin in the urine. This hormone is present in the urine as early as eight days after the first missed period. An early morning specimen of urine is used as human chorionic gonadotrophin is present in higher concentration and is therefore less likely to produce a false negative result.

IMMUNOLOGICAL TESTS

These tests depend on the fact that human chorionic gonadotrophin has antigenic properties.

Gravindex. Latex foam particles are coated with human chorionic gonadotrophin and exposed to the urine to which antiserum has been added. If agglutination occurs, the urine contains no gonadotrophin and the test is negative. If agglutination does not occur, gonadotrophin is present and the test is positive. A single drop of urine gives the result in two minutes and is 92% acurate.

Prognosticon, Prepuerin. Sensitised red cells are added to 8 ml of urine. The test is positive if agglutination does not occur.

Midpregnancy (second trimester)

AMENORRHOEA

This persists; the space between the decidua vera and the decidua capsularis is obliterated by the developing gestational sac and the two layers fuse together. Any bleeding occurring at this stage is pathological and usually indicates threatened abortion (see p. 172).

NAUSEA AND VOMITING

This should disappear before the sixteenth week resulting in a feeling of wellbeing.

BREAST CHANGES

After the sixteenth week of pregnancy a milky secretion can be expressed from the breasts. This is called colostrum and is a precursor of milk which persists until about three days after the birth of the baby.

A secondary areola (Fig. 2.3) may appear in some women at about the twentieth week. This extends to a varying depth beyond the primary areola but is different in that it is a mottled pigmentation which fades after the baby is born.

UTERINE GROWTH

The uterus rises out of the pelvis during the thirteenth week and thereafter continues to rise so that it reaches a point just above the umbilicus at the twenty-fourth week of pregnancy.

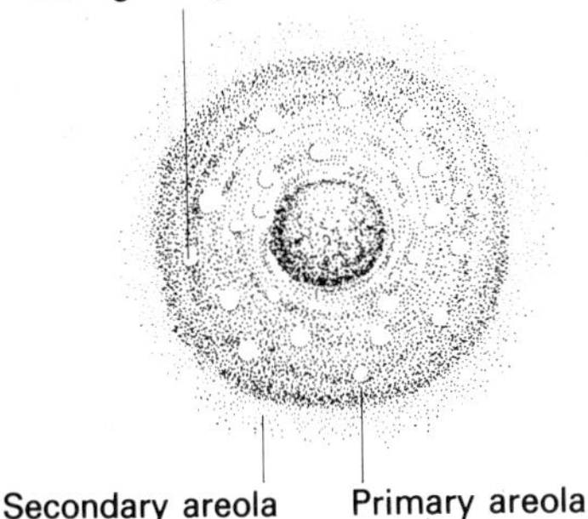

Fig. 2.3 Secondary areola.

BRAXTON HICKS CONTRACTIONS

These are present from about the sixteenth week and increase in intensity as pregnancy progresses. They are painless, irregular, uterine contractions of short duration and have the effect of increasing the uterine blood flow to the placenta.

QUICKENING

Fetal movements will be experienced by the woman during this period of pregnancy and the term quickening is used to describe the first movements felt. A multigravida who has experienced quickening before, may be aware of these movements between sixteen and twenty weeks, but a primigravida who has not experienced quickening may not be aware of them until eighteen to twenty-two weeks. The fetus, however, moves long before sixteen weeks, but it is not until the movements are more vigorous and reflected on the abdominal wall that they are experienced by the expectant mother.

UTERINE SOUFFLE

About the twenty-fourth week the uterine souffle can be heard. It is a blowing sound, synchronous with the maternal pulse, and is due to the blood circulating through the enlarged uterine arteries.

INTERNAL AND EXTERNAL BALLOTTEMENT

Internal ballottement may be demonstrated after the eighteenth week by moving the examining finger sharply upwards in the anterior fornix. The fetus is thus displaced in the amniotic fluid and descends on the examining finger. About the twenty-fourth week external ballottement can be demonstrated.

FETAL HEART SOUNDS

After the twenty-fourth week the fetal heart may be heard. The beat is about 140/min, and not synchronous with the maternal pulse.

X-RAY EXAMINATION

The presence of a fetus can be shown by X-ray at the sixteenth week but in view of the risk of radiation to the fetus and the introduction of ultrasound (see p. 317) this investigation is no longer used.

Late pregnancy (third trimester)

AMENORRHOEA

Amenorrhoea persists. Any bleeding occuring at this stage usually indicates antepartum haemorrhage (see p. 179).

UTERINE GROWTH

The growing uterus now fills the abdominal cavity, displacing the intestines (Fig. 2.4). This accounts for the breathlessness on exertion of which the woman frequently complains. This is relieved when the presentation engages in the pelvis at about thirty-six weeks in a primigravida, and the thirty-eighth week or later in the multigravida. Hence the term lightening is used to describe the lowering of the fundus and the consequent relief from pressure on the diaphragm.

FREQUENCY OF MICTURITION

Pressure of the fetal head on the bladder results in frequency of micturition in late pregnancy.

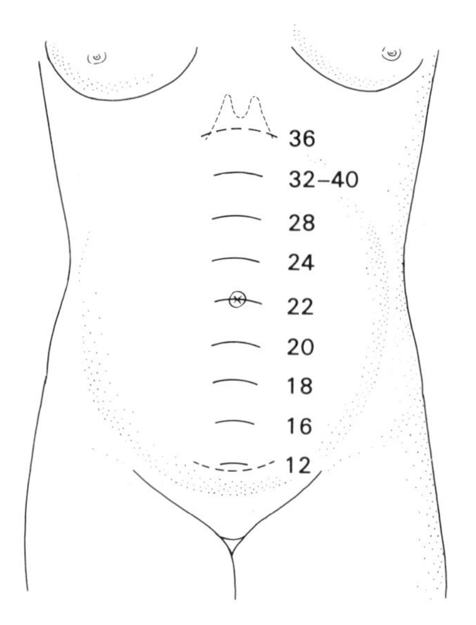

Fig. 2.4 Height of fundus uteri at various weeks of pregnancy.

Summary of signs and symptoms of pregnancy

Possible

Although these signs and symptoms are associated with pregnancy, they also present in association with other conditions and there is therefore, only a possibility that the woman is pregnant. However, a combination of these signs and symptoms in women of childbearing age makes the diagnosis a strong probability.
Amenorrhoea.
Nausea and vomiting.
Breast changes: fullness, tenderness, tingling at four weeks; enlargement, nodular at six weeks; venous network at eight weeks; primary areola, Montgomery's tubercles at the twelfth week; colostrum at the sixteenth week; secondary areola at the twentieth week.
Frequency of micturition: early, sixth to twelfth week; late, from thirty-sixth week.
Quickening: multigravida, sixteen to eighteen weeks; primigravida, eighteen to twenty-two weeks.
Pigmentation of skin: breasts, primary areola at twelve weeks, secondary areola at sixteen weeks; abdomen, linea nigra; vulva; face, chloasma.

Probable

These signs are most likely to be present as a result of pregnancy but may also be found in other conditions.
Cervix: softening, violet discolouration.
Jacquemier's sign.
Osiander's sign.
Hegar's sign: sixth to tenth week.
Uterine growth.
Braxton Hicks contractions: from sixteen weeks.
Internal ballottement: eighteenth week.
External ballottement: twenty-four weeks.
Uterine souffle.
Positive pregnancy test.

Positive

By their very nature these signs are only found in association with pregnancy.
Fetal heart sounds: twenty-four to twenty-six weeks.
Fetal movement felt or seen by observer.

Palpation of fetal parts.
Ultrasonography: pregnancy; fetal heart, eight to nine weeks.
X-ray demonstration of fetal bones; sixteenth week.

Minor disorders of pregnancy

The minor disorders of pregnancy are those which in themselves do not endanger the life of the pregnant woman or fetus. Nonetheless they must not be ignored as they may interfere with sleep and nutrition, and may undermine the woman's general health and wellbeing.

FREQUENCY OF MICTURITION

The bladder is indented by the growing anteverted uterus during the first twelve weeks of pregnancy and cannot therefore contain a normal amount of urine resulting in the necessity for frequent emptying of the bladder. This is spontaneously relieved when the uterus rises out of the pelvic cavity.

An increased fluid intake causing polyuria, and stretching of the urethral sphincter allowing small amounts of urine to escape into the urethra, aggravates the condition. It may recur in late pregnancy when the fetal head descends into the pelvis.

NAUSEA AND VOMITING

The effects and various aspects of morning sickness have already been described above (see p. 17). Vomiting ceases spontaneously before the sixteenth week of pregnancy in nearly all cases, without any treatment. However, many women seek the advice of their general practitioner, and an antiemetic may be prescribed, although where possible the use of drugs in early pregnancy should be avoided.

The woman is advised to eat a dry biscuit or dry toast before rising in the morning and to avoid fatty or highly seasoned food.

The cause of the nausea and vomiting, which is more common in primigravidae, is not known, but it may be related to the increased levels of hormones to which the woman gradually becomes adjusted.

HEARTBURN

This is a burning pain caused by regurgitation into the oesophagus of acid stomach contents. It occurs because of relaxation of the cardiac sphincter of the stomach during pregnancy, due to the effects of progesterone. Small frequent meals and alkaline preparations such as mixture of magnesium trisilicate, Aludrox or Gastrils help to relieve the condition by neutralising the acidity of the stomach contents.

CONSTIPATION

This is due to a reduction in peristalsis caused by the relaxing effect of progesterone on smooth muscle. Common sense advice about regular habits, taking sufficient fluids and fruit and vegetables is often all that is needed. Aperients, if needed, should be mild such as Senokot. Liquid paraffin should not be used as this prevents absorption of the fat-soluble vitamins A, D, E and K.

VARICOSE VEINS

Varicose veins may appear for the first time during pregnancy, or may become worse if already present. They usually develop in the legs, anal canal or on the vulva. General causes include relaxation of smooth muscle in the vein walls due to progesterone, pressure and increased uterine blood flow resulting in pelvic congestion.

Varicose veins of the legs. The venous pressure in the legs is increased during pregnancy and this is aggravated by weight gain as pregnancy advances. The legs ache and oedema and irritation may occur. The woman is advised to avoid standing for long periods, to rest with her legs elevated and wear supportive tights or if more severe, elastic stockings. These women are more prone to thrombophlebitis and phlebothrombosis (see p. 299).

Varicose veins of the vulva. These may be supported and discomfort eased, by a firm pad. Particular care must be taken in labour if an episiotomy is performed as severe bleeding can occur.

Haemorrhoids. These are further aggravated by constipation, therefore, management involves prevention or treatment of the problem. Anusol suppositories and cream may be applied to give relief and nupercaine ointment used if irritation is a problem. Haemorrhoids may prolapse during delivery due to pressure from the fetal head.

BACKACHE

Backache is a common disorder of pregnancy, partly because the changes of posture that occur cause extra stress on the muscles along the spinal column, and partly because of the softening of ligaments round the lower back and sacroiliac region which happens in response to the release of hormones in the later stages of pregnancy.

Most low back problems are related in some way to how the woman carries her weight. During the latter weeks of pregnancy the weight of the gravid uterus tends to cause lordosis, therefore advice regarding correct posture is important preventative treatment. The woman is advised to sleep on a firm mattress, and, when sitting, to use an upright chair.

CRAMP

Muscular cramp in the calves of the legs, feet and sometimes thighs is not uncommon in mid to late pregnancy especially occurring at night. The cause of the cramp is unknown but it has been attributed to deficiency in sodium, calcium and vitamin B. Temporary relief may be experienced in an attack of cramp by dorsiflexing the foot and massaging the cramped muscle.

PRURITIS VULVAE

Irritation of the vulva may occur in pregnancy. The usual cause is vaginal discharge which may be due to an excess of the normal secretions or to an infection with *Candida* or *Trichomonas* (see p. 232). Glycosuria may also cause pruritis vulvae but in many cases no cause can be assigned.

FAINTING

This may occur in early pregnancy due to vasomotor instability, hypoglycaemia or cerebral vasoconstruction due to a low arterial P_{CO_2} caused by over-breathing. In late pregnancy it may be due to the supine hypotension syndrome (see p. 28).

Serious conditions such as anaemia, ectopic pregnancy and heart disease must be excluded.

PALPITATIONS

Awareness of the heart beat because of increased stroke volume may occur in pregnancy. A rise of 15 beats/min is normal but a resting tachycardia greater than this may indicate diseases such as anaemia, thyrotoxicosis or heart disease.

PARAESTHESIA

In late pregnancy tingling and numbness of the hands and fingers, especially on waking, is often observed. Some of these cases are due to carpal tunnel syndrome which is associated with oedema causing compression of the median nerve, and such cases may be relieved by giving a short course of diuretics. In most cases complete recovery takes place after delivery.

BRACHIAL NEURALGIA

Pressure on the lowest part of the brachial plexus may be due to oedema or sagging of the shoulder girdle during pregnancy. The woman should be advised to avoid carrying heavy shopping baskets. Elevation of the arm with a sling may help to relieve the pain.

EXCESSIVE SALIVATION (PTYALISM)

This is a rare condition in which so much saliva is produced it cannot be swallowed. There is in severe cases constant dribbling from the mouth causing great discomfort and loss of sleep. It is a disorder of early pregnancy, appearing about the eighth week, and often disappearing about the twenty-fourth week, but occasionally persisting until term. Atropine or a mixture containing belladonna may relieve the excessive salivation. If severe it causes vomiting, dehydration, hypoprotinaemia, thirst and soreness of the tongue and lips.

Physiology of pregnancy—general

During pregnancy, marked changes take place in the physiology of the woman and nearly every system shows some alteration.

Cardiovascular

BLOOD VOLUME

The circulating blood volume increases gradually until term. This is due to an increase in both the plasma volume and the red cell mass which is hormonal in origin (Fig. 2.5). The number of red cells increases about 20% and the plasma volume by about 50% resulting in a reduction in the red cell count and the haemoglobin concentration.

Cardiac output rises by about 30–40% during pregnancy but falls in late pregnancy when the woman lies on her back causing vena caval compression which may manifest as supine hypotension.

During pregnancy vasodilatation occurs due to the action of progesterone. This causes a decrease in peripheral resistance and an increased blood flow to the skin producing warmth of the extremities.

The colloid osmotic pressure of the plasma falls due to a reduction in the concentration of albumin and this may contribute to oedema.

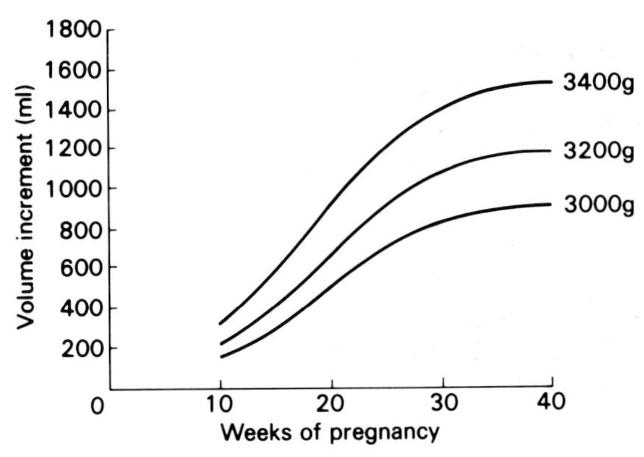

Fig. 2.5 The increase in plasma volume during normal pregnancy (relating to the weight of the baby). Modified from Hytten & Lind (1973) p. 36.

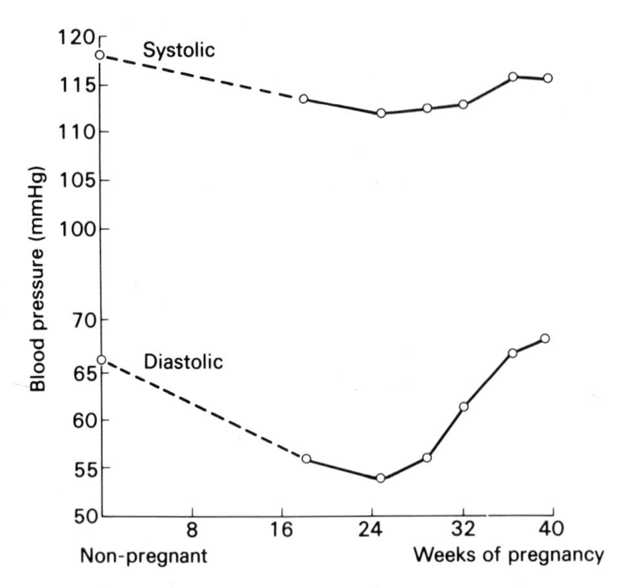

Fig. 2.6 Changes in supine arterial blood pressure during pregnancy. Modified from Hytten & Lind (1973).

HEART RATE

The heart rate and stroke volume are raised causing an increase in cardiac output from about 4 to 6 l/min by term.

BLOOD PRESSURE

Both systolic and diastolic blood pressures fall during pregnancy, reaching their lowest during the sixteenth to twenty-fourth weeks. The fall in the diastolic is greater than that in the systolic and both values return to normal at term (Fig. 2.6).

After the thirtieth week of pregnancy approximately 10% of women can develop a profound fall in blood pressure if allowed to remain supine for more than a few minutes; this is due to a lowered venous return when the uterus compresses the inferior vena cava. This vena caval compression reduces the venous return to the heart resulting in a fall in blood pressure and a feeling of faintness. This is known as the supine hypotension syndrome.

Central venous pressure measured in the right atria is 5–15 cmH_2O during pregnancy.

THE BLOOD

The normal values in pregnancy are:

Red blood cells (erythrocytes), 4–5 million/ml^3;

Reticulocytes, 0.2–2.0% of total red cells;

Erythrocyte sedimentation rate, 4–7 mm in the first hour;
Plasma fibrinogen concentration, 300–50 mg/dl;
White blood cells (leucocytes), 4–10 million/ml^3;
Platelets, 150 000–500 000/ml^3;
Mean corpuscular volume (MCV), 80–92 fl;
Mean corpuscular haemoglobin (MCH), 27–32 pg;
Serum fibrinogen, 0.4 g/dl;
Haemoglobin, 10.5–12.5 g/dl.

Due to the increase in the plasma volume, haemodilution occurs and causes a fall in the amount of haemoglobin per decilitre of blood. Because there is more haemoglobin in the total circulation, the fall in concentration is referred to as physiological anaemia.

Endocrine/hormonal

THYROID GLAND

The thyroid gland becomes visible and palpable in 70% of pregnant women. Total plasma thyroxine is raised in pregnancy, but the proportion which is free is reduced and there is, therefore, reduced thyroid activity.

PITUITARY GLAND

There is enlargement of the pituitary gland during pregnancy and although the gonadotrophic hormones, follicle stimulating and luteinising hormones, are suppressed during pregnancy levels of other anterior lobe hormones namely adrenocorticotrophic hormone and thyrotrophic hormone are raised. The adrenocorticotrophic hormone stimulates the adrenal cortex to secrete corticosteroid hormones and thyrotrophic hormone stimulates thyroid gland to produce thyroxine.

ADRENALS

The suprarenal of the cortex secretes three different kinds of hormone, collectively known as corticosteroids.

1 Mineralocorticoids regulate sodium and potassium balance in the body and aldosterone is the most potent.

2 Glucocorticoids stimulate conversion of protein to carbohydrate and have a diabetogenic effect. The principle one is hydrocortisone.

3 Sex hormones. The suprarenal cortex can supplement the production of sex hormones.

There is an increased concentration of adrenal glucocorticoid hormones in the blood and urine during pregnancy, and also an increase in the excretion of aldosterone. The suprarenal of the medulla secretes adrenaline.

THE PLACENTA

Hormones produced by the placenta are described below (see p. 100).

Metabolic rate

The metabolic rate is raised in pregnancy due to extra maternal and fetal tissue and such activities as increased respiratory and cardiac output. The maternal cells have a slightly reduced metabolic rate because of reduced thyroxine concentration.

Respiratory system

During pregnancy the volume of air breathed in per minute is increased and is achieved by a slight increase in the respiratory rate and increasing movement of the rib cage. The ribs are splayed and the woman breathes by expanding the chest wall sideways. The respirations are deeper, oxygenation is increased and the carbon dioxide content in the blood leaving the lungs falls.

Renal tract

Dilatation of the renal pelvis and ureters occurs during pregnancy. Kinking of the ureters occurs especially on the right side due to the pressure of the gravid uterus which leans and rotates to the right. Blood flow to the kidneys is increased from 800 to 1250 ml/min and glomerular filtration from 85 to 150 ml/min. There is a reduced ability to reabsorb glucose and because of this glycosuria presents not infrequently in pregnancy. Blood urea falls from a non-pregnant level of 20–30 mg% to less than 20 mg%.

Frequency of micturition is discussed above (see p. 18).

Gastrointestinal tract

Relaxation of smooth muscle, due to the effects of progesterone, takes place throughout the gastrointestinal tract.

There is relaxation of the cardiac sphincter of the stomach resulting in reflux of gastric contents causing heartburn. The acidity of the stomach contents is reduced and the residual contents are increased.

The sense of taste alters in pregnancy and many women have aversions or cravings for certain types of foods which may extend at its extreme to pica.

Nausea and vomiting, constipation and ptyalism have been discussed above (see pp. 24, 25, 26).

Weight

The pregnant woman gains approximately 12.5 kg in weight during pregnancy, 3–4 kg in the first twenty weeks and 0.5 kg per week thereafter (Fig. 2.7). In most cases the weight gain is more than that due to fetal structures

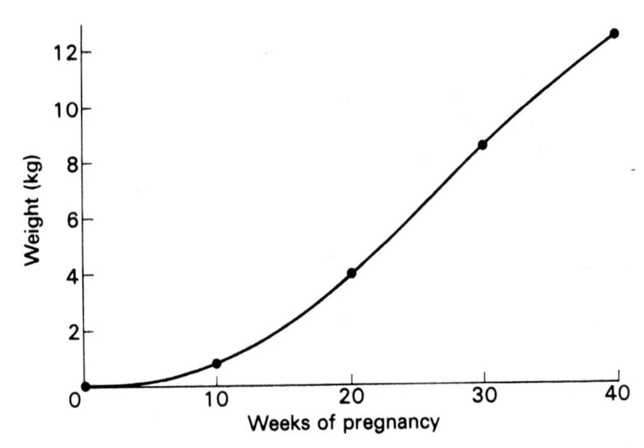

Fig. 2.7 Average weight gain in pregnancy.

Table 2.1 Distribution of weight gain in pregnancy.

Maternal		Fetal	
Uterus	0.9 kg	Fetus	3.3 kg
Breasts	0.4 kg	Placenta	0.7 kg
Blood	1.2 kg	Amniotic fluid	0.8 kg
Extracellular fluid	1.2 kg		
Fat	4.0 kg		
Total	7.7 kg	Total	4.8 kg

and the growth of the uterus and breasts. Part of the maternal weight gain is due to retention of fluid and disposition of adipose tissue (Table 2.1).

Skin

The skin of the abdomen, breasts and thighs is stretched during pregnancy and bluish-red scars called striae gravidarum may appear. These are the result of rupture of some of the deeper layers of the skin and are thought to be due to an excess of glucocorticoids secreted by the suprarenal cortex.

Pigmentary changes have already been described (see p. 19).

Musculo-skeletal

Relaxation of ligaments and joints occurs as a result of the effects of the placental oestrogens. There is an increase in lumbar lordosis in pregnancy which counteracts the weight of the gravid uterus.

Antenatal care

Until 1915, few pregnant women came under the care of a doctor or midwife until they went into labour. Ballantyne held the first antenatal clinic in the Royal Maternity Hospital, Edinburgh in that year. Clinics had previously been held in Boston in 1911 and Sydney in 1912.

Subsequently various Acts of Parliament have had an influence on the provision of antenatal care.

The Maternal and Child Welfare Act, 1918, placed responsibility for making provision for the health and care of expectant mothers and young children with local authorities. This resulted in the setting up of maternal and child welfare clinics.

The National Health Service Act, 1946, which came into being in 1948, provided free care for everyone at the time it was required.

The National Health Service Reorganisation Act, 1973, which had its inception in April 1974, unified the community and hospital maternity services.

Antenatal care is preventative medicine. It aims:

1 To reduce maternal and perinatal mortality and morbidity. At the beginning of the twentieth century the maternal mortality rate was 4–5/1000 registered total births and by 1982 it was reduced to 0.10/1000. During the same period perinatal mortality was reduced from 60–70/1000 to 11.3/1000 registered total births.
2 To promote, maintain or improve physical and mental health.
3 To detect underlying disorders.
4 To ensure a live, mature, healthy baby.
5 To educate expectant mothers and prospective fathers.

The woman usually consults her general practitioner when she has missed one or two periods, and he will refer her to the district general hospital, or if a home confinement is requested, make the appropriate arrangements.

Women should be encouraged to consult their doctor as soon as they suspect that they are pregnant so that advice regarding smoking, alcohol and drugs can be given as early as possible, and the woman referred to the hospital within the first trimester. This enables a history to be taken and examinations and investigations to be carried out at the earliest possible time.

History taking

The history should provide a methodical record of events in a woman's life relevant to the pregnancy. It must be accurate and should give an indication if the woman is in danger of complications of pregnancy, labour and the puerperium. In other words it should identify the 'at risk' woman. It should be obtained in private where the conversation cannot be overheard, and the questions asked using words that the woman will understand.

Although time is at a premium in a busy clinic, history taking cannot be hurried and many questions may need to be phrased in different ways to ensure that the correct answer is obtained. For example, the question, were you well during your last pregnancy? may receive the answer yes, *but* the question, did you come into hospital before labour started? may also bring the answer yes, the reason for admission being hypertension which in most cases does not make the woman feel unwell.

The history

PERSONAL DETAILS

a Full name, for identification purposes.

b Age. If the woman is a primigravida and over thirty or under seventeen years of age, or a multigravida over thirty-five years of age, then she is in the 'at risk' age group.

c Race/country of origin. Certain diseases or conditions can be related to race, e.g. sickle cell disease is common in negroid people.

d Religion. Some religions impose certain restrictions on their members, and these must be taken into consideration.

e Occupation. This information is required when giving advice about the advisability of continuing work.

f Marital status. It is important to know whether the woman is married, single, widowed, separated or divorced.

The same details may be required of the husband/partner in particular the information related to race and occupation. Race is important in terms of characteristics passed on to the child, and occupation in relation to social class and income of the family.

FAMILY HISTORY

Any hereditary or familial diseases or conditions should be recorded. These include a family history of diabetes mellitus, hypertension, psychiatric illness, tuberculosis, multiple pregnancy and congenital malformations.

GENERAL MEDICAL HISTORY

This includes any past or present disease that would have either an adverse effect on the pregnancy or would be adversely affected by the pregnancy. Diabetes mellitus, hypertension and renal diseases fit into both categories, whereas heart disease and thromboembolic disorders fit into the latter.

If the woman has any allergies or is taking any form of medication these should also be recorded.

Infectious diseases, especially those that could have caused damage to vital organs, e.g. rheumatic fever may have resulted in mitral stenosis, or those that may cause fetal malformation if contracted for the first time in pregnancy, e.g. rubella, are also recorded.

It is important to know whether the woman has a history of psychiatric illness as this may recur during pregnancy or following the birth of the baby.

SURGICAL HISTORY

Any operations, excluding obstetric operations, especially those involving the genital tract or vital organs are recorded. Appendicectomy is noted because, although it is not a major operation, appendicitis can then be excluded as a possible cause if the woman presents with acute abdominal pains in pregnancy.

Details of any blood transfusion are noted.

Serious accidents, especially those involving the pelvis and lower limbs, should be noted as alteration in the shape and size of the pelvis may have resulted.

CONTRACEPTION

Details about the type of contraception used and the success of the method are recorded. If oral contraception was used immediately prior to the pregnancy it is important to establish whether or not normal periods had recommenced.

FERTILITY

If the woman has had a period of infertility the following details should be noted. Whether infertility was primary or secondary, and the length and treatment if any.

MENSTRUAL HISTORY

An accurate menstrual history is essential to estimate the expected date of delivery.

Information required

a Age at menarche.

a Cycle. Length of the cycle when not taking oral contraceptives. Regularity of cycle; are the intervals regular from the beginning of one period to the beginning of the next or do they vary from month to month?

c Date of the last normal menstrual period (LMP). To establish the normality of the period, check onset, duration and amount of blood loss. Any deviation indicates that the period was not normal and should be discounted. For example, a period that lasted for two or three days instead of four, with only a slight loss or with clots may indicate a threatened abortion. If counted as the last period, the calculated date of delivery may be incorrect by one month, a potentially dangerous miscalculation.

Calculation of the estimated date of delivery (EDD)

a Based on a twenty-eight day cycle. Add nine months and seven days to the first day of the last normal menstrual period, e.g. LMP, 30th January 1983; EDD, 6th November 1983.

b Based on a thirty-five day cycle. Add nine months and fourteen days to the last normal menstrual period, e.g. LMP, 30th January 1983; EDD, 13th November 1983.

c Based on a twenty-one day cycle. Add nine months only to the first day of the last normal menstrual period, e.g. LMP, 30th January 1983; EDD, 30th November 1983.

Therefore, the number of days in excess of twenty-eight are added to the seven days and those less than twenty-eight are subtracted.

No accurate calculations can be made in the following circumstances: last menstrual period not known; irregular menstrual cycle; last 'period' was withdrawal bleeding following oral contraception. In these circumstances an ultrasonic scan should be performed to establish the period of gestation (see p. 317).

OBSTETRIC HISTORY

Previous pregnancy

The following possibilities should be noted.

a Occurrence of oedema or excessive weight gain.

b Raised blood pressure.

c Abnormal constituents in the urine, e.g. proteinuria.

If any two of the above signs were present this would indicate a history of pre-eclampsia, and a recurrence of hypertensive complications in this pregnancy should be anticipated.

d Vaginal bleeding, if it occurred before the twenty-eighth week, means there is a history of threatened abortion; if after, antepartum haemorrhage.

e Any abnormalities of micturition or abnormal vaginal discharge may indicate previous urinary tract or vaginal infection both of which may present again in this pregnancy.

f Excessive vomiting, necessitating admission to hospital, indicates a history of hyperemesis gravidarum.

Previous labours

a Did the pregnancy go to full term?

b If labour was premature, was it spontaneous or induced?

c If labour was induced, why was this undertaken and what method was used?

d How long did labour last?
e Was the delivery spontaneous or were instruments used?
f If instruments were used, why and what type of instrumentation?
g Was an episiotomy performed or a laceration sustained?
h Was the placenta delivered without any difficulty?
i Was blood loss normal or excessive?

Previous puerperia
a The length of stay in hospital may give an indication of any problems.
b A history of prolonged or heavy lochia and a raised temperature would suggest puerperal infection.
c Excessive bleeding, secondary postpartum haemorrhage.
d Pain or swelling of legs would indicate possible thromboembolic disease.

Previous babies
a Was the baby alive or stillborn?
b The sex of the child.
c The length of pregnancy, indicates whether the baby was mature, immature or postmature.
d The weight in relation to length of pregnancy will indicate a baby whose weight was normal for gestational age or one who was light-for-dates suggesting placental insufficiency, or heavy-for-dates with the possibility of the mother having latent diabetes. The weight is important even though the baby was stillborn.
e Any problems at birth, e.g. asphyxia neonatorum, or later, e.g. jaundice. If the baby was cared for in a special care baby unit, this would indicate a problem.
f How the baby was fed, and if breast fed, for how long?
g Health of child now.

Previous abortions
a Duration of pregnancy.
b Type of abortion, e.g. spontaneous, induced, therapeutic, complete or incomplete.
c If incomplete, what method was used to remove retained products of conception? Dilatation of the cervix sometimes predisposes to cervical incompetence in subsequent pregnancies.
d Was blood loss normal or excessive?

If there is anything abnormal in the previous obstetric history, the woman's full name and address at the time, the place of delivery and hospital number if known, should be obtained. This is so that the hospital can be contacted and full details obtained as the management of this pregnancy may be influenced by the more detailed information.

If the woman has been married before or had a baby before her marriage by a different partner this should be indicated. A change of partner may present problems that did not previously arise, e.g. a Rhesus negative woman previously married to a Rhesus negative man but now with a Rhesus positive husband. There now is a possibility of Rhesus incompatibility complicating pregnancies (see p. 365).

Whilst the history is being obtained, an opportunity to observe the woman's reaction to her previous pregnancies and children and this pregnancy is taken.

If the woman's previous experience of labour was unpleasant and she is looking forward to this labour with fear then help could be offered even at this early stage. For example, it may set the woman's mind at rest to be offered epidural analgesia.

If the pregnancy is unplanned and the baby unwanted, the possibility of child abuse should be considered.

PRESENT PREGNANCY

Enquiries are made as to the progress of the pregnancy so far. The woman should be asked if she has had any bleeding since her last period or if she has an excessive vaginal discharge. Any vomiting is noted and also symptoms such as breathlessness or unusual tiredness.

SOCIAL FACTORS

Information is obtained about the woman's smoking and drinking habits and if she is taking any form of medication. If the woman smokes, a note should be made of the number of cigarettes smoked each day. She is told about the dangers of smoking (see p. 40) and advised to give up, if possible, or to reduce the number of cigarettes smoked to five a day.

A note is made of the amount of alcohol the woman drinks, and advice is given about the risks associated with the consumption of alcohol (see p. 41). She is advised not to take any drugs or tablets of any description unless prescribed for her by a doctor who knows she is pregnant.

History taking provides the midwife with a good opportunity for health education and other subjects may present. For example, if when making enquiries about previous pregnancies, the woman either has several children or the pregnancies are not well-spaced, a preliminary discussion about contraception might be appropriate. The opportunity to give advice about the advantages of breast feeding may present when discussing how previous babies were fed.

If the woman or her family has any social problems, arrangements should be made for her to see a medical social worker.

Midwifery care plan

Childbirth is a very individual experience for the woman and her family, and their expectations and needs may vary considerably. The woman should be asked if she has any preferences about the care she receives during pregnancy, labour and the postnatal period, and in the care of her baby.

The information should form the basis of a midwifery care plan that should be reviewed and modified as necessary during pregnancy. The plan should ensure that the woman's needs are known to all staff involved in her care to avoid unnecessary repetition of questions or some preference being overlooked.

General examination

A complete examination of the woman is necessary. At the first visit a physical examination is made including examination of the heart, lungs, breasts, blood pressure and urine. Oedema and varicosities are also looked for.

HEIGHT

The woman's height is measured because a woman of small stature, 1.52 m or less, may have a small pelvis (see p. 247).

WEIGHT

The weight is estimated and forms a baseline for subsequent measurements. The weight is also compared with the height (Fig. 2.8). Obesity presents many problems in pregnancy, women who are overweight are more prone to pre-eclampsia. Women who are overweight may, by means of diet, have their weight controlled so that they do not gain any weight during their pregnancy.

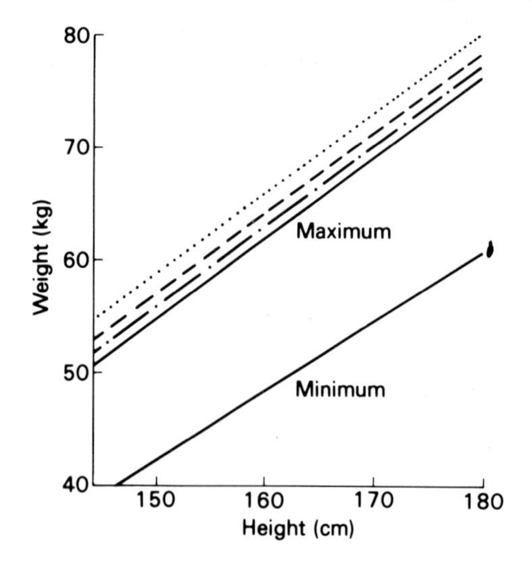

Fig. 2.8 Desirable range of weight for women of differing height; the dotted lines show the upper limit of desirable weight in pregnant women at 10, 15 and 20 weeks.

URINALYSIS

The urine is examined for glucose, proteins and ketones. A midstream specimen of urine is obtained and examined for bacteria. Asymptomatic bacteruria (see p. 202), is not uncommon in women and may predispose to pyelonephritis during pregnancy (see p. 202).

BLOOD PRESSURE ESTIMATION

The blood pressure is recorded and this reading forms the baseline for subsequent recordings. The age and size of the woman and stage of pregnancy (see p. 28) should be taken into account when deciding if the blood pressure is within the normal range.

Obstetrical examination

This includes examination of the abdominal and pelvic organs.

ABDOMINAL EXAMINATION

The purpose of the examination is to exclude abdominal masses, and to ascertain whether or not the uterus can be palpated abdominally. This does not usually occur until about fourteen weeks, but may occur earlier if abnormal growth occurs as in multiple pregnancy or hydatidiform mole.

VAGINAL EXAMINATION

The objectives of this examination are:

a To confirm pregnancy.
b To ascertain the size of the uterus in relation to the period of gestation.
c To exclude any soft tissue masses.
d To examine the adnexa to ensure normality.
e A preliminary estimation of the general shape and size of the pelvis.

A speculum examination is performed prior to the digital examination. The state of the cervix is noted and, unless contraindicated, a cervical smear is obtained.

Investigations: blood

ABO GROUP AND RHESUS FACTOR

It is essential to know the ABO group and Rhesus factor of the woman's blood. If bleeding occurs at any time during the pregnancy, labour or the puerperium, blood can then be crossed-matched without unnecessary delay.

ANTIBODY SCREENING

The blood is also examined for antibodies especially if the woman has Rhesus negative blood.

HAEMOGLOBIN ESTIMATION

The haemoglobin is estimated and in some hospitals a full blood count is carried out. This is important to detect anaemia and the cause, and enables early appropriate treatment to be commenced.

BLOOD ELECTROPHORESIS

If the woman is of African, Asian or Southern European origin the blood is examined for abnormal haemoglobin, e.g. sickle cell disease and thalassaemia.

SEROLOGY

All pregnant women have a serological test for syphilis performed. These tests include the Reiter Protein Complement Fixation test (RPCFT), Venereal Disease Reference Laboratory Slide test (VDRL), Wasserman and Kahn tests.

RUBELLA ANTIBODIES

If contracted in early pregnancy, rubella can result in fetal abnormalities but protection is given to the fetus by maternal antibodies. If antibodies are not present vaccination is offered in the puerperium.

MATERNAL SERUM ALPHA–FETOPROTEIN LEVELS

This estimation may be made routinely or selectively where there is an increased risk of neural tube abnormality. Levels above the 95th centile—twice the median value, are an indication to investigate the amniotic fluid alpha-fetoprotein levels (see p. 475).

Advice

The woman should be given an opportunity to ask questions and time allowed to answer her queries.

The importance of attending for antenatal care is stressed as is the need to report immediately any abnormal occurrence, particular stress being placed on reporting any vaginal bleeding.

SMOKING

The woman is advised to discontinue smoking if possible or if not, to reduce the number of cigarettes to five per day. In addition to the dangers of smoking in relation to the mother's health there are other dangers in pregnancy. Carbon monoxide reduces transport of oxygen and nicotine causes vasoconstriction of maternal and fetal vessels. The result is placental insufficiency and retarded fetal growth.

ALCOHOL

The woman should be advised not to consume alcohol during her pregnancy as this readily crosses the placenta and circulates in the fetal blood in the same concentrations as in the maternal blood, and is potentially harmful to the fetus.

DRUGS

The woman is advised not to take any form of medication unless prescribed for her by a doctor.

DIET

The dietary intake in pregnancy has to provide for the needs of the growing fetus, maintenance of maternal health and preparation for successful lactation (see p. 51).

SLEEP AND REST

The woman is encouraged to rest for an hour or two during the day. This of course cannot be achieved if she is working or if she has an active toddler. If she does not have someone who can look after the child she may be able to take her rest when the child rests although this may not be the most convenient time.

She should spend eight hours in bed each night, she may not sleep but she is resting.

EXERCISE

The woman should avoid strenuous activity during pregnancy but moderate accustomed exercise in the fresh air is encouraged.

WORK

Unless contraindicated by ill health or unsuitable employment the woman is usually able to continue working until the end of the twenty-eighth week of pregnancy.

CLOTHING

Comfortable non-restrictive clothing is advised. Shoes should be sensible and not put the woman at risk of falling or produce strain of ligaments.

DENTAL CARE

The woman is advised to visit her dentist as dental caries may progress very rapidly in pregnancy and result in septic foci which are potentially dangerous.

Dental care is free during pregnancy and for one year after the birth of the baby.

GENERAL HYGIENE

Advice is given about general hygiene stressing that, due to increased activity of the sweat glands, the woman perspires more freely during pregnancy. In addition there is an increase in vaginal secretions and colostrum may leak from the nipple. Therefore, there is a need for more attention to personal hygiene.

BREAST CARE

Advice is given about a suitable brassiere which should be large enough not to compress the breast tissue but give good support to the enlarging breasts. Broad straps prevent cutting into the shoulder as the weight of the breasts increases. The woman is advised to give particular attention to the nipple area when washing to clean away the crusts of colostrum that may form.

COITUS

This should be avoided in early pregnancy if there is a history of bleeding or if the woman has a history of abortion. In late pregnancy, there is an increased risk of infection and early rupture of membranes.

Maternity benefits

Maternity benefits are available to most women during pregnancy.

MATERNITY GRANT

A sum of twenty-five pounds can be claimed from fourteen weeks before the week containing the expected date of delivery, and three months after. The grant is a non-contributory benefit that is intended to contribute towards the expense of having a baby (see p. 439).

MATERNITY ALLOWANCE

This is a weekly sum of money payable to the woman who has been employed and is paid on her national insurance contributions. It is payable from eleven weeks before the week containing the expected date of delivery and seven weeks after, providing the woman is not working. The purpose is to encourage the woman to give up work in late pregnancy. If the woman has to discontinue work prior to the twenty-ninth week then sickness benefit is claimed until she is eligible for the maternity allowance. The amount changes frequently and the student is advised to familiarise herself with the latest figure (see p. 439).

MATERNITY PAY (see p. 439)

OTHER BENEFITS

The pregnant woman is entitled to free dental care and chiropody, and is exempt from prescription charges. These benefits continue for one year after the birth of the baby. The expectant and nursing mother is entitled to one pint of free milk a day. This also applies if the family is in receipt of supplementary benefits, family income supplement or is of low income.

Preparation for parenthood classes

The woman is advised to attend these classes especially if this is her first pregnancy (see p. 51).

Booking arrangements

Arrangements are now made regarding type of antenatal care, place of confinement and length of stay in hospital.

These arrangements take into consideration social, medical and obstetric factors as well as the woman's preferences. When discussing the plans with the woman it must be explained that subsequent events may necessitate changes being made in the arrangements.

ANTENATAL CARE

1 Care may be completely undertaken by the hospital staff.
2 Care may be shared between the hospital staff and the general practitioner and community midwife.
3 Care may be completely undertaken by the general practitioner and community midwife as occurs when a home confinement is arranged.

PLACE OF CONFINEMENT

1 Consultant obstetric unit.
2 Maternity hospital or home with no resident medical staff.
3 General practitioner unit.
4 Home.

LENGTH OF STAY IN HOSPITAL

1 Full stay of about ten days.
2 Early transfer home to the care of the community midwife and general practitioner.

High risk groups

Women who fit into these categories should be booked for antenatal care and confinement in a major obstetric unit. A full stay in hospital following delivery may also be indicated.

Primigravida
Thirty years of age or over; seventeen years of age or under.

Multigravida
Thirty-five years of age or over; para four or more; any abnormality occurring during previous pregnancy, labour or puerperium; previous perinatal death or low birth weight baby.

All women
Single or unsupported; height less than 1.52 m; obesity; pre-existing medical disorders; infertility; previous gynaecological surgery; pelvic deformity.

Women who during pregnancy present with:
Threatened abortion; antepartum haemorrhage; hypertension; anaemia; Rhesus antibodies; multiple pregnancy; polyhydramnios; persistent malpresentation; premature labour (less than thirty-seven weeks); non-engagement of the fetal head at term (primigravida); post dates (seven days).

Dangers of high parity
Anaemia; abnormal uterine action; hypertension; malpresentation; haemorrhage; cord prolapse; prematurity; embolus; congenital malformation, e.g. Down's Syndrome.

Home assessment

If arrangements are made for a home confinement or early transfer home following delivery, a home assessment is undertaken before the arrangements are finalised.

Suitability of the home for early transfer includes:

a Adequate standard of cleanliness.
b Adequate accommodation with no overcrowding.
c Indoor bathroom and toilet.
d Hot and cold running water.
e Adequate heating day and night.
f Help available until the tenth postnatal day to undertake household chores and shopping.
g Household pets under control.

In addition to the items mentioned above the following would be noted when assessing the home for a home confinement.

a Adequate lighting as the delivery may take place at night.
b Telephone in case of an emergency.
c Toilet and bathroom on same floor as mother's room.

d Working surface for delivery pack.
e Access for ambulance, summer and winter.

All details are recorded in the case notes and the cooperation card which is retained by the woman, and an appointment is made for the next visit to the hospital or general practitioner. The woman is given a month's supply of tablets containing iron and folic acid and asked to take one each day.

Subsequent care

FREQUENCY OF VISITS
During pregnancy the woman should be seen and examined every four weeks until the twenty-eighth week, then every two weeks until the thirty-sixth week and then weekly until the birth of the baby.

If at any time there is a deviation from normal, visits should be more frequent.

At each visit the following will be undertaken:

URINALYSIS
The urine is tested for reaction, glucose, proteins, ketones and blood.

WEIGHT
The woman is weighed and the weight compared with previous recordings to ensure that she is gaining weight but not excessively.

BLOOD PRESSURE ESTIMATION
The blood pressure is recorded and compared with previous recordings. A recording of 140 systolic and 90 diastolic is the upper limit of normal.

General examination

OEDEMA
The fingers and pretibial areas and ankles are examined for oedema. Oedema, if present, may be a cause of excessive weight gain and if combined with hypertension and/or proteinuria is a sign of pre-eclampsia.

VARICOSE VEINS
The legs and vulval area are examined for varicosities.

Abdominal examination

The purpose of this examination is:

a To ascertain the size of the uterus in relation to the period of gestation.

b To ascertain the size of the fetus in relation to the period of gestation.

c To determine the lie, presentation and position of the fetus in the uterus.

d To detect abnormalities such as multiple pregnancy and polyhydramnios.

The abdominal examination comprises three aspects; inspection, palpation and auscultation.

INSPECTION

a The size and shape of the uterus is observed in relation to period of gestation.

b The skin of the abdomen is examined for the linea nigra, striae gravidarum and scars.

c Braxton Hicks contractions and fetal movements may be observed as pregnancy progresses.

PALPATION

The size of the uterus (see p. 76). The fundus can be felt by deep palpation at the level of the symphysis pubis at the end of the twelfth week of pregnancy. At the sixteenth week it is halfway between the symphysis pubis and the lower border of the umbilicus.

At twenty weeks it has reached a point just below the level of the umbilicus, and by the twenty-fourth week it is just above the level of the umbilicus.

At twenty-eight weeks it is at a level one-third of the distance between the umbilicus and the xiphisternum, and at thirty-two weeks, two-thirds of that distance.

At thirty-six weeks, the fundus is at the level of the xiphisternum. After the thirty-sixth week of pregnancy lightening occurs; the abdomen becomes more pendulous, and in the primigravida the fetal head engages in the pelvis.

At the fortieth week the height of the fundus is equivalent to that of thirty-two.

This is only a guide and it must be appreciated that the distance between the symphysis pubis and umbilicus, and umbilicus and xiphisternum is not standard. A woman of small stature may appear to have a uterus that is large-for-dates, whereas in a tall woman the uterus may appear comparatively small. Therefore, the height of the woman must be taken into account as well as the contents of the uterus.

The height of the fundus can be more accurately measured using callipers or a tape measure.

Size of the fetus. During the subsequent examination, the fetus within the uterus is palpated and its size in relation to the period of gestation can be assessed. The amount of amniotic fluids is also noted. This increases gradually until late pregnancy when it tends to diminish.
Lie of the fetus. The lie of the fetus is the relation of the long axis of the fetus to the long axis of the mother's uterus. The lie is normal when it is longitudinal, abnormal if transverse or oblique.
Presentation of the fetus. The presentation is that part of the fetus in the lower pole of the uterus. It is the part of the fetus to enter the pelvis when engagement occurs.

When the lie is longitudinal the presentation is either, cephalic (vertex, brow or face) or breech. If the lie is transverse or oblique the shoulder presents. The vertex however, is the normal presentation.
Presenting part. When the presentation is known the presenting part can be determined.

The presenting part is the lowest point on the presentation.
Vertex—the presenting part is the anterior parietal bone.
Face—the presenting part is the anterior malar bone.
Breech—the presenting part is the anterior buttock.
The denominator. The denominator is a fixed point on the presentation used to determine the position.
Vertex—the denominator is the occiput.
Face—the denominator is the mentum.
Breech—the denominator is the sacrum.
Position of the fetus. This is the relationship of the denominator to six points on the mother's pelvis, e.g. left and right anterior, lateral and posterior (Fig. 2.9).
Positions:
Left or right occipito/mento/sacroanterior.
Left or right occipito/mento/sacrolateral.
Left or right occipito/mento/sacroposterior.
Attitude of fetus. The attitude of the fetus refers to the relation of different parts of the fetus to each other, e.g. attitude of flexion—the head, back and limbs are flexed; attitude of deflexion—the head, back and limbs are only partially flexed; attitude of extension—the head, back and limbs are extended.

In relation to the head, attitudes of partial flexion and extension can also be applied.
Engagement. Engagement occurs when the widest diameter on the presentation has passed through the plane of the pelvic brim, e.g.
Vertex—engaging diameter is the biparietal diameter of 9.5 cm.
Face—engaging diameter is the bitemporal diameter of 8.5 cm.
Breech—engaging diameter is the bitrochanteric diameter of 10 cm.

Note that there is no presenting part, denominator, position or engaging

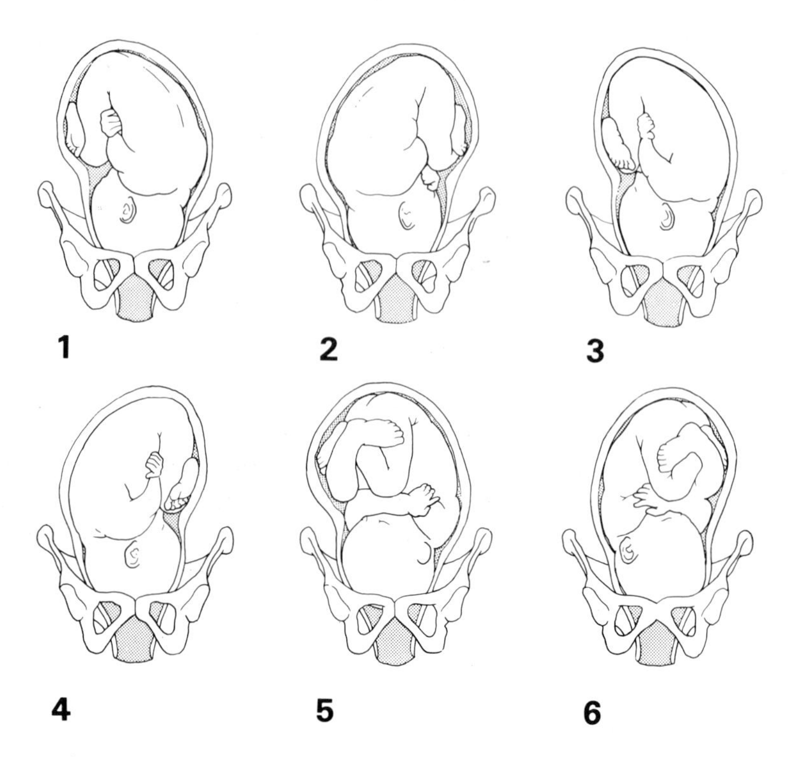

Fig. 2.9 The pelvis brim showing the six positions: 1, left occipitoanterior; 2, right occipitoanterior; 3, left occipitolateral; 4, right occipitolateral; 5, left occipitoposterior; 6, right occipitoposterior.

diameter for a brow or shoulder presentation. This is because vaginal delivery is not possible in either case.

The lie and presentation can be determined from quite early in pregnancy but it is not until after the thirty-fourth week that they become important. By then the lie should stabilise to longitudinal and the presentation should be the vertex. The reason for this is that beyond this time the fetus is less likely to change its lie and presentation and therefore any abnormalities if not corrected would persist. Also labour may start at any time and, therefore, complications arise.

Engagement is relevant after the thirty-sixth week in a primigravida but may not occur until term or onset of labour in a multigravida.

AUSCULTATION

The fetal heart can be auscultated using a Pinard (monaural) stethoscope from about the twenty-fourth week of pregnancy, but earlier using the ultrasonic detector.

The placing of the stethoscope depends on the lie, position and presentation of the fetus and whether or not engagement has taken place.

The fetal heart is auscultated, through the posterior chest wall of the fetus if the position is anterior or lateral, and through the anterior chest wall in a posterior position.

The normal fetal heart beats between 120 and 160 beats/min and is regular and of good volume.

In addition to the routine examinations undertaken at each visit to the doctor, midwife or antenatal clinic the following will be performed.

Twenty-eighth and thirty-fourth weeks

Haemoglobin estimation and antibody screening are carried out. If the woman has Rhesus negative blood a specimen of blood may be obtained from the husband to determine his genotype. This will indicate whether his blood is Rhesus positive or negative and, if positive, whether heterozygous or homozygous. If homozygous the fetus will be Rhesus positive, and therefore incompatible with the mother, if heterozygous there is a 50% chance of Rhesus incompatibility (see p. 365).

Thirty-sixth to thirty-eighth week

Haemoglobin estimation and antibody screen will be repeated. The breasts will be examined and if the woman is going to breast feed she may be shown how to express colostrum to clear the ducts in preparation for lactation. She is encouraged to do this daily. There is, however, evidence to suggest that expression of colostrum not only does not have any beneficial effect, but may, in fact, be harmful. The stimulation of the nipple may cause the release of oxytocin from the posterior lobe of the pituitary gland and this may cause the uterine muscle to contract and the woman to go into premature labour.

The doctor may examine the woman's heart and lungs to ensure that she is fit to receive an inhalational analgesia in labour.

Abdominal examination is performed with special emphasis on the lie, presentation and engagement of the head. If the head is not yet engaged it is important to determine whether it can be made to engage in order to exclude cephalopelvic disproportion. An attempt is made to push the head into the pelvis in a backward and downward direction.

VAGINAL EXAMINATION

A vaginal examination may be performed at this stage of pregnancy to assess the pelvic capacity in relation to the size of the fetal head, as it is necessary at this time for a decision to be made regarding the mode of delivery. Although a preliminary examination was made at the first visit, certain changes will have occurred during pregnancy. The softening and relaxation of the pelvic floor will allow for easier examination. The softening and relaxation of the pelvic ligaments will have resulted in an increase in the pelvic diameters. The fetal head is now almost fully grown and an accurate assessment of cephalopelvic proportion can be made.

If the woman is a multipara the size of previous babies may give an indication of pelvic capacity. If the babies were of average or above average size the pelvic assessment may not be made.

The examination includes:

a Noting the state of the vagina and cervix. The cervix should be soft and may be partially effaced.

b The presentation can be felt through the anterior fornix and if there was doubt following abdominal examination it can be determined vaginally.

c Palpation in an upward and backward direction will determine whether the promontory of the sacrum is palpable. This measurement, from the lower border of the symphysis pubis to the sacral promontory is the diagonal conjugate which measures 12.5 cm. The true conjugate is estimated by deducting 1.5 cm.

d The length and anterior curvature of the sacrum are estimated.

e The bony walls are examined and should be parallel.

f The angle of the pubic arch is assessed and is normally 90°.

g The ischial spines are palpated and the interspinous diameter assessed. It should be approximately 10.5 cm.

h The distance between the inner margins of the ischial tuberosities is assessed by placing four knuckles against the perineum between the ischial tuberosities. This measurement is normally 11 cm.

At all visits to the clinic, midwife or general practitioner advice and reassurance should be given and queries answered. All details of examinations and investigations are recorded in the case notes and on the cooperation card. The cooperation card is returned to the woman at the end of each visit and she is asked to keep it with her at all times and to produce it at each visit to the doctor or hospital. The purpose of the cooperation card is liaison between the hospital staff, the general practitioner and community midwife. An additional use is that should the woman be admitted to a hospital other than the one in which she is booked for confinement, information is immediately available to the staff who have to care for her.

At each visit the woman is reminded about the importance of taking iron tablets and a check is made to ensure that she has an adequate supply to last until her next attendance.

As pregnancy nears term, the woman is reminded of the signs of the onset of labour and when to come into hospital or send for the midwife. It is ensured that she has the telephone number of the hospital and either transport available or knows how to call for an ambulance.

Preparation for parenthood

The midwife has an important role to play in preparing expectant mothers and their husbands for parenthood. All midwives should be prepared to participate in these classes and the teaching of parentcraft is included in the syllabus for the training of student midwives.

Suggested topics to be included in a series of talks, and the period of pregnancy at which they should be given are outlined.

Twelve to sixteen weeks

SESSION 1: DIET IN PREGNANCY

Ideally, the talk should be given by a dietitian who has an important role as a member of the extended team caring for women during their pregnancy. This talk should include advice about the importance of a well balanced diet to meet the needs of the growing fetus as well as maintenance of the health of the expectant mother.

The energy requirement is increased by about 400 kcal (1680 kJ) in pregnancy.

Daily requirements

Proteins: 90 g = 1.512 MJ (360 cal).
Fats: 100 g = 3780 J (900 cal).
Carbohydrates: 320 g = 5376 J (1280 cal).
Minerals: iron, 3–4 mg; calcium, 150 mg; phosphorus, 1 g; iodine, 0.1 mg.
Vitamins.

Proteins are essential for building up body tissues, and are found in cheese, milk, eggs, fish and meat.

Fats if taken excessively will produce weight gain. Fats are found in the dairy produce mentioned above.

Carbohydrates are usually taken in excess. Abnormal weight gain in pregnancy may be due to too many carbohydrates. Carbohydrates are found in sweets, biscuits, bread and potatoes.

Minerals: iron is important to prevent anaemia and for normal blood formation. It is found in red meat, eggs and fresh green vegetables. Supplementary iron is usually given in pregnancy. Calcium is found in milk and 1.15 l provides the daily requirement. Calcium is essential for ossification of bones and teeth, and clotting of blood. Phosphorus is necessary for bone formation and carbohydrate metabolism. It is contained in fish, meat, eggs and milk. Iodine is required for the functioning of the thyroid gland. Sea fish are a source of iodine.

Vitamins: it is most important that the diet should contain a supply of vitamins. Vitamins A and D promote growth and raise resistance to bacterial infections. They are found in milk, butter, cheese and fresh green vegetables. Vitamin B is important in maintaining general health and nutrition and is found in milk, wholemeal bread, red meats and fresh green vegetables. Folic acid, a constituent of the vitamin B complex is often given in conjunction with iron in pregnancy. Vitamin C is essential for normal blood formation and is found in fresh fruit especially oranges and lemons.

When giving advice about diet and the source of nutrients an account must be taken of the woman's financial means and religious and cultural preferences. When advising about red meat as a source of iron for example, liver and the less expensive cuts of beef should be recommended to the woman who is of low income.

Sixteen to twenty-two weeks

SESSION 2: PREGNANCY

This talk should include a brief outline of the anatomy of the reproductive organs, ovulation, fertilization and the development and growth of the embryo and fetus. Audiovisual aids in the form of charts, slides or flannel graft can be used to demonstrate this clearly and simply. The changes that take place in the general physiology and how to cope with the minor disorders that present as a result of these changes should be discussed. Antenatal care is outlined and its importance stressed, and advice about general care and health is given.

From the thirty-fourth week of pregnancy

SESSION 3: LABOUR

An outline of the three stages of labour is given, what to expect, how to recognise the stages and the care that will be given. This session should include information about methods of pain relief including epidural analgesia, and the inhalational analgesia apparatus should be demonstrated. An anaesthetist might like to take part in this session and join in the discussion relating to epidural analgesia.

Procedures such as induction of labour and episiotomy and abnormal deliveries should be introduced and an obstetrician may be invited to give this part of the session.

A tour of the labour ward is arranged to follow this talk.

SESSION 4: POSTNATAL CARE AND INFANT FEEDING

This talk is aimed at familiarising the expectant mother with the changes that take place during the puerperium and with the daily routine and procedure of the postnatal ward. Emphasis should be given to the teaching the mother is given regarding the care of her baby.

Infant teaching is discussed and the advantages of breast feeding explained without making women who elect to bottle feed their babies feel in any way guilty. Equally, it is important not to make breast feeding appear too easy because then when the mother is faced with problems in the early stages of breast feeding she becomes depressed and tends to discontinue it. If she appreciates that there may be difficulties initially but they can usually be overcome with time and patience she will be encouraged to persevere. Preparation of artificial feeds and the sterilisation of feeding equipment is demonstrated (see p. 341). A health visitor may be invited to attend this session to give advice about protection against infectious disease and prevention of accidents.

SESSION 5: DEMONSTRATION OF BABY BATHING

Ideally a baby, not a doll, should be used for this demonstration. The equipment is explained and also ways the woman can adapt to her own preference, i.e. the woman may prefer to put the bath on a board across the bath rather than use a bath stand. The technique of bathing is explained and demonstrated with emphasis on safety and prevention of chilling. Although many women may have bought baby clothes and equipment by this time, a discussion regarding these items can be included in this session.

A tour of a postnatal ward is arranged to follow this talk.

SESSION 6: FILM

An ideal way to complete the series of talks is to show a film that covers all the subjects included in the talks.

Ideally the husbands should be invited to accompany their wives to the classes but sometimes due to lack of facilities or the time the classes are held this is not always possible. In these circumstances the film session could be arranged at a time to enable the majority to attend and a special session could also be arranged to give the prospective father an opportunity to have his questions answered.

Preparation

When preparing a talk or a series of talks to be given to a group of expectant mothers, consideration should be given to the following.

a The type of audience. The group of expectant mothers will come from varying educational and cultural backgrounds and this must, therefore, be taken into account. You need to adapt the content of a talk to the needs of the individual woman so that she may understand within her own intellectual capacity.

b The purpose of the classes. You are attempting to help the woman through the experience of pregnancy and childbirth; therefore, everything must be relevant to the woman and not too technical.

c Emphasising important points. Decide upon the important points you wish to leave with your audience and include these at the beginning or end of your talk when the attention of the group is at its maximum.

d Plan. Although these talks should be as informal as possible and questions and discussion encouraged, it is important to have an outline plan to ensure that important facts are not omitted.

e Audience reaction. Note the things that hold their interest, what makes them restless and the questions they ask. Their reaction will assist you in planning future talks.

f Updating information. It is important to be well informed about the latest procedures and to be aware of items relating to pregnancy that have appeared in the press or on radio or television. It is these that stimulate questions and a little forethought can help you to deal more effectively with the questions.

g Use of words. There should be a balance between using words which are too technical and oversimplification with the risk of talking down to your audience. The woman will hear medical terms used and, therefore, it is helpful to include them. It is, however, better not to presuppose knowledge and technical terminology should always be prefixed by the lay terms.

PSYCHOLOGICAL PREPARATION

It is the midwife's duty to familiarise herself with the current methods of preparation for childbirth so that she knows what has been taught and can offer support to the woman in labour. Lack of knowledge on the part of the midwife may lead to conflicting advice being given and unnecessary anxiety to the mother.

'NATURAL CHILDBIRTH'

In the 1930's, Dr Grantly Dick-Read popularised the theory that fear leads to tension, which in turn causes pain in childbirth. His teaching was based on the idea that by educating expectant mothers the fear of the unknown and, therefore, tension would be removed and a 'natural childbirth' would result.

PSYCHOPROPHYLAXIS

The word psychoprophylaxis was introduced by a Russian, Nicholaiev, in 1949. In 1951, with two colleagues, he explained and demonstrated the method which was adapted and used in many countries.

This method of preparation is based on the Pavlov theory of conditioned reflexes. It provides constructive activity by teaching a set of reactions which need to be practised repeatedly so that they can be performed without conscious thought. The woman is taught to coordinate controlled breathing with muscular activity, and to adapt her reactions to changing situations.

Four levels of controlled breathing are taught and range from slow deep breathing to rapid shallow breathing and finally no active respiratory movement but the mouthing of the words of a song, the tune of which is being tapped out by the fingers. Practical sessions include teaching the expectant mother an awareness of important muscles, such as the pelvic floor muscles, how to relax these muscles as well as exercises to improve muscle tone.

This method requires considerable practice so that the woman is able to respond appropriately to the painful stimulus of labour. She is often supported by her husband who has usually helped her with the practice sessions.

If the woman is able to cope successfully with her labour she derives considerable pleasure and satisfaction from her achievement. However, if she does not feel satisfied with the way she reacted in labour, a sense of failure can result.

PSYCHOPHYSICAL

This method of preparation has evolved from the methods previously mentioned and is based on prenatal instruction designed to give the woman confidence, with consequent easing of tension, to deal with any situation that might arise. The woman is taught controlled breathing and relaxation and how to relax and exert her muscles in the right way at the right time.

HYPNOSIS

Antenatal preparation for childbirth by hypnosis is not widely practised. Hypnosis is induced by repeated, rhythmical, monotonous stimulation and requires careful individual teaching during pregnancy. The depth of hypnosis may be light, medium or deep.

The advantage of this method of preparation is that there is relief of pain without the use of narcotics and their adverse effect on the fetal respiratory centre.

LEBOYER METHOD

This method advocates that the stimuli to which the baby is subjected at birth are reduced to a minimum. The delivery is conducted in a room with subdued lighting. At birth, the baby is placed on the mother's abdomen and gently stroked. The baby is then placed in a bath and the water is lapped over the baby's body.

Concern regarding this method includes an inability to observe the baby's colour adequately in the subdued light, the danger of inhalation of secretions when mucus extraction is omitted, perfusion of the placenta with the baby's blood when the baby's body is higher than the placenta and clamping of the cord is delayed and chilling of the baby due to exposure.

Further reading

CHERTOK L. (1959) *Psychosomatic Methods of Painless Childbirth*. Pergamon, Oxford.
HEARDMAN H. (1982) *Relaxation and Exercise for Childbirth*. Churchill Livingstone, London.
HYTTEN F.E. & LIND T. (1973) *Diagnostic Indices in Pregnancy*. CIBA-GEIGY, Basle, Switzerland.
KITZINGER S. (1972) *The Experience of Childbirth*. 3rd edn. Penguin, Harmondsworth.
LAMAZE F. (1958) *Painless Childbirth—Psychoprophylactic Techniques*. Burke, London.
LEBOYER F. (1975) *Birth Without Violence*. Wildwood House Ltd., London.
SNAITH L. & COXON A. (1968) *Dick-Read's Childbirth Without Fear*. 5th edn. Heinemann, London.
VELLAY P. (1959) *Childbirth Without Pain*. Allen & Unwin, London.
WILLIAMS M. & BOOTH D. (1980) *Antenatal Education—Guidelines for Teachers*. Churchill Livingstone, London.

Chapter 3
Anatomy and Physiology

Anatomy defines the structures of the body and physiology describes how they function.

The plain facts of anatomy and the speculations of physiology may seem far removed from the role of the midwife but intelligent midwifery practice requires an anatomical knowledge of those organs in which changes occur during pregnancy, labour and the puerperium.

In an attempt to demonstrate the importance of this knowledge in practice the physiological changes are described in relation to the anatomy rather than in a separate chapter.

The genital tract

The female genital tract comprises the external genitalia or vulva, and the internal genitalia, which includes the vagina, uterus, Fallopian tubes and ovaries.

The external genitalia

The vulva is made up of the following structures (Fig. 3.1):

THE MONS VENERIS

A rounded prominence in front of the pubes, due to an accumulation of fat under the skin. After puberty the mons veneris is covered with hair which, in the female, extends about one-third of the distance up to the umbilicus with a straight hairline.

LABIA MAJORA (singular, labium majus)

Two folds of fatty tissue and skin which extend downwards and backwards from the mons veneris, enclosing the urogenital cleft, and merge into the perineal body. The outer surface is covered with hairs and the inner surface, which contains numerous sweat and sebaceous glands is smooth.

LABIA MINORA (singular, labium minus)

These are two small folds of skin lying longitudinally within the labia majora enclosing the vestibule. They are smooth and devoid of hair but contain a few sweat and sebaceous glands and are very vascular. Anteriorly the labia

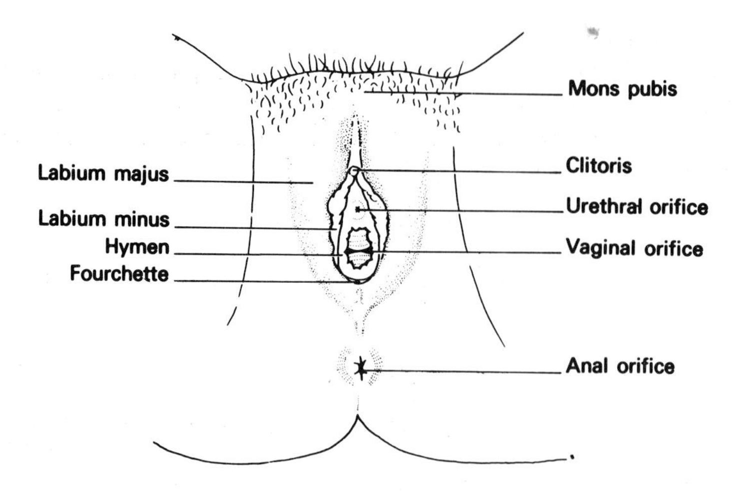

Fig. 3.1 The external genitalia.

minora divide into two folds, the upper fold forms the prepuce or hood over the clitoris, and the lower fold forms the frenulum which is attached to the under surface of the clitoris. Posteriorly the labia minora unite at the fourchette.

When an episiotomy is performed it is from the fourchette that the incision is made.

THE CLITORIS

A small sensitive structure situated within the preputial and frenular folds. It is about 2.5 cm long and is composed of two corpora cavernosa. They are two erectile bodies lying side by side and extending backwards to be attached to the underlying pubic bone by the crura of the clitoris. The rounded apex of the clitoris, which is highly sensitive, is known as the glans clitoris.

THE VESTIBULE

The narrow cleft lying between the labia minora and containing the openings of the urethra and the vagina.

THE VAGINAL INTROITUS (or orifice)

This occupies the lower two-thirds of the vestibule. In the virgin it is covered by an incomplete membrane known as the hymen. The hymen is ruptured during coitus and further lacerations occur during childbirth. The remnants of the hymen which surround the vaginal introitus are called the carunculae myrtiformes. A small depression between the vaginal introitus and the fourchette is known as the fossa navicularis.

THE VESTIBULAR BULBS

Two small collections of vascular erectile tissue lying on either side of the vaginal introitus anterior to the Bartholin's glands and deep to the labia minora and majora. Anteriorly they unite above the urethral orifice to become continuous with the clitoris (Fig. 3.2).

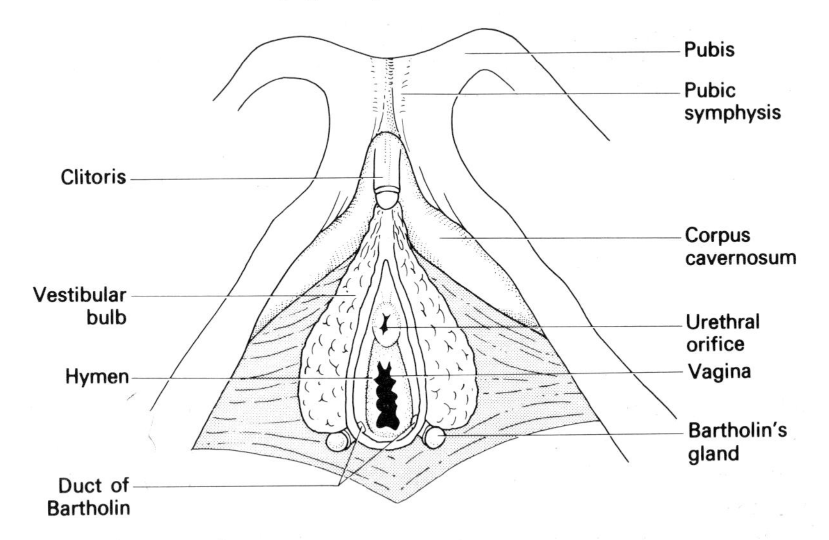

Fig. 3.2 The clitoris, vestibular bulbs and Bartholin's glands.

BARTHOLIN'S GLANDS

These are two compound racemose glands about the size and shape of small beans which lie on either side and posteriorly to the vaginal introitus, behind the vestibular bulbs. They are situated deep to the labia and ducts open on the surface, external to the vaginal introitus and medial to the labia minora. Their function is to excrete mucus to moisten and lubricate the external genitalia.

When performing a mediolateral episiotomy care must be taken to avoid this structure.

The external genitalia is supplied with blood from two main arteries.

1 The femoral artery. Blood reaches the vulva via the superficial and deep external pudendal arteries.

2 The internal pudendal artery via the posterior labial and the deep and dorsal arteries of the clitoris.

Venous return is to corresponding veins.

Lymphatic drainage is into the inguinal glands and the external iliac groups.

The skin of the vulva is supplied by the ilioinguinal nerve, branches of the genitofemoral, posterior cutaneous nerve of the thigh and the pudendal nerve.

During pregnancy there is an increased blood supply to the external genitalia and the skin may become pigmented.

During the second stage of labour the structures of the external genitalia become flattened, and displaced and stretched by the presentation of the fetus. Oedema, bruising and laceration may occur if adequate care is not taken during delivery of the baby. An episiotomy may be required to enlarge the vaginal introitus and, therefore, prevent damage to the surrounding structures (see p. 158–9).

The internal genitalia

The vagina

The upper two-thirds of the vagina develops from the Mullerian ducts and the lower third from the urorectal septum.

The vagina is a fibromuscular canal connecting the uterus above with the external genitalia below. It is situated partly in the perineum and partly in the pelvis.

The long axis of the vagina is directed upwards and backwards almost parallel with the plane of the pelvic brim and almost at right-angles to the long axis of the body of the uterus (Fig. 3.3).

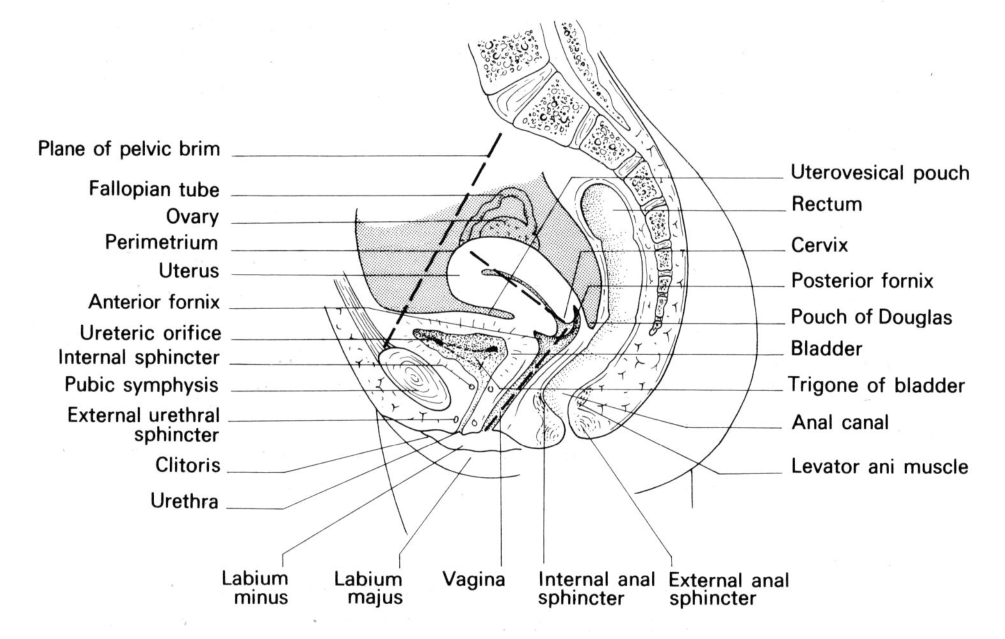

Fig. 3.3 Sagittal section of the pelvis.

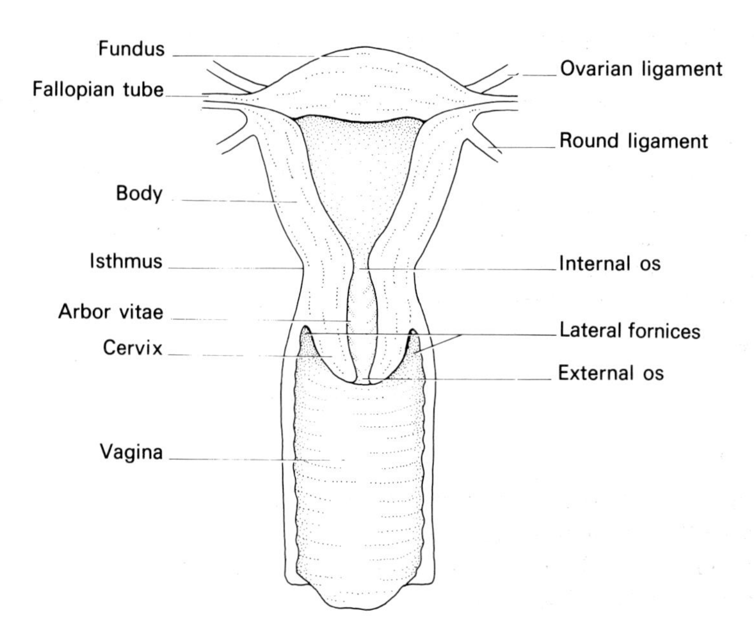

Fig. 3.4 Cross section of vagina and uterus.

The anterior vaginal wall measures approximately 7.5 cm and the posterior wall 10 cm. The reduction in the length of the anterior wall is the result of the cervix projecting into its upper aspect (Fig. 3.3).

The vaginal walls are in close contact in the lower part of the vagina but in the upper part they are separated by the cervix into four recesses, the anterior, posterior and lateral fornices (Figs. 3.3 and 3.4). The lower part of the vagina is the introitus.

Structure

The vagina has four layers.

1 Epithelial. The vagina is lined by stratified squamous epithelium thrown into folds or rugae to allow for stretching. These folds tend to become obliterated with multiparity resulting in a smoother surface.

2 The subepithelial layer is composed of vascular connective tissue.

3 The muscular layer consists of an inner circular and an outer longitudinal layer of non-striated muscle.

4 The fibrous outer layer is a vascular connective tissue containing blood and lymphatic vessels and nerves. It forms part of the pelvic fascia.

VAGINAL SECRETIONS

There are no active secretory glands in the vagina. Vaginal secretions are partly derived from vascular transudation and desquamation of cells and partly from cervical secretions.

The pH of the vagina is 4.5. This high acidity is due to the bacterial action of the Doderlein's bacillus, non-pathogenic bacteria which are normal inhabitants of the vagina during the reproductive phase. They act on the glycogen in the vaginal cells and produce lactic acid which protects against vaginal infections.

RELATIONS OF THE VAGINA

Anteriorly. The lower two-thirds of the vagina is in relation to the urethra, and the upper third to the base of the bladder, separated only by connective tissue (Fig. 3.3).

Posteriorly. The lower third of the vagina is related to the perineal body, the middle third to the rectum and the upper third to the pouch of Douglas. The peritoneum is reflected from the posterior surface of the uterus on to the upper two-thirds of the vagina, before passing on to the anterior wall of the rectum (Fig. 3.3).

Laterally. The vagina is related to the two halves of the levatores ani and the ureters and uterine blood vessels laterally.

Superiorly and inferiorly. The vagina is in relation to the cervix uteri superiorly and the introitus and the structures of the vulva inferiorly.

BLOOD SUPPLY

Three arteries supply the vagina with blood.

1 The cervical (descending) branch of the uterine arteries supply the upper third.
2 The vaginal artery which is a branch of the inferior vesical artery.
3 The middle haemorrhoidal and terminal branches of the pudendal artery.
The corresponding veins flow into the internal iliac veins.

Lymphatics

The lymphatics drain into the inguinal glands from the lower third, and the iliac glands from the upper two-thirds.

Nerve supply

The nerve pathways are via the second, third and fourth sacral nerves.

CHANGES IN THE VAGINA DURING PREGNANCY

Jacquemier's sign. Due to an increased blood supply and venous engorgement the vagina becomes bluish in colour.

Osiander's sign. Pulsation of the uterine artery felt through the lateral fornices.

Leucorrhoea. There is an increase in the vaginal secretions during pregnancy due to increased vascular transudation.

Decreased acidity. The pH of the vagina tends to be higher in pregnancy and this decreased acidity encourages vaginal infections (see p. 231).

CHANGES IN THE VAGINA DURING LABOUR

During the second stage of labour the vagina is distended and elongated by the presentation of the fetus.

INDICATIONS FOR VAGINAL EXAMINATION

1 Prenatal: at booking (see p. 39); at thirty-six weeks (see p. 49); prior to and following amniotomy (see p. 238); examination under anaesthesia (see p. 147).

2 Labour (see p. 147): on admission to assess progress in labour; following rupture of membranes to exclude cord prolapse; to confirm full dilatation of the os uteri; following delivering of each baby in a multiple delivery; prior to a forceps delivery.

TECHNIQUE OF VAGINAL EXAMINATION (see p. 147)

CHANGES IN THE VAGINA DURING THE PUERPERIUM

The vagina, which is smooth-walled and capacious at the end of labour, diminishes in size and at the end of three weeks the rugae of the pre-pregnant state are present.

The uterus

The uterus develops from the Mullerian ducts.

The non-pregnant uterus is a hollow, muscular, pear-shaped organ situated in the pelvis. It is anteverted, i.e. tilted forwards, and anteflexed, i.e. slightly bent on itself, and lies at right-angles to the vagina and the plane of the pelvic brim (Figs. 3.3 and 3.5).

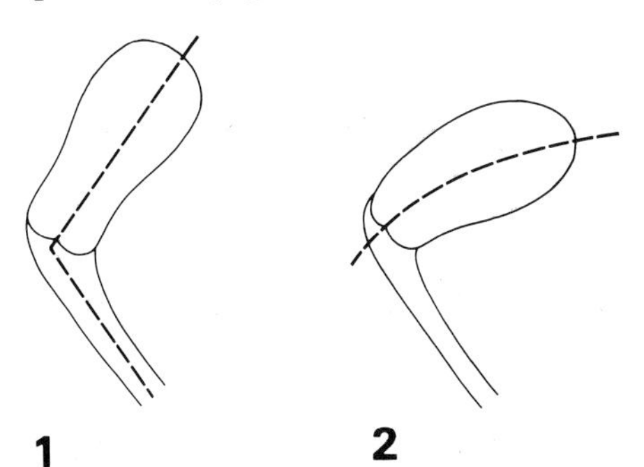

Fig. 3.5 The uterus in relation to the vagina; 1, anteverted; 2, anteflexed.

The external measurements of the uterus are 7.5 cm long, 5 cm wide, and 2.5 cm thick, and it weighs about 60 g. The cavity of the uterus is 6.25 cm long.

The uterus consists of:

The body. This forms the upper two-thirds of the uterus. The Fallopian tubes enter the lateral aspects at the area known as the cornua, and the upper rounded part of the body above the Fallopian tubes is described as the fundus (Fig. 3.6).

The isthmus. This is the area approximately 7 mm long situated between the body of the uterus and the cervix. It is here that the uterine arteries enter the uterus, the peritoneum is reflected off the bladder on to the anterior aspect of the uterine body, and the ureters cross on the way to the bladder (Fig. 3.6).

The cervix. This forms the lower third of the uterus. It comprises the internal os opening into the cavity of the uterine body, and the external os opening into the vagina and a spindle-shaped cervical canal. The cervix lies partly within the vagina, the vaginal portion and partly above, the supravaginal portion (Fig. 3.6).

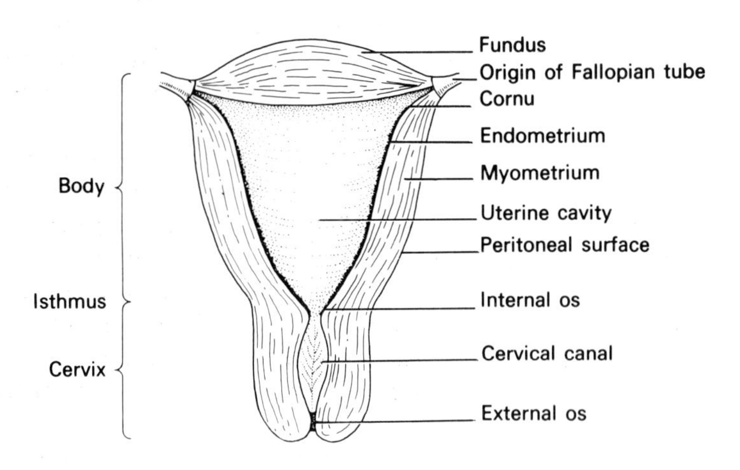

Fig. 3.6 The divisions of the uterus.

STRUCTURE

The uterus has three layers; the endometrium, myometrium and perimetrium (Fig. 3.6).

The endometrium. The lining of the body of the uterus differs from that of the cervix.

The lining of the body comprises:

a A single layer of ciliated cubical epithelium.

b Simple mucus secreting tubular glands, lined with non-ciliated cubical cells. The bases of the glands extend down to the muscle coat. The glands open into the cavity of the uterus.

c A vascular connective tissue called stroma which lies between the tubular glands.

The endometrium varies in thickness and vascularity according to the phase of the menstrual cycle.

The cervical mucosa comprises:

a Columnar epithelium.

b Compound racemose glands which branch into the muscle layer. Their function is to produce mucus.

c Collagen, a fibrous connective tissue.

The vaginal portion of the cervix is covered with stratified squamous epithelium continuous with that of the vagina. The junction of the two epithelia forms the squamocolumnar junction an important area for carcinoma *in situ*.

Changes occur in the endometrium lining the body of the uterus during each of the three distinct phases of the menstrual cycle.

1 Menstrual phase. The endometrium is shed down to its basal layer.

2 Proliferative phase. Under the influence of oestrogens from the developing Graaffian follicle the endometrium regenerates from the basal layer. It becomes thicker, the blood vessels increase in size, the tubular glands become taller, and the cells in the stroma become more densely packed and spindle-shaped.

3 Secretory phase. There is a further increase in the thickness and vascularity of the endometrium during this phase. Under the influence of oestrogens and progesterone from the corpus luteum the stromal cells enlarge and become closely packed together, forming the compact layer. The glands become elongated, more tortuous, and filled with secretions. The deeper portions of the glands are more dilated than the superficial and form the spongy layer. The basal layer resting on the muscle coat, remains unchanged. Menstruation occurs when the arterioles in the deepest layer of the endometrium contract strongly and occlude the blood flow, so that ischaemic necrosis occurs. Disintegration of the superficial part of the endometrium and escape of blood and mucus occurs as the result of a fall in the levels of oestrogens and progesterone. The stroma becomes infiltrated with blood and the tension produced leads to rupture with escape of blood and detachment of the superficial layers of the endometrium. These fragments are carried away in the blood and mucus which passes out of the uterus as the menstrual flow.

The myometrium. This is the muscle coat and is composed of plain muscle fibres. In the non-pregnant uterus the muscle layers are not well defined. The uterine blood vessels enter the substance of the uterine wall and branch within the myometrium. In the deep layers, connective tissue and elastic fibres are intermingled with the muscle fibres, especially in the cervix.

The perimetrium. This is the peritoneal coat and covers the posterior surface and the upper two-thirds of the anterior surface. The loose double fold of peritoneum, leaving the uterus at each lateral border, and containing the Fallopian tubes in the upper border, is the broad ligament.

BLOOD SUPPLY

The uterus, together with the ovaries and Fallopian tubes are supplied both from the uterine and ovarian arteries.

The uterine arteries are branches of the internal iliac arteries. They run along the broad ligament and at the level of the isthmus give off descending branches to the cervix and vagina. The main branch of the uterine artery is coiled and tortuous, and ascends in the lateral borders of the body of the uterus, and anastomoses with the ovarian artery just below the cornua.

The veins from the fundus, ovaries and tubes drain into the ovarian veins which join the inferior vena cava on the right and the renal vein on the left. The veins from the cervix and lower part of the body drain into the uterine veins.

LYMPHATICS

The lymphatic drainage from the body of the uterus is into the internal iliac glands and from the cervix, into the internal iliac and sacral glands via the parametrial and obturator glands.

NERVE SUPPLY

Sympathetic fibres from eleventh and twelfth thoracic nerves and parasympathetic fibres from the second, third and fourth sacral nerves supply the uterus.

UTERINE LIGAMENTS

The uterus is maintained in its normal position of anteversion and anteflexion by the uterine ligaments (Fig. 3.7).

The two transverse cervical ligaments pass from the cervix laterally to the side walls of the pelvis. The two uterosacral ligaments pass from the cervix

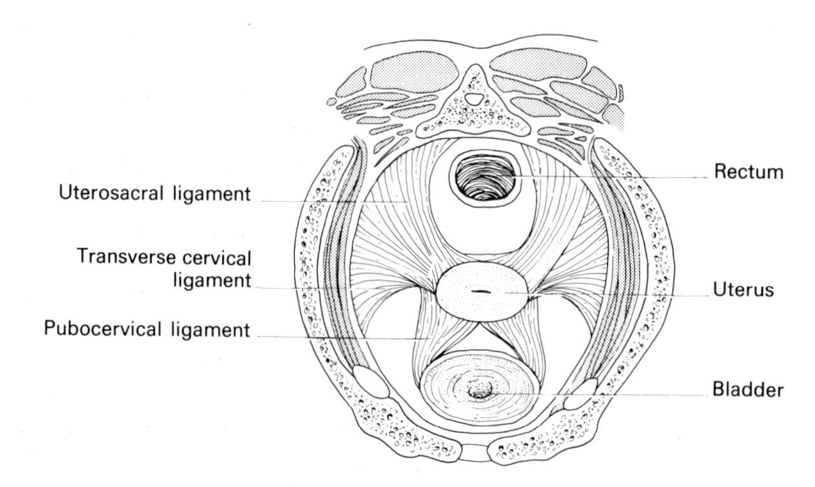

Fig. 3.7 The uterine ligaments (seen from above).

backwards, one on either side of the rectum to the sacrum. The two pubocervical ligaments pass from the cervix forwards under the bladder to the symphysis pubis. The two round ligaments pass from the cornua in the broad ligament, down and forwards through the inguinal canal to the labia majora. The two ovarian ligaments pass from the ovaries to the cornua. The broad ligaments have already been described (see p. 65).

RELATIONS

Anteriorly, the cervix is related to the bladder, the uterovesical pouch and the pubocervical ligaments. Posteriorly, the uterus is related to the peritoneal cavity, the pouch of Douglas, and the uterosacral ligaments; laterally, to the Fallopian tubes, ovaries and the broad, ovarian and round ligaments; and superiorly, to the intestines. Inferiorly, the uterus is related to the vagina and the anteverted body of the uterus to the bladder.

Physiological changes in the uterus during pregnancy

CHANGES IN SIZE AND SHAPE

At the end of pregnancy, the uterus measures approximately 30 cm long, 22.5 cm wide and 20 cm thick (see p. 22, Fig. 2.4). The weight of the uterus increases to about 1 kg. Uterine growth which occurs as the result of the action of the oestrogenic hormones, takes place by hypertrophy and hyperplasia. Hypertrophy describes the growth of the individual muscle fibres of the uterine wall which become ten times longer and three times thicker, and hyperplasia the development of new muscle fibres.

In the early months of pregnancy the walls thicken, but in the later months they are stretched and thinned.

During the first three months of pregnancy the shape of the uterus becomes globular, but after the fifth month it is ovoid and maintains this shape until term.

These alterations in the shape of the uterus are due to varying rates of growth which occur in its different parts. The blastocyst normally embeds in the body and this part of the uterus becomes uniformly enlarged and is called the upper uterine segment. At the same time growth occurs in the isthmus. As this does not normally contain the blastocyst it does not become wider but increases in length, growing from 7 mm to 25 mm (Fig. 3.8[1]). The empty isthmus lying between the expanded upper uterine segment above and the cervix below, forms the basis of Hegar's sign of pregnancy (see p. 19).

By about the twelfth week of pregnancy, the gestation sac fills the cavity of the upper segment of the uterus and the isthmus opens out and receives the developing embryo into its cavity. The expanded isthmus may now be referred to as the lower uterine segment (Fig. 3.8[2]).

The uterus now comprises the upper uterine segment which has developed

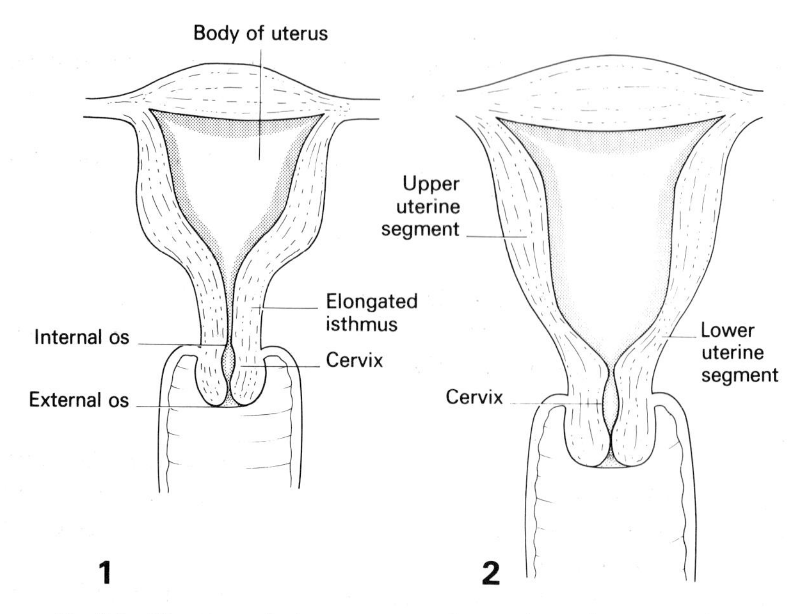

Fig. 3.8 The uterus during pregnancy; 1, at eight weeks; 2, at twelve weeks.

from the uterine body, the lower uterine segment which has developed from the isthmus and the virtually unchanged cervix.

Enlargement of the uterus may be observed clinically (see p. 22). As the uterus grows into the abdominal cavity it leans towards and becomes slightly rotated to the right. This uterine obliquity and rotation is caused by the descending colon occupying the left side of the abdominal cavity.

CHANGES IN THE CERVIX

The cervix maintains a length of 2.5 cm during pregnancy. However, it increases in width and becomes much softer after the twelfth week. This is due to its increased vascularity, to the relaxing effect of oestrogen on the connective tissue ground substance, and to proliferation of the cervical mucosa and compound racemose glands. These glands excrete a mucus to form a mucoid plug, known as the operculum, which occupies the cervical canal during pregnancy and effectively prevents the entry of harmful substances into the uterus. Changes occur in the connective tissue (collagen) of the cervix which makes it resistant to stretch, and causes the cervix to remain closed. As pregnancy progresses, changes in the property of the collagen takes place causing the cervix to be less resistant to stretch. This allows for the formation of the lower uterine segment (see p. 75) and effacement and dilation of the cervix. Those changes are probably due to rising levels of oestrogens in early pregnancy and increasing levels of naturally produced prostaglandins in late pregnancy.

CHANGES IN THE ENDOMETRIUM

The ovarian and menstrual cycles prepare the endometrium for the reception of the fertilised ovum. It becomes known as the decidua and is divided into three parts.

1 The decidua basalis is the part of the decidua which lies between the developing blastocyst and the myometrium.

2 The decidua capsularis covers the blastocyst and separates it from the uterine cavity.

3 The decidua vera lines the remainder of the uterine cavity.

The blastocyst usually embeds in the decidua lining the fundus of the uterus or the upper part of the anterior or posterior wall.

CHANGES IN THE MYOMETRIUM

The three layers of the myometrium become more clearly defined. The outer layer is composed of longitudinal fibres which pass over the fundus from front to back, starting and ending at the internal os (Fig. 3.9[1]). They help to pull up and dilate the cervix and os.

The middle layer is the thickest and the fibres are arranged in bundles which cross and recross each other obliquely (Fig. 3.9[2]). They are arranged around the arteries and veins and have a vital function in the control of bleeding from the placental site following separation of the placenta.

The innermost layer consists mainly of circular fibres, encircling the lower uterine segment and the Fallopian tubes (Fig. 3.9[2]). The structure of the uterine muscle is therefore adapted to take up and dilate the cervix and os, expel the fetus and the placenta and membranes and arrest bleeding from the placental site.

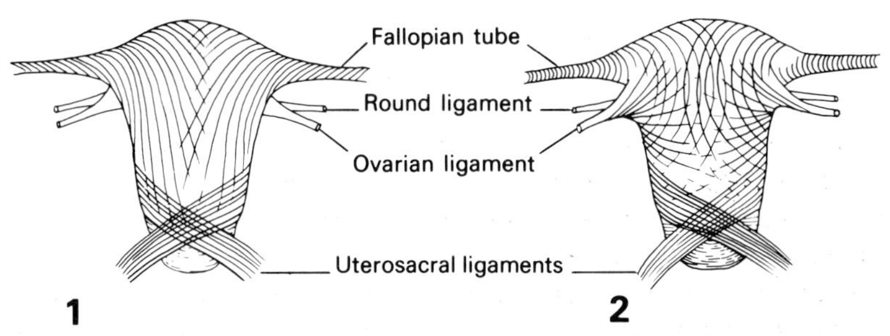

Fig. 3.9 The direction of muscle fibres in the uterine wall; 1, outer (longitudinal) layer; 2, inner (circular and oblique) layers.

CHANGES IN THE BLOOD SUPPLY

During pregnancy, the uterine and ovarian blood vessels become greatly enlarged. The main vessels are convoluted and the branches of the arteries run a corkscrew-like course through the uterine muscles. The blood supply of the uterus is estimated to increase twenty-fold during pregnancy.

OTHER CHANGES IN THE UTERUS

The uterine ligaments, which contain smooth muscle, become thickened during pregnancy, and the lymphatic vessels are greatly enlarged.

As already mentioned uterine growth occurs as a result of stimulation by oestrogens, which are derived from the ovary and subsequently the placenta. Progesterone from the same sources, stimulates the conversion of the endometrium into the decidua, and brings about relaxation. However, from about the sixteenth week of pregnancy periodic waves of contraction occur. These are the Braxton Hicks contractions already described (see p. 21). These contractions are part of the physiological growth process of uterine muscle, in preparation for labour. They increase the blood flow to the placenta, and towards the end of pregnancy they become stronger and more frequent, and are responsible for the taking up of the cervix.

Physiological changes in the uterus during normal labour

Labour is the process by which the products of conception are expelled from the uterus after the twenty-eighth week of pregnancy.

Normal labour starts spontaneously at or about term. The fetus presents by the vertex, and labour is completed spontaneously within twenty-four hours without injury to mother or child.

The progress of labour is influenced by three factors:

1 The powers.
   - **a** The contractions and retraction of uterine muscles (primary powers).
   - **b** The action of abdominal muscles and diaphragm (secondary powers).
2 The passages.
   - **a** The cervix, vagina and pelvic floor.
   - **b** The pelvis.
3 The passengers.
   - **a** The fetus.
   - **b** The placenta and membranes.

CAUSES OF ONSET

The precise stimulation which initiates labour is not known. Regulation of myometrial function and activity depends on mechanical and neural factors which are set in a complex background of hormonal activity.

Modern evidence suggests that the onset of labour is controlled by the fetus itself. Increasing activity in the fetal pituitary-adrenal axis leads to a rise in oestrogen production by the fetoplacental unit associated with increasing production of prostaglandin $F_{2\alpha}$ and perhaps a fall in progesterone, a balance of hormones and prostaglandin which promote myometrial contraction. When the fetal pituitary-adrenal axis is defective as in some anencephalics, labour may not occur spontaneously. The same endocrine activity probably leads to surfactant production in the fetal lung, thus preparing it for air breathing.

The role of oxytocin is not entirely clear but its capacity to cause uterine contraction is related to the concentration of prostaglandin present and it is therefore only permitted to act when the fetus is 'ready'.

Prostaglandins are present in the decidua in late pregnancy and local secretion of prostaglandins occurs if a finger is inserted into the cervix and the chorion separated from the decidua.

STAGES OF LABOUR

There are three stages of labour.

First stage. From the onset of regular uterine contractions accompanied by effacement and dilatation of the cervix and os to full dilatation of the os uteri. This is the longest stage of labour and lasts approximately twelve to fourteen hours in primigravidae (Fig. 3.10) and six to eight hours in multigravidae (Fig. 3.11).

Second stage. From full dilatation of the os uteri to the birth of the baby. This stage lasts approximately forty-five minutes in primigravidae and thirty minutes in multigravidae.

Third stage. From the birth of the baby to expulsion of the placenta and membranes. This stage may last about twenty to thirty minutes if not actively managed. Active management of the third stage of labour has reduced the length of the stage to between five and fifteen minutes.

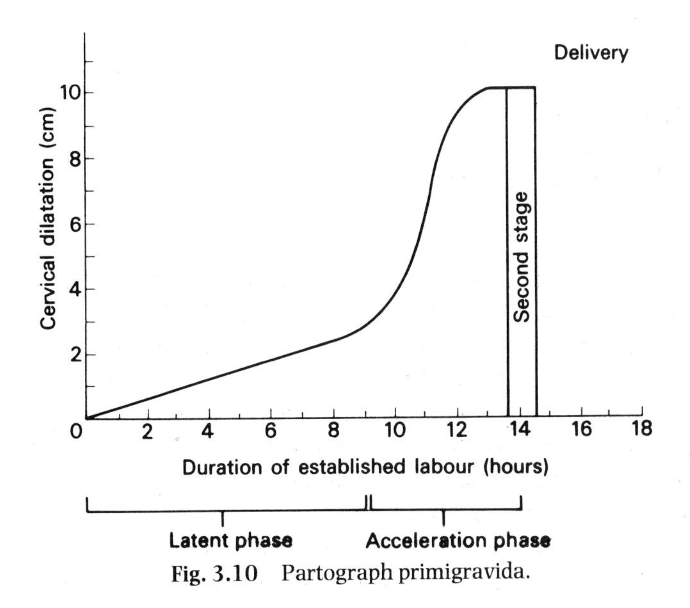

Fig. 3.10 Partograph primigravida.

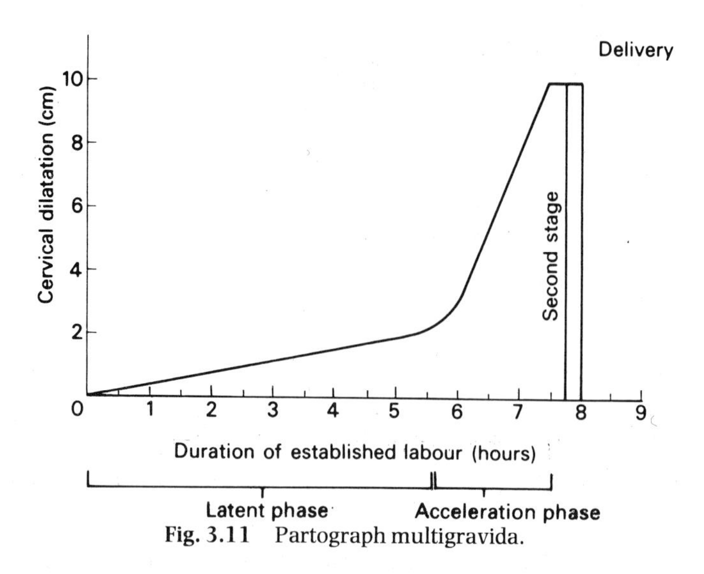

Fig. 3.11 Partograph multigravida.

Physiology of the first stage of labour

CONTRACTIONS OF UTERINE MUSCLE

During pregnancy, the uterine muscle is constantly contracting and relaxing. The contractions become stronger and more frequent towards the end of pregnancy, but they remain painless and do not result in dilatation of the os (see p. 21).

At the onset of labour the contractions change and usually become painful and the os uteri begins to dilate. At the onset of labour the contractions are weak (20 mmHg), infrequent (every twenty to thirty minutes) and of short duration (twenty to thirty seconds). As labour progresses the contractions become stronger, more frequent and last longer, until by the end of the first stage of labour they are strong (40–60 mmHg), frequent (every two or three minutes) and lasting forty-five to sixty seconds. This progressive increase in strength, length and frequency of uterine contractions is an indication that labour is progressing normally.

Pacemaker. In the uterus, just as in the heart, there is a pacemaker, a zone where the contraction begins and from which it spreads to the rest of the uterus. The normal contraction starts near one of the cornua and the wave takes ten to thirty seconds to spread over the uterus as a whole. The two cornua may act alternately.

Descending gradient. Not only does the contraction spread downwards from the fundus, but in the upper part of the uterus the contraction is more sustained and stronger than in the lower part of the uterus. This is referred to as the descending gradient (Fig. 3.12).

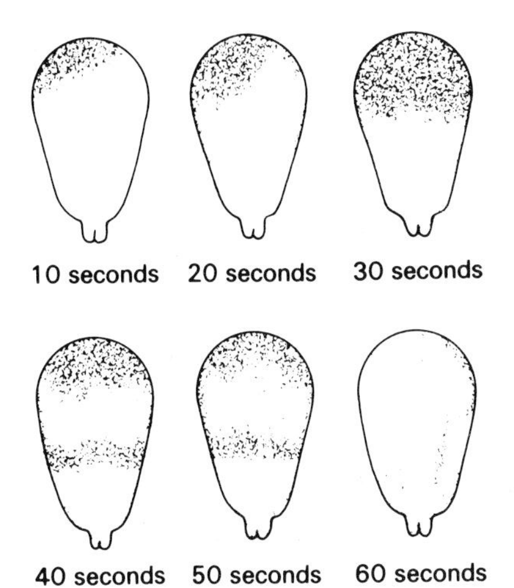

Fig. 3.12 Descending gradient.

Fundal dominance. The longer and stronger contraction of the upper part of the uterus is called fundal dominance. Hence, when making observations of the length and strength of the uterine contractions the hand, or external transducer if monitoring apparatus is being used, is placed on the fundus.

During uterine contractions there is interference with the blood flow to the placenta, and a reduction in the oxygen and an increase in the carbon dioxide content of the placental blood. When the contractions are weak the interference is minimal but as the contractions increase in strength the blood flow is further diminished.

Resting tone. Between contractions the tone of the uterine muscle returns to normal, below 10 mmHg (Fig. 3.13). The placental blood flow is now unimpeded and the exchange of oxygen and carbon dioxide between the fetal and maternal blood resumes.

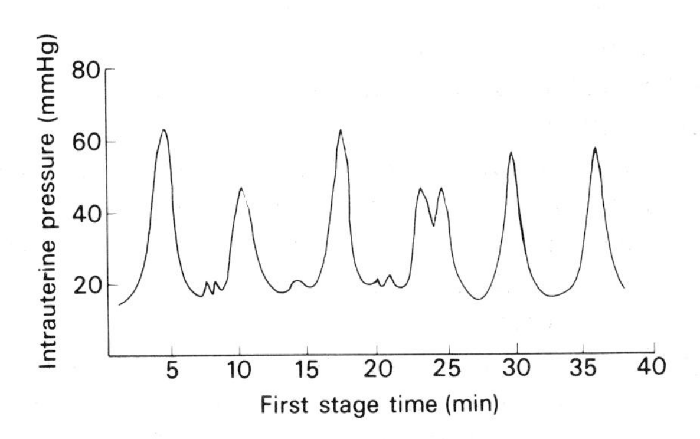

Fig. 3.13 Uterine contraction.

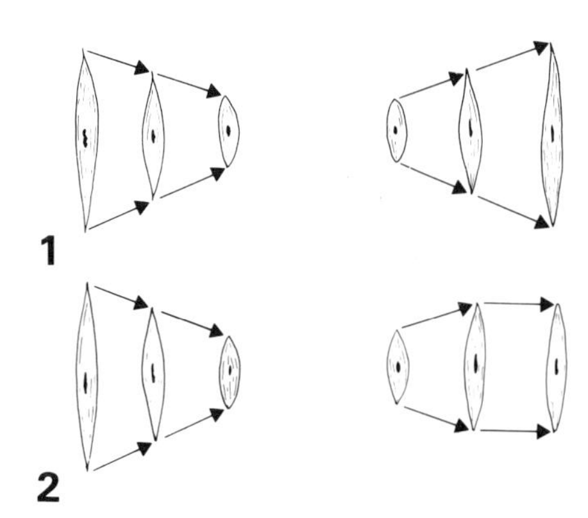

Fig. 3.14 Contraction of muscle fibres followed by 1, normal relaxation; 2, retraction.

Contraction. The temporary increase in tone and shortening of muscle fibres is called contraction. It is usually followed by an equal degree of relaxation and lengthening, i.e. the muscle fibres are isotonic, they have the same strength, and isometric, they have equal dimensions as prior to the contraction. Contractions alone would not therefore expel the fetus from the uterus without another factor called retraction.

Retraction. A process of progressive and maintained shortening and thickening of the muscle fibres which accompanies and succeeds contraction is called retraction. It retains some of the advantages gained by the previous contraction, and is essential for dilatation of the os uteri and descent of the fetus through the birth canal. Therefore, although there is an equal degree of relaxation following a contraction, i.e. the muscle fibres are isotonic, there is not an equal degree of lengthening, i.e. the muscle fibres are not isometric (Fig. 3.14).

The upper uterine segment. This is the active contractile and retractile part of the uterus during labour. The muscle fibres become shortened as labour progresses, hence the upper uterine segment becomes shortened, the walls become thickened and the cavity reduced in size.

The lower uterine segment. During labour, the lower uterine segment is passive. It contracts weakly and relaxes and is drawn upwards, lengthened, thinned out and dilated. The cavity becomes larger and accommodates the fetus as it is progressively being expelled for the upper uterine segment.

Polarity. The neuromuscular harmony between the upper and lower uterine segments is termed polarity and describes the contrasting but harmonious activity between the two parts of the uterus, i.e. the upper uterine segment contracts strongly and retracts and the lower uterine segment contracts less strongly and relaxes.

Retraction ring. The term given to the line of demarcation between the upper and lower segments is the retraction ring (Fig. 3.15). This physiological junction develops as a result of retraction of the upper uterine segment producing progressive thickening of the walls of the upper segment and at

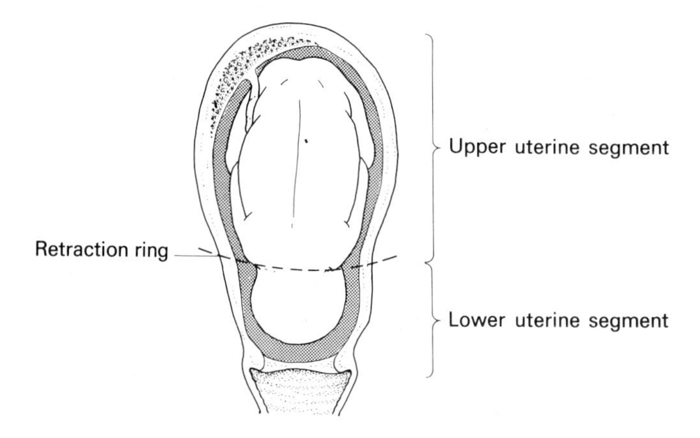

Fig. 3.15 The retraction ring.

the same time progressive thinning of the walls of the lower uterine segment.

Effacement and dilatation of the cervix and os uteri. As the muscle fibres of the upper uterine segment become shorter, traction is exerted on the less active lower uterine segment. This completes the process of effacement of the cervix which usually starts in the last four weeks of pregnancy. The internal os dilates and the spindle-shaped cervical canal now becomes funnel-shaped. The cervix is pulled up and becomes incorporated into the lower uterine segment. The degree of effacement of the cervix is noted during vaginal examination in labour (Fig. 3.16).

The external os is now known as the os uteri and is dilated by the continuing traction exerted by the retracting upper uterine segment. Dilatation

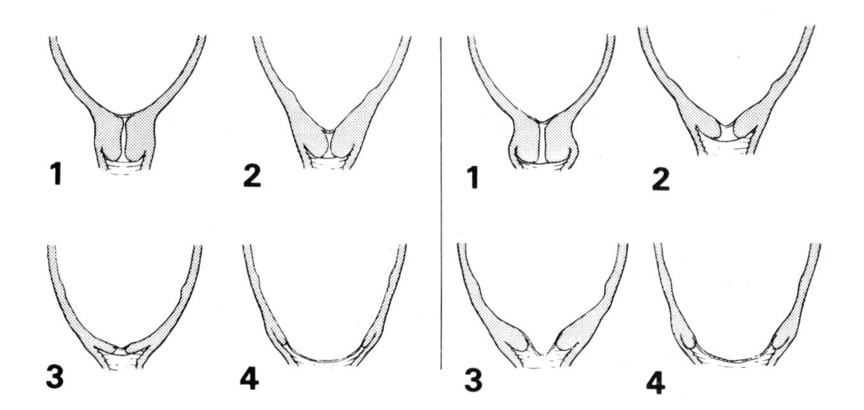

Fig. 3.16 Cervical effacement and dilatation; (left) primigravida, 1, before labour; 2, early effacement; 3, complete effacement; 4, complete dilatation; (right) multigravida, 1, before labour; 2, effacement and beginning dilatation; 3, dilatation; 4, complete dilatation.

of the os uteri is measured in centimetres and, although it may vary according to the size of the fetal head, full dilatation of the os uteri is usually defined as 10 cm. In multigravidae, dilatation of the external os often accompanies effacement of the cervix rather than following it as is more usual in primigravidae.

Formation of the forewaters and hindwaters. As the cervix is being effaced the chorionic membrane attached to the decidua vera above the internal os becomes detached and the loosened bag of membranes containing a small quantity of amniotic fluid, protrudes into the cervical canal. As effacement of the cervix continues, the fetal head descends on to the cervix and separates the amniotic fluid in the bag of membranes from the remainder. The collection of amniotic fluid in front of the fetal head is known as the forewaters and the remainder as the hindwaters.

The forewaters. Pressure builds up within the forewaters during a uterine contraction and even pressure is applied on the cervix aiding effacement and early dilatation of the os uteri. Beyond 4 cm dilatation however, the forewaters may delay rather than encourage dilatation, and the membranes are usually ruptured, if this has not occurred spontaneously, to allow the head to come into close contact with the os uteri and assist further dilatation.

Hindwaters. The amniotic fluid retained in the uterus behind the fetal head forms the hindwaters and acts as a buffer protecting the fetus and placenta from the full force of contractions. Pressure within the forewaters and hindwaters increases during a contraction.

'*Show.*' As effacement and dilatation of the cervix and os uteri takes place the operculum becomes displaced from the cervical canal and is shed *per vaginum* as the 'show'. The mucus is usually slightly bloodstained due to bleeding from capillaries of the decidua vera as the chorion became detached.

Physiology of the second stage of labour

Contraction. During the second stage of labour the nature of the uterine contractions changes and they become expulsive. The contractions are strong, 60–80 mmHg and increased in amplitude by the secondary powers (Fig. 3.17).

Secondary powers. When the diaphragm is lowered and fixed at the height of inspiration and the abdominal muscles are contracted, a very strong pressure is applied to the uterus considerably increasing the expulsive force of the uterine contractions.

Fetal axis pressure. This refers to the force exerted by the contracting uterus and the secondary powers and transmitted via the fetal long axis to the head. It causes descent of the fetus through the birth canal.

Descent of the fetus is also brought about by extension and elongation of the fetus as its body unfolds from its previously flexed attitude.

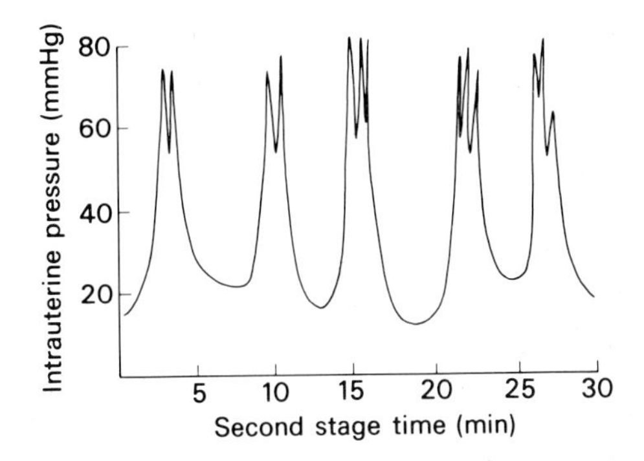

Fig. 3.17 Intrauterine pressure in the second stage of labour.

Retraction. In the second stage of labour retraction of the muscle fibres continues and advances more rapidly as the fetus is gradually expelled.

Physiology of the third stage of labour

The third stage of labour is the time of maximum risk to the mother and is concerned with the separation and descent of the placenta and membranes and the control of haemorrhage.

SEPARATION OF THE PLACENTA AND MEMBRANES

Separation of the placenta commences with the contraction that delivers the baby's trunk and is usually completed with the first contraction after the birth of the baby.

Separation occurs at the deep spongy layer of the decidua basalis and occurs due to continuing contraction and retraction of the uterine muscle causing diminution of the placental site. The placenta has no power of contraction and therefore becomes separated from its site of attachment.

Methods of separation. There are two methods by which placental separation takes place.

1 Schultze method. The centre of the placenta becomes detached first, the placenta becomes inverted as it descends and the fetal surface presents at the vulva with the membranes trailing behind. The retroplacental clot is retained in the inverted placenta with minimal blood loss (Fig. 3.18).

2 Mathews Duncan method. The lower edge of the placenta separates first and presents at the vulva, the placenta slides out folded longitudinally on itself with some of the membranes preceding it and some trailing behind. The retroplacental bleeding escapes before the placenta (Fig. 3.19).

Signs of placental separation and descent. As the placenta separates and descends, signs that this process has taken place can be observed.

1 The uterus rises to the level of the umbilicus. This indicates that the placenta has descended into the lower uterine segment and the upper uterine segment has been displaced upwards.

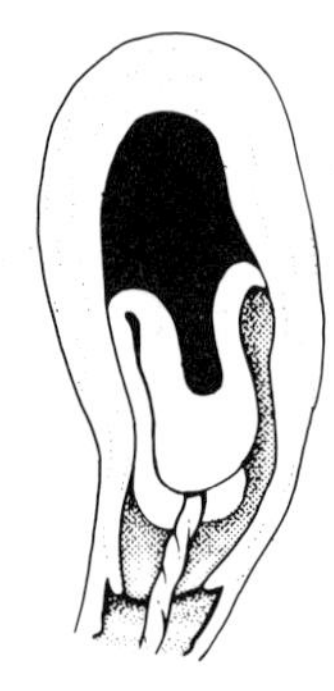

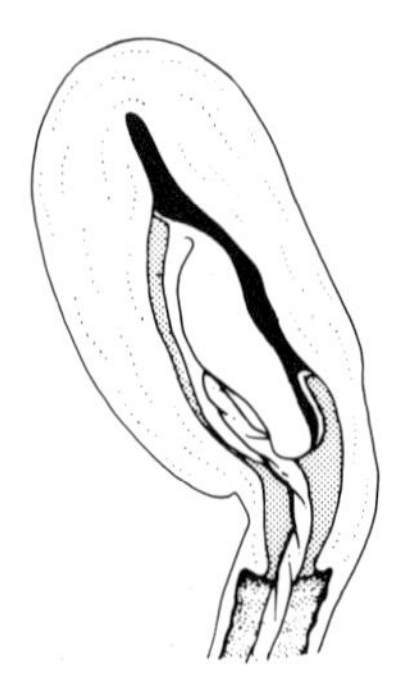

Fig. 3.18 (left) Schultze method of placental separation.
Fig. 3.19 (right) Mathews Duncan method of placental separation.

2 The uterus becomes smaller and more mobile. This indicates that the placenta has been expelled from the uterus and the empty uterus is now able to contract and retract.
3 The length of the umbilical cord outside the vulva increases, indicating descent of the placenta.
4 A show of blood denoting separation of the placenta, is seen *per vaginum*.

The signs of placental separation and descent must be awaited before an attempt is made to deliver the placenta and membranes when some methods of delivery are used, i.e. maternal effort and fundal pressure.

Control of haemorrhage. The control of haemorrhage is by:
1 The constriction of the blood vessels by contraction and retraction of the oblique muscle fibres (Fig. 3.20).
2 The clotting of the blood which is activated by separation of the placenta.
3 The collapse of the blood vessels.

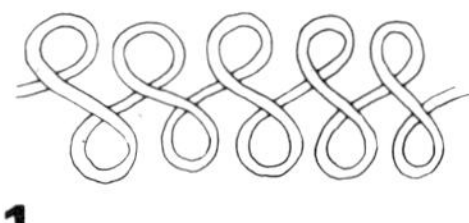

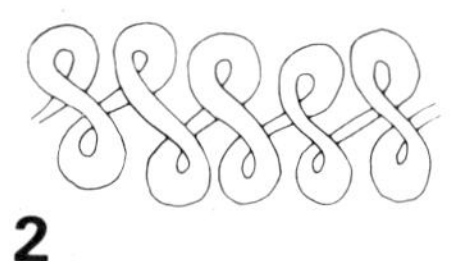

Fig. 3.20 The action of the oblique muscle fibres; 1, relaxed; 2, retracted.

Changes in the uterus during the puerperium

After delivery a series of changes takes place known as involution, which restores the uterine body and cervix, together with the ligamentary and muscular supports to approximately the same condition as before pregnancy.

INVOLUTION OF THE UTERUS

There are two main reasons for involution of the uterus.

1 Ischaemia. The blood supply to the uterus is reduced due to contraction. Deprived of their blood supply the muscle fibres diminish in length and in breadth.

2 Autolysis. The protoplasm of the muscle cells is broken down by proteolytic enzymes in a process known as autolysis and the end products are excreted by the kidneys as urea.

Uterine size. After delivery, the uterus weighs about 1 kg and measures 20 cm in length. The process of involution is most rapid during the first week of the puerperium, the uterus at the end of this time being about 11.5 cm in total length and about 0.5 kg in weight. By about ten days after delivery the uterus has descended into the pelvis and the fundus can only just be palpated behind the symphysis pubis.

The uterus returns to its position of anteversion and anteflexion.

Reforming of the cervix. For several days after delivery the cervix remains patulous, but by the end of the first week it is reformed. The cervical canal closes and the external os, which is seen as a transverse slit and referred to as a multiparous os, may not admit a finger.

Shedding of the decidua. At the beginning of the puerperium the uterine cavity is lined by remnants of the spongy layer of the decidua. Degeneration occurs due to ischaemia and the decidua is shed as the lochial discharges. Lochia consist of blood, mainly from the placental site, remnants of the decidua, leucocytes, vaginal epithelium and secretions. For the first three to four days the discharges are red, lochia rubra, changing to pinkish brown in colour, lochia serosa, and finally white, lochia alba, as the preponderance of blood diminishes.

Regeneration of the endometrium. The new endometrium regenerates from the basal layer of the decidua. Regeneration begins about the tenth day after delivery and is completed in about a month except at the placental site, where the process of regeneration takes six to seven weeks.

Menstruation. The ovarian and menstrual cycles resume and menstruation takes place between forty-nine and fifty-six days following delivery, unless lactation is taking place in which case the process is delayed by a few weeks due to high prolactin levels.

The Fallopian tubes (uterine tubes)

The Fallopian tubes are derived from the Mullerian ducts. They are two muscular tubes extending, one on either side, from the cornua of the uterus to the peritoneal cavity. One end of the tube opens into the uterine cavity and the other into the peritoneal cavity.

The function of the uterine tubes is to convey ova from the ovary to the uterus and spermatozoa to the ova. Fertilisation of an ovum normally takes place in the tube.

The tubes are about 10 cm long and for the purpose of description are divided into four parts (Fig. 3.21).

1 Interstitial. The narrowest part of the tube which lies within the uterine wall.

2 Isthmus. The part lying adjacent to the uterus.

3 Ampulla. The widest part of the tube. It is in this part that fertilisation of the ovum normally takes place.

4 Infundibulum. The fimbriated lateral extremity. This part of the tube turns backwards and downwards. The fimbriae surrounding the opening of the tubes serve to enlarge the receiving area for the ova expelled from the ovary and become engorged with blood around the time of ovulation. One fimbria is elongated and connects with the ovary below and is known as the fimbria ovarica.

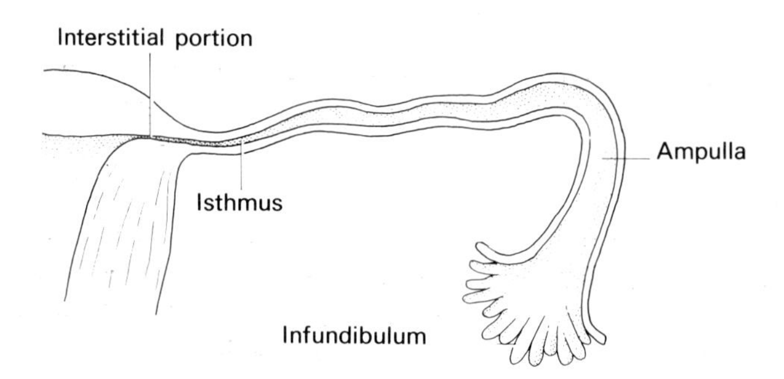

Fig. 3.21 The parts of the Fallopian tube.

STRUCTURE

The Fallopian tube is composed of three layers.

1 An inner layer of mucous membrane composed of a single layer of columnar epithelium. The membrane is thrown into a series of complicated longitudinal folds called plicae, which become more complex towards the fimbriated end where the lining is thicker than at the uterine end (Fig. 3.22). Some columnar cells are ciliated and the cilia maintain a constant movement which propels the ovum along the tube towards the uterus. The non-ciliated

cells are secretory and produce protein rich secretions which provide nourishment for the ova. These cells are known as the goblet cells and when collapsed, as peg cells. There is no submucous layer.

2 The middle muscular layer forms the main thickness of the tube and consists of an inner layer of circular muscle fibres which are most numerous in the isthmus, and an outer layer of longitudinal fibres. The muscle layers become progressively thinner from isthmus to infundibulum while the lumen becomes progressively wider (Fig. 3.22).

Peristaltic movements of the muscular layer reinforces the ciliary movement in propelling the ovum along the tube.

3 The outer or peritoneal layer is formed by the upper fold of the broad ligament which is absent from the inferior surface.

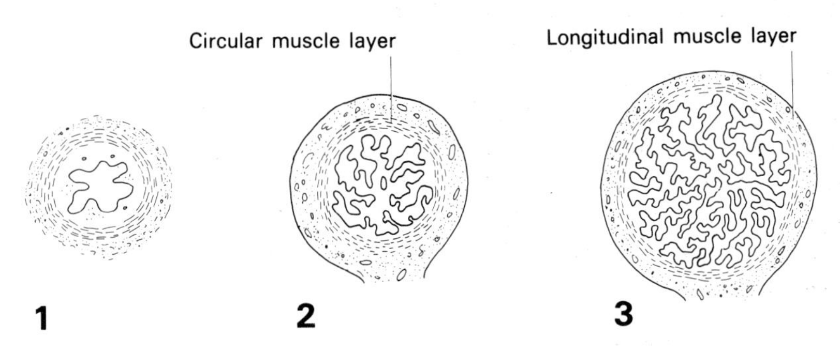

Fig. 3.22 A section through the Fallopian tube at; 1, interstitial portion; 2, isthmus; 3, ampulla.

RELATIONS

Medially, the Fallopian tubes are related to the uterus, laterally, to the infundibulopelvic ligament and side walls of the pelvis, and inferiorly, to the ovaries and broad ligaments. Anteriorly, posteriorly and superiorly are the contents of the peritoneal and abdominal cavities.

BLOOD SUPPLY

The blood supply of the uterine tubes is from the ovarian and uterine arteries with venous drainage into the corresponding veins.

LYMPHATIC DRAINAGE

The drainage of lymph is into the lumbar glands.

NERVE SUPPLY

The tubes are supplied by both motor and sensory parasympathetic and sympathetic nerves.

When the fertilised ovum remains within the tube and continues to develop, rupture of the tube may be the sequel (see p. 178, ectopic pregnancy). This may occur as a result of ciliary damage due to inflammation. If blockage of the tube is complete which may occur as a result of scarring after inflammation, the woman will be sterile.

CHANGES IN PREGNANCY

The musculature of the Fallopian tubes undergoes hypertrophy during pregnancy.

CHANGES IN THE PUERPERIUM

The musculature of the Fallopian tubes shares in the general process of involution.

The ovaries (the female gonads)

The ovary is an almond-shaped organ whose structure and function varies according to the age of the woman.

The ovaries are dull white in colour and measure approximately 2.5 cm in length, 2 cm in width, 1.25 cm in thickness and weigh about 6 g. Prior to ovulation the ovary appears smooth and shining, it then becomes increasingly scarred and irregular due to the presence of Graafian follicles, corpora lutea and corpora albicantia. The ovaries are situated on the posterior surface of the broad ligament with the long axis lying horizontally (Fig. 3.23).

Attachments. The ovary is attached by the mesovarian to the broad ligament, by the ovarian ligament to the cornua of the uterus and by the infundibulo-pelvic ligament to the side wall of the pelvis. It is brought into contact with the Fallopian tube by the fimbria ovarica.

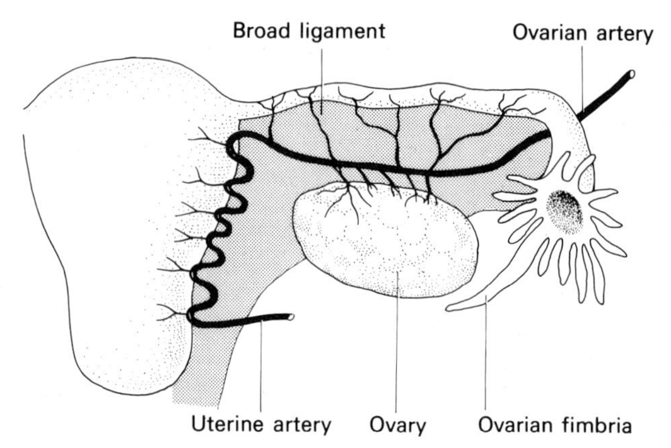

Fig. 3.23 The position of the ovary in relation to the Fallopian tube and the broad ligament.

STRUCTURE

The ovary consists of an inner medulla and an outer cortex.

The medulla is attached to the broad ligament by the mesovarian. It consists of fibrous tissue and transmits the ovarian vessels, lymphatics and nerves which enter and leave the ovary via the mesovarian and infundibulo-pelvic ligament.

The cortex is the functional part of the ovary. It consists of a dense stroma containing and supporting ovarian follicles and corpora lutea at various stages of development. The outer part of the cortex is formed by a fibrous layer, which is known as the tunica albuginea. The germinal epithelium covers the tunica albuginea. It is a layer of cubical cells which is continuous with the broad ligament at the mesovarian and from which the ova are derived.

RELATIONS

Anteriorly, the ovaries are related to the broad ligament and mesovarian, posteriorly, to the peritoneal cavity and intestines, medially, to the body of the uterus and the ovarian ligament and laterally, to the infundibulopelvic ligament, ureter, internal iliac artery and side wall of the pelvis.

BLOOD SUPPLY

The ovaries are supplied with blood by the ovarian arteries which are branches of the aorta, and venous drainage is into corresponding veins. The left vein drains into the left renal vein, and the right into the inferior vena cava.

LYMPHATIC DRAINAGE

The lymph is drained into the lumbar glands.

NERVE SUPPLY

The nerve supply to the ovaries is derived from the ovarian plexus.

THE OVARIAN FOLLICLES

An ovary at birth contains about 200 000 primordial follicles, i.e. an ovum enveloped in a single layer of cells (Fig. 3.24).

As the follicle develops the layer of cells proliferates and there is an increase in the number of capsular cells. Fluid, liquor folliculi, appears between the cells and divides those surrounding the ovum from the outer layer. This structure, which is known as the Graafian follicle, remains small until puberty (Fig. 3.25).

At puberty the Graafian follicle ripens and enlarges to about 8 mm in diameter and comprises:

1 The ovum with a large nucleus.
2 The perivitelline space immediately beyond the ovum.

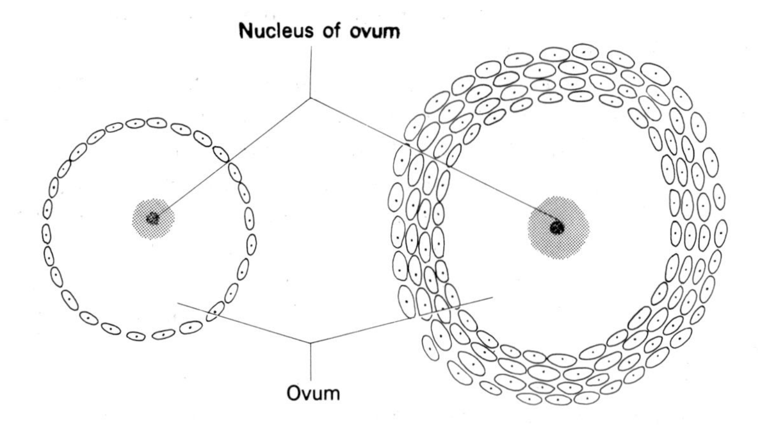

Fig. 3.24 (left) Primordial follicle.
Fig. 3.25 (right) Graafian follicle prior to puberty.

3 The zone pellucida, a membrane adjacent to the perivitelline space.
4 Granulosa cells surrounding the ovum and forming the discus proligerus. The cells of the discus next to the perivitelline space are arranged in such a manner that they appear to radiate from the ovum. The formation is known as the corona radiata, and these cells contain amorphous material which forms a translucent membrane, the zona pellucida.
5 The follicle is lined with granulosa cells, similar to those of the discus proligerus, and they form the membrana granulosa (Fig. 3.26).
6 The follicle is filled with fluid, the liquor folliculi which lies between the discus proligerus and the membrana granulosa. It is thought to be derived from the granulosa cells.
7 Membrana limitans externa is a basement membrane which encloses the follicle.

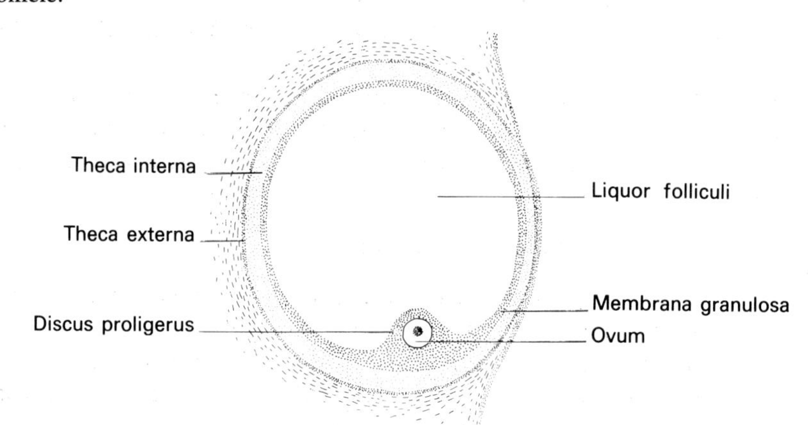

Fig. 3.26 Graafian follicle.

8 The theca interna and externa are layers of compressed stroma cells.
9 The stroma of the ovary.

Ovulation. At ovulation the ripe Graafian follicle reaches the surface of the ovary and ruptures, discharging the ovum, surrounded by the discus proligerus, and the liquor folliculi into the peritoneal cavity.

Corpus luteum. Following ovulation, the cells of the membrana granulosa begin to proliferate and grow inwards. The cells develop a yellowish pigment, and the name corpus luteum is given to the structure which marks the site of the recently ruptured follicle. The corpus luteum grows for fourteen days after which time hyaline material is deposited between its cells and it begins to atrophy.

Corpus albicans. The cells of the corpus luteum undergo degeneration, the colour gradually changing from yellow to white. The cells of the corpus luteum disappear, and after nine months it becomes converted into a small hyaline nodule, known as the corpus albicans.

The ovarian and menstrual cycles are described elsewhere (see p. 13).

CHANGES IN THE OVARY DURING PREGNANCY

If fertilisation of the ovum ocurs, the corpus luteum continues to grow slowly until the third or fourth month. Its function is to maintain the pregnancy by producing oestrogens and progesterone until the placenta takes over. The corpus luteum persists throughout pregnancy beginning to regress before parturition.

CHANGES IN THE OVARY DURING THE PUERPERIUM

The corpus luteum continues to regress completing the process of degeneration a considerable time after parturition. Following expulsion of the placenta, the levels of oestrogens and progesterone fall and a negative feedback stimulates recommencement of the ovarian-menstrual cycle.

Ovulation takes place thirty-five to forty-two days after the birth of the baby.

It is important to note that ovulation may precede menstruation, and, therefore, it is possible for a woman to conceive before menstruation recommences. Contraceptive advice must therefore take this fact into account.

Fertilisation and implantation of the ovum

Following ovulation, the ovum surrounded by the discus proligerus is received into the Fallopian tube. It passes slowly along the tube towards the uterine cavity propelled by ciliary movements and peristaltic contractions. During its journey along the tube the ovum is nourished by the cells of the discus proligerus and secretions from the goblet cells.

Spermatozoa are deposited in the upper vagina during intercourse. Each ejaculation of human semen contains 200–300 million spermatozoa, many of which are killed by lactic acid in the vagina. The remainder pass through the cervical canal to the uterine cavity and the Fallopian tube.

The spermatozoon

The mature male gamete capable of fertilising the mature ovum.

MATURATION OF THE SPERMATOZOON

Primary spermatocytes develop in the seminiferous tubules of the testes. They undergo a reduction division (meiosis) in which the number of chromosomes is halved, forming secondary spermatocytes (see p. 468). The secondary spermatocyte divides to form spermatids (mitosis). These develop without further division into ripe spermatozoon in the epididymis and vas deferens by a process of spermatogenesis (Fig. 13.2).

STRUCTURE

The spermatozoon is a small structure, 60 μm in length, comprising:

1 A head which contains the nucleus and is covered by two caps, one the acrosome, containing hyaluronidase.

2 A neck, the narrow constricted area next to the head containing the centriole of the cell.

3 A middle piece or body consists of fibrils surrounded by mitochondria which use fructose as a source of energy.

4 A tail or flagellum which is very active and propels the spermatozoon along the female genital tract covering its own length in three seconds (Fig. 3.27).

The male genital system (see p. 420).

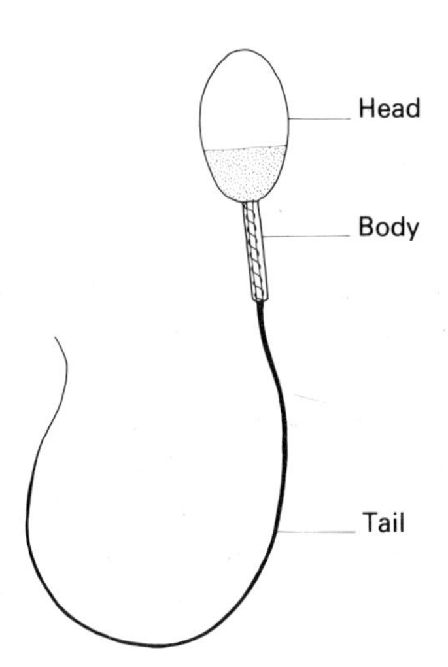

Fig. 3.27 A spermatozoon.

Fertilisation

Fertilisation of the ovum takes place within the outer third of the Fallopian tube and is possible usually only within twenty-four hours of ovulation and forty-eight hours of intercourse. This is because an ovum remains capable of being fertilised for only twenty-four hours and because spermatozoon retain their fertilising capacity for only forty-eight hours. These facts are of importance when giving advice regarding the 'safe' period method of contraception.

At fertilisation the spermatozoon penetrates the discus proligerus by means of an enzyme hyaluronidase contained in the acrosome. The head of the spermatozoon becomes detached from the tail and the sperm nucleus travels to the centre of the ovum where it meets the nucleus of the ovum. The two nuclei fuse, thus re-establishing the number of chromosomes at forty-six. The resultant cell is called a zygote. After penetration by a spermatozoon other spermatozoa are unable to enter the ovum due to chemical alteration in the discus proligerus.

SEX DETERMINATION

The nucleus of the ovum contains twenty-two autosomes and the X sex chromosome. The nucleus of the spermatozoon carries twenty-two autosomes and an X or a Y chromosome. If fertilisation is by a spermatozoon carrying the X chromosome the zygote will contain forty-four autosomes plus two X chromosomes and will develop into a female; if by a spermatozoon carrying the Y chromosome the zygote will contain forty-four autosomes plus X and Y chromosomes, and will develop into a male. Thus the sex is determined at the time of fusion of the nuclei and is solely dependent upon the father.

Segmentation of the fertilised ovum

After fertilisation the zygote passes along the Fallopian tube reaching the uterus in about four days. During this time the zygote divides firstly into two cells, then into four and eight and so on. This process is known as segmentation of the fertilised ovum, and the mass of cells produced, as the morula (Fig. 3.28). The zona pellucida binds the cells together and prevents adherence to the walls of the tubes, but it disappears by the time the cavity of the uterus is reached. Each cell division produces two equal sized cells half the size of the original cell. Thus the cells become progressively smaller and there is no increase in the overall size of the resultant mass of structure.

Fluid appears between the cells of the morula and a small cystic structure known as the blastocyst is formed. It is at this stage of development that the uterine cavity is reached, four days after fertilisation and five to six days after ovulation.

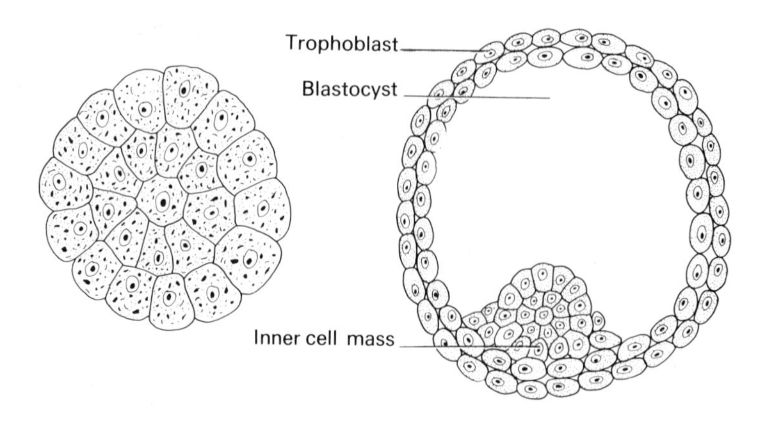

Fig. 3.28 (left) A morula.
Fig. 3.29 (right) A blastocyst.

BLASTOCYST

The blastocyst consists of a capsule of cells known as the trophoblast, which will develop into the placenta and chorion, and a mass of cells at one pole known as the inner cell mass, which will give rise to the embryo and amnion (Fig. 3.29).

Implantation of the blastocyst

About two days after entering the uterine cavity the blastocyst becomes attached to the endometrium, and embeds in it. This is called implantation and usually takes place seven to eight days after fertilisation. It is the cells of the trophoblast, by means of excreting ferments, which digest the endometrial cells and so form a depression in which the blastocyst rests. The digestive process continues and the blastocyst sinks deeper into the lining of the uterus which is now known as the decidua. The deepest cells constitute the entering pole and contain the inner cell mass. Finally, the blastocyst is completely embedded in the decidua, the last part to enter being the closing pole (Fig. 3.30). The superficial part of the decidua closes over the blastocyst, its site being marked by a small fibrin plug.

The blastocyst usually embeds in the decidua lining the fundus of the uterus or the upper part of the anterior or posterior walls. The blastocyst is now nourished by the secretions from the tubular glands which have a high content of glycogen.

The blastocyst forms a small nodule in the decidua and as it enlarges it bulges progressively into the uterine cavity.

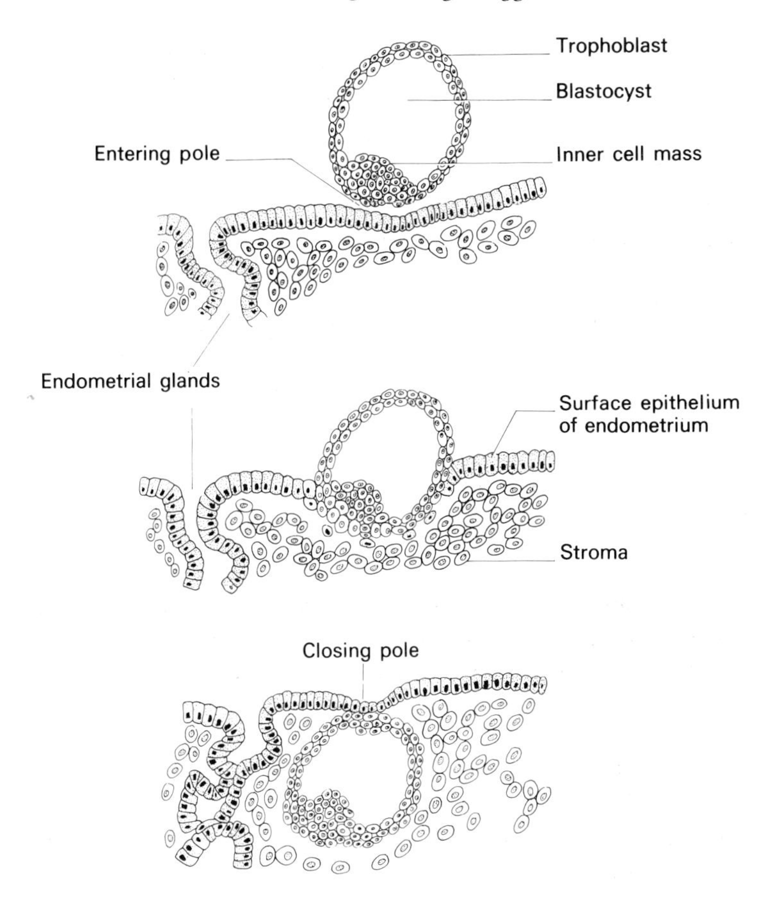

Fig. 3.30 Implantation of the blastocyst.

FORMATION OF THE DECIDUA

The decidua becomes divided into three parts (Fig. 3.31).

1 The decidua basalis, being that part of the decidua which lies between the blastocyst and the myometrium.

2 The decidua capsularis, covers the blastocyst and separates it from the uterine cavity.

3 The decidua vera, lines the remainder of the cavity.

As the cells of the trophoblast digest the endometrial cells they also grow into the arterioles and destroy the muscle walls. Bleeding occurs and occasionally blood escapes into the uterine cavity and is lost *per vaginum*. This blood loss, known as implantation bleeding, is very slight and appears a few days before the menstrual period would be expected. It is important, therefore, to obtain a clear history of the bleeding to ensure that it is not confused with the last menstrual period.

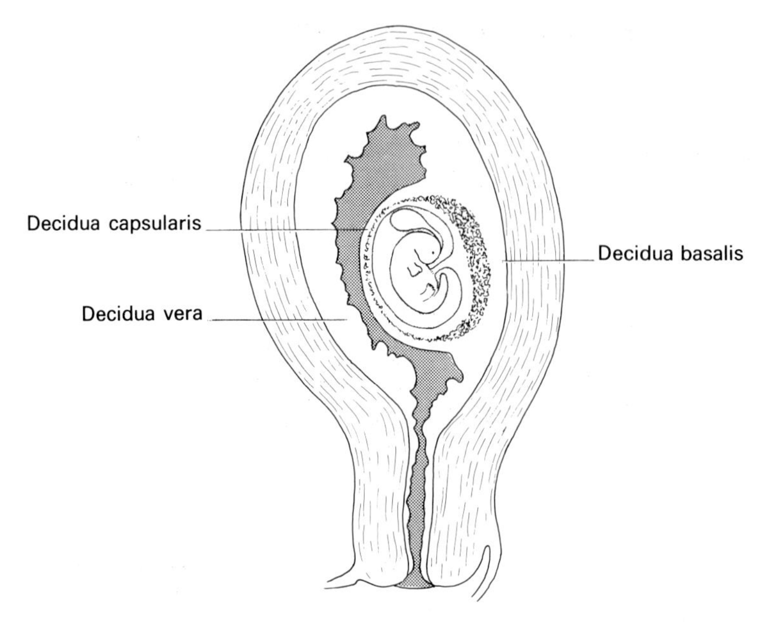

Fig. 3.31 The parts of the decidua.

Development of the placenta

As the blastocyst is implanting in the decidua a continuous process of growth and development is taking place in both the trophoblast and the inner cell mass.

The trophoblast becomes differentiated into three layers (Fig. 3.32).

1 An outer layer known as the syncitiotrophoblast or syncitium. This layer develops rapidly and the cell boundaries are not formed. The tissue is composed of masses of small nuclei scattered throughout a layer of protoplasm.

2 An inner layer known as the cytotrophoblast or Langhan's layer. This is composed of a single layer of cells with complete cell membranes, known as Langhan's cells.

3 Lying below the cytotrophoblast is a layer of primitive mesenchyme. This is continuous with similar tissue in the inner cell mass. The point where they join is known as the body stalk.

Every part of the surface of the trophoblast is in contact with the glands of the congested and oedematous decidua which provides secretions rich in glycogen and protein for the cells of the invading trophoblast.

Spaces appear in the syncitiotrophoblast. These vacuoles are known as the choriodecidual spaces and they are filled with blood from the eroded decidual capillaries. The embedded blastocyst is completely surrounded by a pool of maternal blood. This is the earliest phase of uteroplacental circulation.

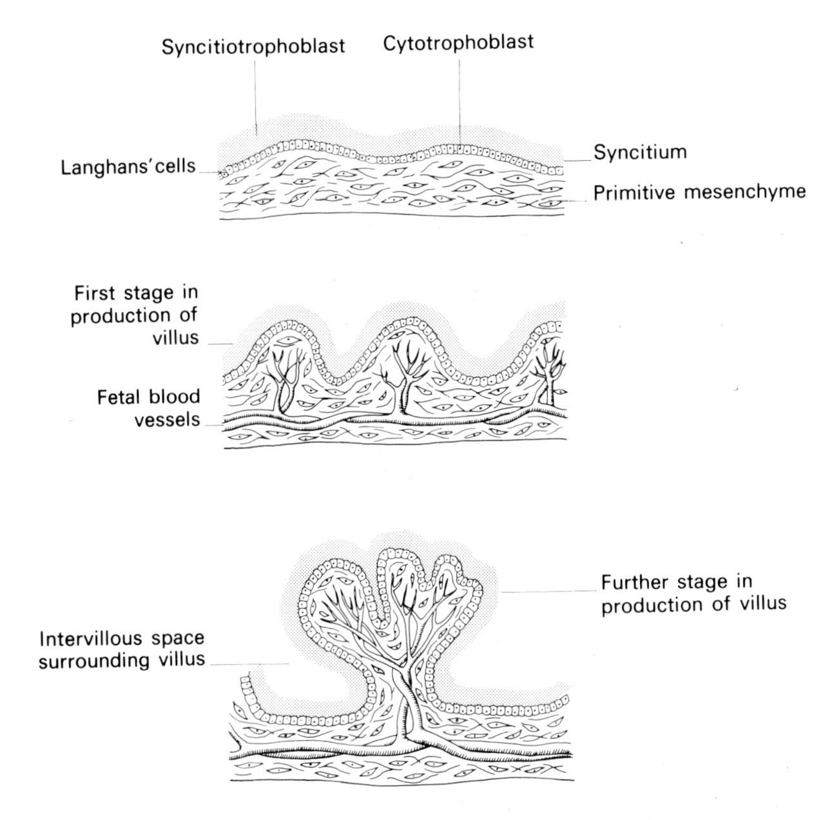

Fig. 3.32 The three layers of the trophoblast and stages in the formation of primitive villi.

Finger-like processes of the trophoblast grow outwards in all directions into the decidua and choriodecidual spaces (Fig. 3.32). These are the primitive villi; they contain all three layers of the trophoblast, having an outer layer of syncitiotrophoblast, an inner layer of cytotrophoblast and a core of mesenchyme, and are bathed in maternal blood (Fig. 3.33).

The trophoblast is now known as the primitive chorion. Approximately three weeks after fertilisation the villi begin to branch, and the finger-like processes develop until a branching tree-like structure is formed. These villi penetrate deeply into the decidua, but however complicated their structure they contain the original three layers of the trophoblast and are bathed in maternal blood. The blood-filled spaces between the villi are now known as intervillus spaces.

A new system of blood vessels is being formed in the mesenchymal core of the villi. The structures are now known as chorionic villi (Fig. 3.34).

Blood vessels have appeared in the mesoderm of the embryo, yolk sac and

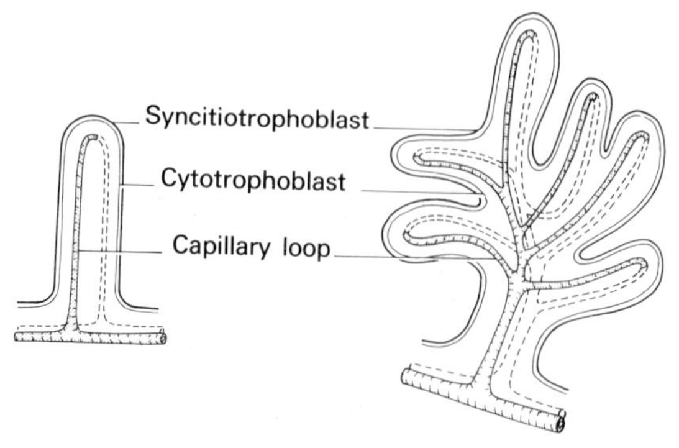

Fig. 3.33 (left) A primitive villi.
Fig. 3.34 (right) A chorionic villi.

the connecting body stalk. A fetal circulatory system continuous with that of the chorionic villi is complete by twenty-one days.

Oxygen and food substances, derived from maternal blood, pass through the walls of the villi into the fetal blood vessels, which carry them via the body stalk to the inner cell mass where the fetus is developing.

During the third month of pregnancy some of the villi continue to proliferate whilst others atrophy. Those villi which invaded the decidua basalis develop into complicated arborescent structures and form the chorion frondosum.

The villi which penetrated the decidua capsularis become smaller as the decidua stretches, and by about the twelfth week of pregnancy they disappear leaving a smooth layer of chorion known as the chorion laeve (Fig. 3.35).

The chorion frondosum develops into the fetal part of the placenta, and the chorion laeve into the chorion. Thus the placenta and chorion are both derived from the primitive chorion which is a derivation of the trophoblast.

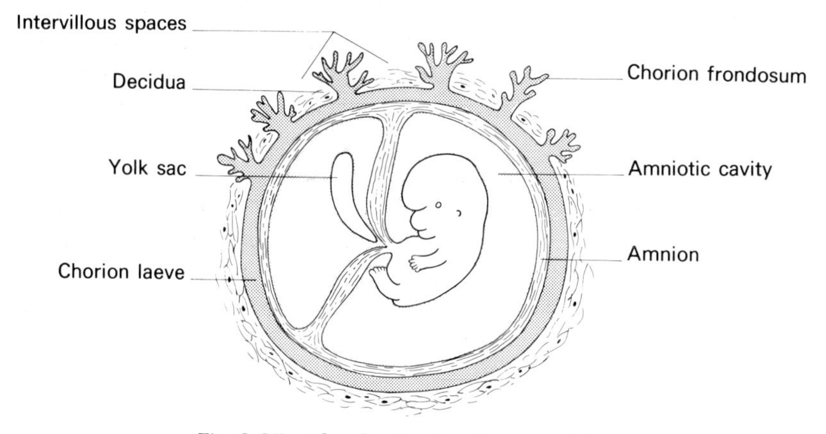

Fig. 3.35 The chorion frondosum and laeve.

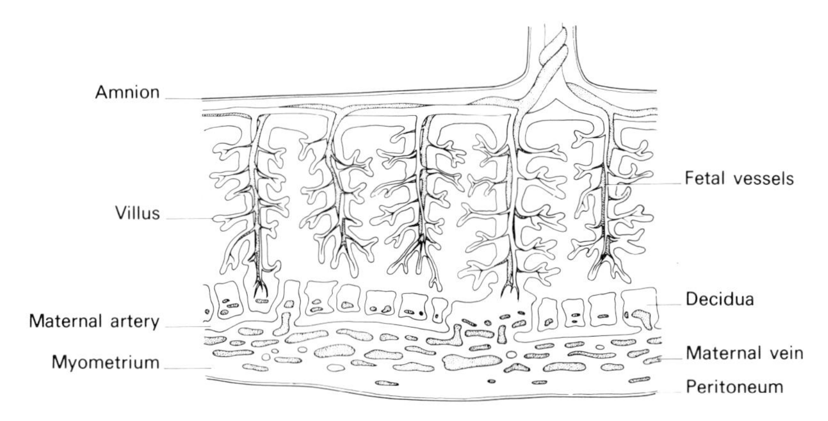

Fig. 3.36 A section of the placenta.

By the twelfth week of pregnancy, the uterine cavity is obliterated by the meeting and fusion of the decidua capsularis and the decidua vera.

After the fourth month of pregnancy, the villi become thinner but more numerous. The inner layer of cytotrophoblast disappears leaving only the syncitium. The mesenchyme in the villi is reduced in amount but the capillaries increase in size. The tissue barrier between the fetal and maternal circulations is therefore diminished and exchange of substances from one circulation to the other facilitated.

As the placenta grows, the blood flow from the coiled uterine arteries to the decidual capillaries increases and large blood sinuses form at the placental site (Fig. 3.36).

The villi which form the placenta are of two types.

1 Nutritive villi. These do not reach the decidual surface, they branch repeatedly, their tips remain free and lie in the maternal blood in the intervillus spaces. They are concerned with nutritive processes.

2 Anchoring villi. These grow down into the decidua and are attached by cellular growth at their tips to the deeper layers of the decidua. Therefore, in addition to their nutritive function they stabilise the placenta through their attachment to the decidua.

Stability is also achieved by decidual septa which pass into the placenta between clumps of villi and around the edge. Under normal circumstances the villi are prevented from invading the basal layer of the decidua or the muscle of the uterine wall by a layer of fibrinoid material which is present in the deeper part of the spongy layer of the decidua. This is known as the layer of Nitabuch.

The placenta at term

The placenta is developed from the chorion frondosum of the trophoblast. At term, the placenta is a circular, spongy, disc-shaped structure about 20 cm in diameter, with a maximum thickness of about 2.5 cm at its centre and diminishing in thickness towards the periphery. The average weight is about 480 g, however, this varies according to the size of the child, the weight being about one-sixth of that of the baby.

The placenta has two surfaces (Fig. 3.37).

1 The maternal surface is attached to the decidua basalis. It is uneven, spongy, and divided into a number of lobes, composed of cotyledons, each separated from the other by a groove or sulcus. There are approximately twenty lobes although the number varies considerably and may be as few as five. The cotyledons are made up of masses of minute villi and the dark red colour of this surface is due to the fetal blood contained in the villi and maternal blood contained in the intervillus spaces.

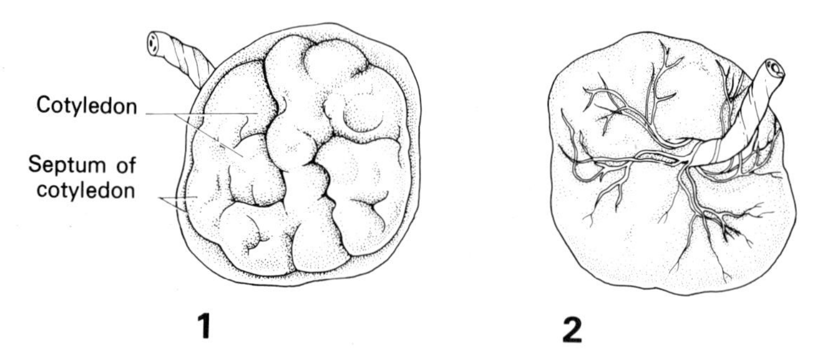

Fig. 3.37 The two surfaces of the placenta; 1, maternal; 2, fetal.

2 The fetal surface lies adjacent to the amniotic cavity and is covered by the translucent amnion which is reflected on to the umbilical cord. Beneath the amnion can be seen the branches of the umbilical vessels, radiating from the point of insertion of the umbilical cord.

Although the placenta has grown considerably since the twelfth week, it has not essentially changed its structure. Its main mass is composed of villi enclosed in a choriodecidual space with a marginal sinus. The space is bounded on the fetal side by the chorionic plate from which the villi arise, and on its basal side by a decidual plate, composed of that part of the decidua to which the anchoring villi are attached, and which separates with the placenta at delivery. The villi, with the chorionic plate, form the fetal placenta, and constitute the greater part of the placenta, the decidual plate, the material placenta is a thin layer, which is often incomplete.

Attached to the placenta are two membranes.

1 The chorion is derived from the chorion laeve of the trophoblast. It is continuous with the placenta at its edge and lines the decidua vera to which it is loosely attached. Its inner surface is lined with amnion. The chorion is thicker and less translucent than the amnion, but more friable. If care is not taken when delivering the membranes, the chorion may become torn and retained, resulting in an increased blood loss. On inspection the chorion may be seen to have tiny irregular attached fragments of decidual tissue.

2 The amnion is derived from the ectoderm of the inner cell mass. It is a translucent membrane which lines the chorion and covers the fetal surface of the placenta. It can easily be separated from the chorion and peeled off the placenta as far as the attachment of the cord with which it becomes incorporated.

The amnion consists of five layers.

1 Epithelium; an inner layer of non-ciliated cuboidal cells.

2 Basement membrane; firmly fused to compact layer.

3 Compact layer; acellular and resistant to infiltration by inflammatory leucocytes.

4 Fibroblast layer.

5 Spongy layer; composed of a network of collagen and mucus which permits movement of amnion over chorion and the layer to alter shape. It is capable of great distension.

The amnion varies in thickness from 0.2 to 0.5 mm according to amount of fluid and mucus in the spongy layer.

The umbilical cord

The umbilical cord develops from the body stalk. It is usually about 50 cm long but may vary considerably. It is usually 1.25 cm in thickness but varies according to the amount of Wharton's jelly. It is normally inserted into the centre of the fetal surface of the placenta. The cord is dull white in colour, composed of Wharton's jelly derived from mesoderm and covered by a layer of stratified cuboidal cells continuous with the fetal epidermis at one end and the amniotic epithelium at the other. Localised accumulations of Wharton's jelly produce irregularities in the cord known as false knots. These may contain an umbilical vein. True knots occur as the result of movements of the fetus.

The umbilical cord contains three vessels. One umbilical vein, formed by the fusion of two veins, carrying oxygenated blood from the placenta to the fetus, and two umbilical arteries, derived from the iliac arteries of the fetus, carrying venous blood from the fetus to the placenta (Fig. 3.38). The arteries spiral around the vein in an anticlockwise direction.

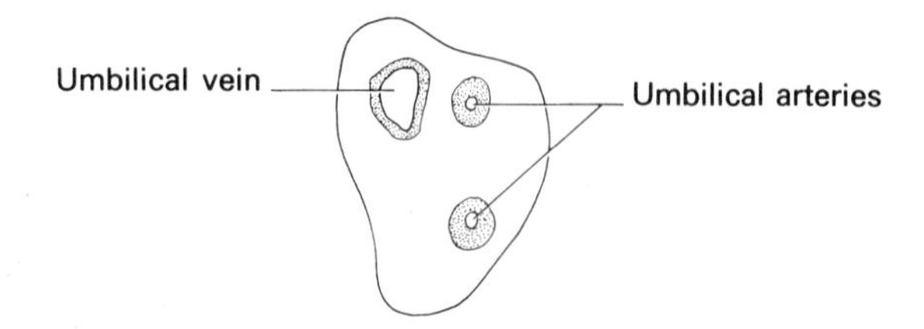

Fig. 3.38 Section of the umbilical cord.

Abnormalities of placental development and cord insertions

Placental abnormalities

Placenta succenturiata. An accessory lobe is present at some distance from the margin of the placenta, and is connected to it by membranes containing branches of the umbilical vessels (Fig. 3.39). This occurs due to hypertrophy of chorionic villi in the chorion laeve. Placenta succenturiata is of considerable importance on account of the tendency for it to be retained *in utero* after the placenta has been expelled. This may cause a primary postpartum haemorrhage.

Placenta bipartita or tripartita. A placenta divided into two or three main lobes connected by membranes conveying branches of the umbilical vessels which unite when joining the cord (Fig. 3.40).

Placenta circumvallata. The centre part of the fetal surface is depressed and around it, at some distance from the margin, appears a thick band (Fig. 3.41). This is a fold of amnion and chorion.

Placenta membranacea. This is a rare condition in which the whole of the chorion has developed into placental tissue.

Placenta accreta. The chorionic villi extend into the basal layer of the decidua.

Placenta increta. The chorionic villi extend into the myometrium.

These abnormalities of invasion may be due to imperfect development of the decidua basalis where the layer of Nitabuch is absent or marked invasive properties of the chorionic villi. These conditions are very rare.

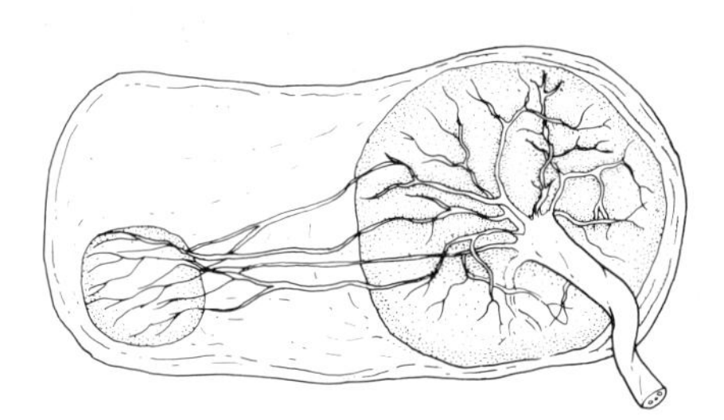

Fig. 3.39 A placenta succenturiata.

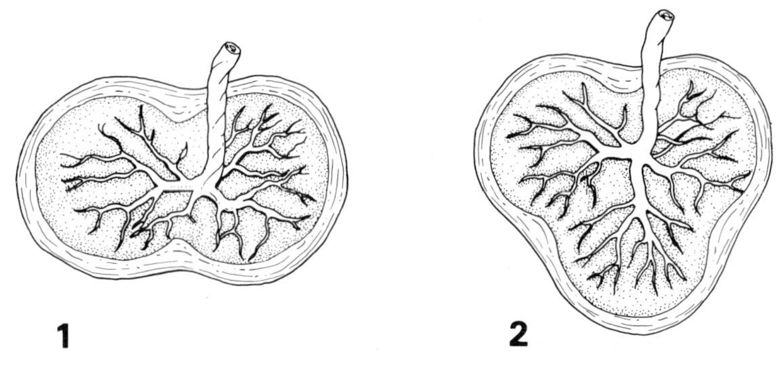

Fig. 3.40 1, a placenta bipartita; 2, a placenta tripartita.

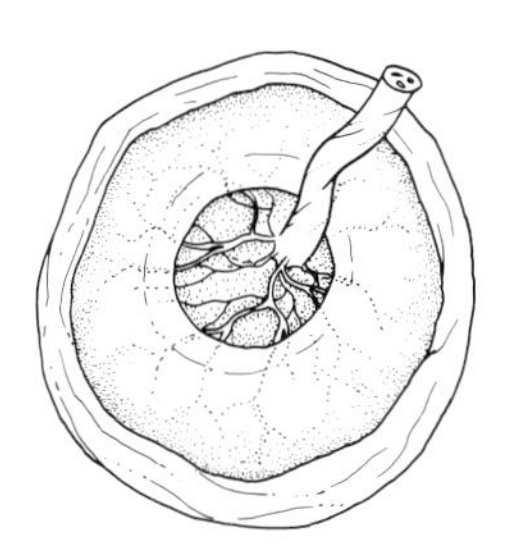

Fig. 3.41 A placenta circumvallata.

CHANGES IN PLACENTAL TISSUE

Placental infarctions. Necrosis of chorionic villi due to ischaemia. These are red if examined at an early stage in their development but later they become white. They are often associated with pre-eclampsia and if very extensive may cause fetal death.

Calcification. Calcareous nodules on the surface of the placenta are very common. They are probably due to deposits of chalky material in the necrotic tissue around the anchoring villi and in the superficial layer of the decidua basalis.

PLACENTAL DISEASES

Syphilis. A typical syphilitic placenta is large and pale. The chorionic villi are enlarged and avascular. This type of placenta is only seen in an untreated case when the fetus dies *in utero*.

Erythroblastosis fetalis. In this condition the placenta resembles that of the typical syphilitic placenta. It may weigh more than the baby.

Diabetes mellitus. In untreated cases or where the treatment fails to control the disease, the placenta is enlarged, pale and oedematous.

Hydatidiform mole. Cystic degeneration of the chorionic villi occurring before the twelfth week of pregnancy (see p. 176).

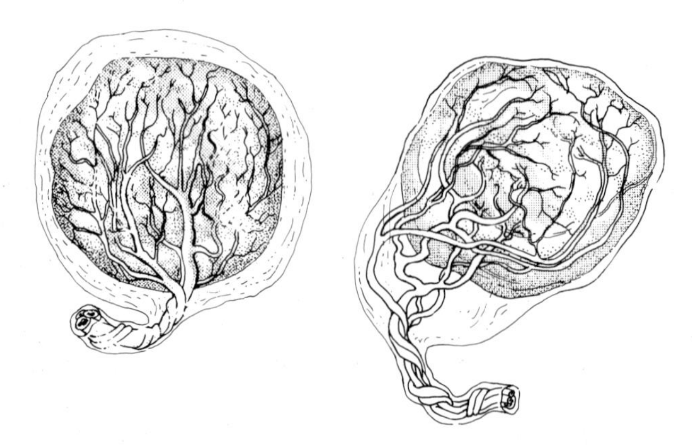

Fig. 3.42 (left) A battledore placenta.
Fig. 3.43 (right) A velamentous insertion of the cord.

Abnormalities of cord insertions

Battledore placenta. The umbilical cord is inserted at or near the margin of the placenta (Fig. 3.42). It is without clinical importance.
Velamentous insertion of the cord. The umbilical cord is inserted into the membranes some distance from the edge of the placenta with the umbilical vessels passing through the membranes to and from the placenta (Fig. 3.43).

It is of great clinical importance if the placenta is situated low in the uterus and the velamentous portion of the umbilical vessels crosses the membranes covering the internal os. This condition is known as vasa praevia, and it is inevitable that the vessels will be compressed by the presentation, causing fetal hypoxia and later rupture which in turn causes fetal bleeding and death.

Functions of the placenta

The placenta is the means through which the fetus obtains its requirements. It selects from the maternal blood the substances necessary for fetal life and growth. It also stores some of these and changes some so that the fetus can utilise them. There is no mixing of fetal and maternal blood. The two are separated by the epithelium of the villi and the thickness of the walls of the fetal capillaries within the villi. Through this very thin intervening partition, diffusion of gases and of nutritive and waste products occurs.

Carbon dioxide and waste products pass from the fetal blood to the maternal blood, while oxygen and nutritive substances pass in the reverse direction.

The main functions of the placenta can be considered under the following headings.

Respiratory function

The fetus derives its oxygen supply from the oxygenated maternal blood. Oxygen is carried to the placenta in the form of oxyhaemoglobin. In the intervillus spaces, the oxyhaemoglobin dissociates into haemoglobin and oxygen. The oxygen diffuses through the walls of the villi and combines with the reduced fetal haemoglobin to form fetal oxyhaemoglobin. The maternal haemoglobin returns to the lungs for reoxygenation, whilst the fetal oxyhaemoglobin is carried in the fetal circulation to the fetal tissues (see p. 312–5). Here it dissociates, gives up oxygen to the growing cells of the tissues, and the reduced fetal haemoglobin then returns to the placenta for oxygenation.

The fetal blood contains more red blood cells and more haemoglobin than the maternal blood and the fetal heart beats faster (120–160 beats/min). This enables the fetus to compensate for the fact that maternal blood contains less oxygen than atmospheric air.

Another factor of importance is that the haemoglobin of the fetus has a slightly different chemical composition from that of adult haemoglobin. It has the property of combining with oxygen more readily than adult haemoglobin. The fetus must have a low P_{O_2} to avoid switching on adult mechanisms, i.e. closing umbilical vessels and so on, and takes elaborate steps to keep the P_{O_2} low, while ensuring a large supply of O_2. Carbon monoxide, from cigarette smoking, also crosses freely and is avidly bound by fetal haemoglobin so that the fetus of a woman who smokes may have 15–20% of its haemoglobin rendered useless for oxygen transport.

Placental transfer

NUTRITIVE FUNCTION

Everything needed by the fetus for growth and development traverses the placenta but a wide range of mechanisms is employed. Gases, water and some electrolytes cross freely to the fetus by diffusion. More complex nutrients cross by more elaborate methods; glucose by 'facilitated diffusion' (a process in which part of the transfer mechanism is active and requires oxygen) amino acids and fatty acids by carrier mechanisms and micronutrients such as vitamins by elaborate transport systems which are one-way, e.g. folate travels only from mother to fetus, the fetus cannot send any back to the mother even if she is grossly deficient.

From these components the fetus builds its own large molecules. Formed fats such as triglycerides or cholesterol do not cross; nor do proteins with the single important exception of gammaglobin which has a specific carrier mechanism and ensures that the infant is born with a full complement of its mother's antibodies.

BARRIER FUNCTION

The placenta has a protective role and acts to some extent as a barrier which generally prevents cells, including bacteria from reaching the fetus. It is likely that micro-organisms and cancer cells only reach the fetus by causing damage to the placenta first. But any substance of small molecular weight (less than 1000) can be assumed to cross quite readily and that includes almost all drugs and anaesthetic agents.

Excretory function

Waste metabolic substances, in addition to carbon dioxide, pass through the walls of the villi by diffusion. The substances enter the maternal blood and are then excreted by the mother. Although the fetal metabolism is mainly anabolic, there are considerable amounts of waste products including heat to be transferred to maternal circulation.

Endocrine function

The placenta is the most versatile endocrine organ in the body. Many placental hormones are also produced elsewhere in the body, e.g. the ovary which produces oestrogens and progesterone.

CHORIONIC GONADOTROPHIN

Only placental tissue can produce chorionic gonadotrophin, therefore the discovery of this hormone in the blood or urine is diagnostic of pregnancy, although not necessarily a normal pregnancy.

Chorionic gonadotrophin is produced by the cells of the cytotrophoblast from the time the blastocyst begins to embed until term. The production of this hormone rises rapidly to a peak about sixty days after the last menstrual period after which it is maintained at a low level (Fig. 3.44). Chorionic gonadotrophin has a luteotrophic action, i.e. it stimulates the corpus luteum and prolongs its life. By the time the placenta has formed and its steroid hormones have taken over the function of the corpus luteum there is no longer any need for chorionic gonadotrophin. In spite of the disappearance of gonadotrophins the production of chorionic gonadotrophin persists throughout pregnancy and may have other functions.

OESTROGENS

These are steroid hormones of which more than twenty different kinds have been isolated from pregnancy urine. For the most part they are metabolites of one or two precursors. Oestrogens in the form of oestriol, oestrone and oestradiol are produced by the corpus luteum during the first three months of pregnancy and by the syncitium of the placenta during the final six months.

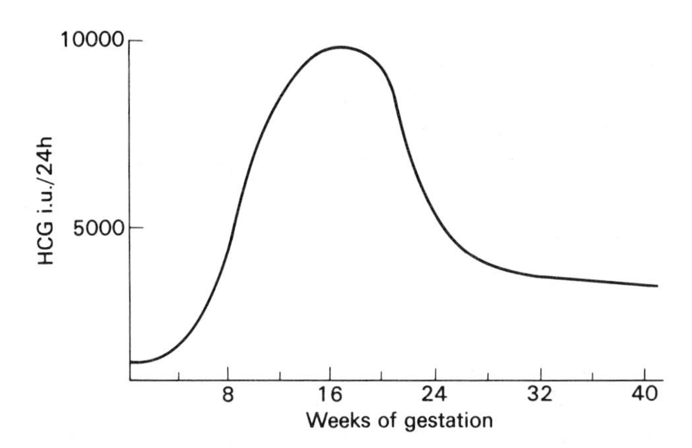

Fig. 3.44 Chorionic gonadotrophin levels in normal pregnancy.

They are also derived from the cortex of the fetal and maternal adrenal glands. In the non-pregnant woman oestriol results from the metabolism in the liver of more active oestrogens produced by the ovaries. In pregnancy it is present in large amounts and is produced by the fetoplacental unit. Total oestrogens or oestriol may be measured and used as an index of fetal wellbeing and placental efficiency (see p. 322).

PROGESTERONE

Like oestrogens, progesterone is a steroid hormone which is secreted in early pregnancy by the corpus luteum stimulated by chorionic gonadotrophin. Later in pregnancy the syncitium of the placenta produces progesterone which at first reinforces, and then gradually takes over the function. Its excretion product pregnanediol is present in the urine and can be measured and used as an index of placental efficiency (see p. 324).

HUMAN PLACENTAL LACTOGEN (human chorionic somatomammotrophin)

This is a protein hormone produced by the syncitiotrophoblast. It has mammotrophic activity and has immunological and biological resemblance to human growth hormone and, therefore, is thought to facilitate maximum fetal growth (see p. 322). It may also amplify the function of other hormones such as erythropoietin.

THYROID STIMULATING HORMONE

This hormone is produced by the placenta but its role is unknown.

Amniotic fluid

Amniotic fluid is the pale straw-coloured fluid which fills the amniotic sac and surrounds the fetus. It is present as soon as the amniotic sac is formed.

The amount of amniotic fluid varies with the period of gestation. In early pregnancy it is closely related to the weight of the fetus. The quantity of amniotic fluid increases as pregnancy advances, reaching a maximum of 500–1500 ml by thirty-five weeks, after which time it gradually diminishes. At term the amniotic fluid contributes about 0.9 kg to the total weight gain.

COMPOSITION

The amniotic fluid is composed of approximately 98.8% water and 1.2% solid matter. The constituents are:

1 Normal: glucose; protein and amino acids; electrolytes—sodium, potassium and chlorides; urea, uric acid and creatinine; lipids and phospholipids, e.g. sphingomyelin and lecithin; enzymes, e.g. renin; hormones, e.g. oestriol, human placental lactogen, human chorionic gonadotrophin and prostaglandins; solid constituents—desquamated cells from the fetus and amnion, lanugo and vernix caseosa.

2 Abnormal: meconium—a sign of fetal hypoxia; bilirubin is normally present but if increased is associated with haemolytic disease; blood which may be of fetal or maternal origin.

The amniotic fluid is thought to be derived from the following sources:

1 Secretions from the cells of the amnion.
2 Transudate from fetal vessels in the cord and placenta.
3 Transudate from maternal vessels in the decidua.
4 Micturition by the fetus.

In early pregnancy the amniotic fluid closely resembles plasma and suggests that this is the main source in the first twenty weeks of pregnancy. After midpregnancy the volume of fetal urine is increased and it is thought that this is then the main source.

CIRCULATION

The amniotic fluid is not a static fluid, water and electrolytes exchange rapidly by diffusion with maternal extracellular fluid. The fetus swallows the fluid which is then absorbed through the gut into the circulation and transferred to the maternal blood at the placenta. Therefore, there is total replacement of the water (but not the solid) content every three hours.

FUNCTIONS

The functions of the amniotic fluid during pregnancy:

a To provide a distension growth stimulus to meet the needs of the growing fetus.

b To maintain a stable environmental temperature for the fetus.

c To allow the fetus to move freely without expenditure of energy which can then be used for growth and development. Early movement of muscles stimulates their further growth.

d To protect the fetus from trauma.

e To equalise pressure over the fetus and cord. This ensures symmetry of growth.

f To prevent adhesions between the fetus and amnion.

g To provide nourishment by means of its nutritive substances.

h To provide weightlessness which aids circulation of blood.

i To provide a reservoir for urine.

The functions of the amniotic fluid during labour:

a To aid effacement and dilation of the cervix and os uteri by means of the hydrostatic pressure transmitted from the uterine muscle through the amniotic fluid.

b To prevent excessive diminution of the placental site during retraction of the uterine muscle.

c To equalise the pressure of the uterine contractions on the fetus.

d When the membranes rupture the birth canal is flushed from above downwards by a sterile fluid.

Polyhydramnios

Polyhydramnios is an excess of amniotic fluid.

CLINICAL FEATURES

The uterus is globular and large for the period of gestation. The skin of the abdominal wall may appear tense and shiny with marked striae gravidarum. Fetal parts may be difficult to palpate and there is excessive ballottement. Malpresentation and unstable lie may be noted. A fluid thrill can be elicited by placing a hand against one side of the abdomen and flicking the thumb against the other. The fetal heart is muffled and pressure symptoms are increased.

AETIOLOGY

As the exact origin of amniotic fluid is uncertain, the cause of polyhydramnios is not clearly understood. However, several fetal and maternal conditions are commonly associated with it, and they can be considered as follows:

Increased secretions. Fetal—anencephaly, hydrocephaly, spina bifida and multiple pregnancy. Maternal—pre-eclampsia, diabetes mellitus, congestive cardiac failure and chorioangioma, a rare vascular tumour of the placenta.

Diminished removal. Fetal—oesophageal atresia and severe haemolytic disease. The oedematous fetus is unable to swallow the fluid.

ACUTE POLYHYDRAMNIOS

This type is very rare, occurring about once in every 12000 pregnancies. It usually occurs before the twentieth week and is usually associated with uniovular twins or gross fetal abnormality.

Differential diagnosis. Hydatidiform mole may present with undue enlargement of the uterus in early pregnancy. However, there will be no fluid thrill, no ballottement or fetal parts felt.

Management. The rapid onset of pressure symptoms and the distress of the woman requires immediate treatment. The woman is admitted to hospital and a straight abdominal X-ray is taken to exclude multiple pregnancy and fetal abnormality, although a normal radiograph does not necessarily exclude the latter.

Paracentesis may be attempted if no fetal abnormality is seen. However, the results are not very satisfactory as the amniotic fluid rapidly increases again and abortion may occur. It is usually necessary to terminate the pregnancy by rupturing the membranes.

CHRONIC POLYHYDRAMNIOS

This type is more common occurring about once in 200 pregnancies. There is a gradual increase in the amniotic fluid from midpregnancy and signs and symptoms usually present after the thirtieth week.

Differential diagnosis. Multiple pregnancy, may present with signs and symptoms similar to those of chronic polyhydramnios but, there will be no fluid thrill, no ballottement, and fetal parts are more easily identified. One or two fetal hearts will also be heard distinctly.

Management. In the majority of cases rest in bed is the only treatment necessary. However, if an X-ray reveals a gross fetal abnormality, artificial rupture of membranes is indicated.

If the pregnancy is near term labour is usually induced by hindwater rupture of the membranes. This allows the amount of amniotic fluid withdrawn to be controlled, and reduces the risk of placental abruption which may occur if there is a rapid decrease in the volume of the uterus.

COMPLICATIONS OF POLYHYDRAMNIOS

During pregnancy:

a Pressure symptoms.

b Malpresentation and unstable lie due to the increased space available. There is a risk of cord prolapse when the membranes rupture, and obstructed labour if contractions commence in the presence of an abnormal lie.

c Placental Abruption due to diminution of the placental site when the membranes rupture.

During Labour:

a Premature labour may ensue due to overdistension of the uterus.

b Prolonged labour may result due to malpresentation and hypotonic uterine action.
c Cord prolapse when the membranes rupture.
d Postpartum haemorrhage or retained placenta may occur due to atonic uterus.

Because of the high incidence of oesophageal atresia in association with polyhydramnios, a Number 8 Jacques catheter should be passed on the baby at birth to exclude this abnormality.

Oligohydramnios—rare

Oligohydramnios is a gross deficiency in the normal amount of amniotic fluid in the amniotic cavity. This condition is associated with renal agenesis and causes deformities of the fetus due to pressure, e.g. talipes. Amputation of limbs due to adhesions of amnion have been reported.

The bony pelvis

A knowledge of the pelvis is of great importance to the student of midwifery. It forms a bony canal through which the fetus must pass during the process of birth, and if the canal is of average size and shape, the fetus of normal size will negotiate it without difficulty. However, if the pelvis is abnormal in size and shape, or the fetus is of above average size, difficulties will be encountered.

The normal female pelvis is called the gynaecoid pelvis and is found in about 50% of women.

The pelvis is composed of four bones; the two innominate bones, the sacrum and the coccyx.

THE INNOMINATE BONES

The two innominate (no name) bones form the sides and front of the pelvis. They are made up of three bones fused together (Fig. 3.45).

1 The ilium comprises the largest part of the innominate bone. It has a smooth, concave inner surface forming the iliac fossa. The prominent ridge lying below the fossa is known as the iliopectineal line which terminates anteriorly in a bony prominence called the iliopectineal eminence. It is here the ilium fuses with the superior ramus of the pubic bone. The outer aspect of the ilium is gently curved and has a roughened surface. The iliac crest is the name given to the ridge which surmounts the two surfaces. Anteriorly, the iliac crest terminates in a bony prominence called the anterior superior iliac spine whilst posteriorly it ends at the posterior iliac spine. Below the spines are situated smaller bony prominences the anterior and posterior inferior iliac spines. At its lowest part the ilium forms two-fifths of the acetabulum, where

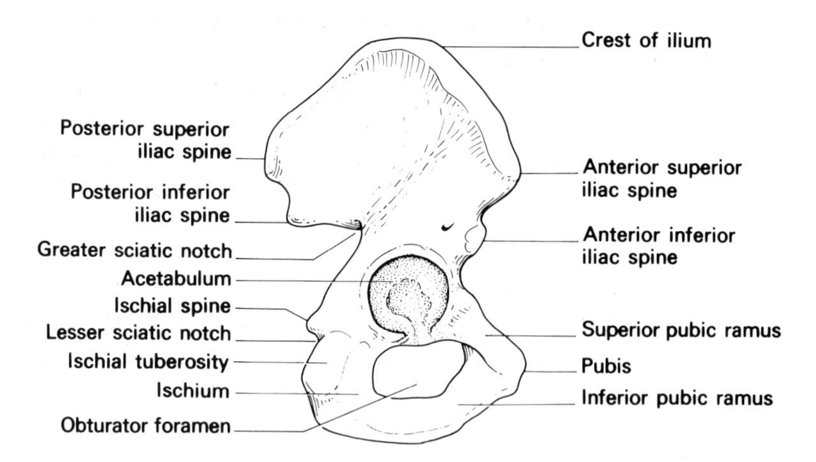

Fig. 3.45 The innominate bone.

it fuses with the ischium and the pubis. Behind the acetabulum the ilium forms the upper part of the greater sciatic notch.

2 The ischium is the lowest part of the innominate bone, and forms the lowest two-fifths of the acetabulum where it fuses with the ilium and the pubis. The ischial tuberosity is the irregular part of the bone on which the weight of the body rests when sitting. Passing up and inwards from the ischial tuberosity the bone becomes continuous with the inferior pubic ramus, so forming the pubic arch. The ischium forms the lower border of the obturator foramen. The inner aspect of the ilium forms the side walls of the true pelvis. About 5 cm above the ischial tuberosity is a projection of bone known as the ischial spine. This separates the greater sciatic notch above from the lesser sciatic notch below.

3 The pubis is the smallest of the three bones forming the innominate bone and is the only one to articulate with the corresponding bone on the opposite side. The body of the pubic bone is square and articulates with the body of the other pubic bone to form the symphysis pubis (Fig. 3.46). Passing from the body of the pubic bone are two rami. The superior ramus passes upward to the acetabulum of which it forms one-fifth, and where it fuses with the ilium and the ischium. It forms the upper border of the obturator foramen. The inferior ramus passes downward to join the ischium, so forming the upper part of the pubic arch.

THE SACRUM

The sacrum forms the posterior wall of the true pelvis, and consists of five sacral vertebrae which are fused together to form one bone. The inner surface is smooth and concave, and forms the hollow of the sacrum, whilst the outer surface is irregular and convex.

The sacral alae articulate with the iliac portions of the two innominate bones at the sacroiliac joints (Fig. 3.46).

The first sacral vertebra, which articulates with the fifth lumbar vertebra, overhangs the sacral hollow and the central point of the upper projecting margin is known as the sacral promontory. The fifth sacral vertebra articulates with the upper border of the coccyx at the sacrococcygeal joint.

THE COCCYX

The coccyx consists of four fused coccygeal vertebrae. The first coccygeal vertebra articulates with the fifth sacral vertebra at the sacrococcygeal joint.

Ossification of the bones of the pelvis is not completed before the age of twenty-five.

THE PELVIC JOINTS

The four bones comprising the pelvis are bound together by four pelvic joints.

The two sacroiliac joints are formed by the articulation of the ilium to the sacrum. The articular surfaces are on the inner surface of the ilium above the greater sciatic notch and the lateral surface of the sacrum, extending for the length of the first two sacral vertebrae. The supporting ligaments pass anteriorly and posteriorly to the joint from the fifth lumbar vertebra to the ilium.

The symphysis pubis consists of a disc of fibrocartilage which is interposed between the bodies of the pubic bones. The symphysis is reinforced by ligaments which pass from one pubic bone to the other in front, behind, above and below the disc of cartilage.

The sacrococcygeal joint is situated between the lower border of the sacrum and the upper border of the coccyx. The slight backward movement that normally occurs at this joint is greatly increased during labour and increases the space available to the fetal head at the anteroposterior diameter of the pelvis.

The pelvic joints become modified in pregnancy to allow increased movement. Under the influence of the hormone progesterone the ligaments supporting the joints become softened. This results in a slight increase in pelvic diameters and therefore assists the passage of the fetal head through the pelvis (see pp. 49–50, pelvic assessment).

THE PELVIC LIGAMENTS

The four ligaments supporting the pelvic joints have already been described above.

The two sacrotuberous ligaments pass from the posterior superior iliac spines and the lateral borders of the sacrum and coccyx to the ischial tuberosities. They bridge the greater and lesser sciatic notches.

The two sacrospinous ligaments pass from the lateral borders of the sacrum and coccyx across the greater sciatic notch to the ischial spines. They lie in front of the sacrotuberous ligaments. The length of the sacrotuberous and sacrospinous ligaments give an indication of the angle of the greater sciatic notch and therefore an assessment of their length forms part of the examination when a pelvic assessment is performed in the latter weeks of pregnancy.

The two inguinal ligaments pass from the anterior superior iliac spines to the upper borders of the pubic bones.

Gimbernat's ligaments occupy the angle between the inner end of the inguinal ligaments and the upper part of the pubic bones.

The obturator membranes are ligaments partially closing the obturator foramen.

The pelvis

Although a knowledge of the constituent parts of the pelvis is important it is the pelvis as a whole that must be understood in order to appreciate its significance and its relationship to the fetal head.

The female pelvis is adapted to provide a birth canal for the fetus and therefore differs from the male pelvis (see p. 247). The inlet is oval rather than heart-shaped and more capacious, the cavity is shallower, more roomy, and less funnel-shaped and the outlet is wider.

The features of the pelvis and their significance will now be discussed in more detail.

The pelvis is divided by the iliopectineal line into a false and a true pelvis. Above the iliopectineal line is the false pelvis which is of little importance in midwifery. The true pelvis lies below the iliopectineal line. It has an inlet, a cavity and an outlet.

THE PELVIC INLET

The inlet is bounded by:

1 The promontory of the sacrum which projects inwards reducing the length of the anteroposterior diameter.

2 The alae of the sacrum are wide and flat and assist in increasing the transverse diameter.

3 The upper part of the sacroiliac joints. These form the posterior point from which the oblique diameters are measured.

4 The iliopectineal lines curve gently outward and forward increasing the transverse diameter of the inlet.

5 The iliopectineal eminences. These mark the terminal points of the iliopectineal lines and are the anterior landmarks to which the oblique diameters are measured.

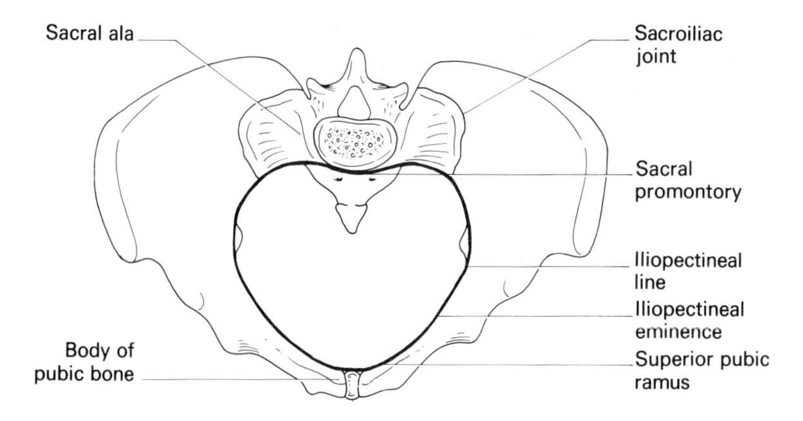

Fig. 3.46 The inlet of the pelvis and its landmarks.

6 The upper inner border of the superior pubic rami. They continue the curve of the iliopectineal lines and create a roomy fore-pelvis.
7 The upper inner border of the body of the pubis (Fig. 3.46).
The diameters of the pelvic inlet. The anteroposterior diameter of the inlet is measured from an inward projecting eminence on the posterior border of the upper surface of the symphysis to the centre of the promontory of the sacrum. This measurement is also known as the obstetrical conjugate and measures approximately 11 cm. The length of the obstetrical conjugate is calculated by deducting 1.25 cm from the diagonal conjugate. This is the distance between the lower border of the symphysis pubis and the promontory of the sacrum which is measured when the pelvis is assessed in late pregnancy (Fig. 3.47).

A second anteroposterior diameter is described. This is measured from the centre of the upper surface of the symphysis to the promontory of the sacrum. This is the anatomical conjugate and is slightly longer than the obstetrical conjugate (Fig. 3.47).

The transverse diameter of the inlet is the distance between the two points farthest apart on the iliopectineal lines and measures approximately 13 cm. It intersects the obstetrical conjugate slightly posterior to its central point. The transverse diameter divides the inlet into the anterior and posterior segments (Fig. 3.48).

The oblique diameters of the inlet are measured from the sacroiliac joints to the opposite iliopectineal eminences (Fig. 3.48). The right oblique from the right joint and the left oblique from the left. The oblique diameters measure approximately 12 cm.

The sacrocotyloid diameters are measured from the centre of the sacral promontory to the iliopectineal eminences on either side (Fig. 3.48). These diameters measure approximately 9 cm.

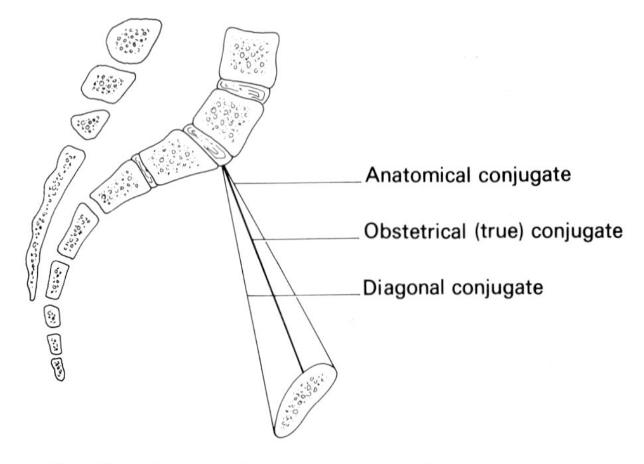

Fig. 3.47 The obstetrical, anatomical and diagonal conjugates.

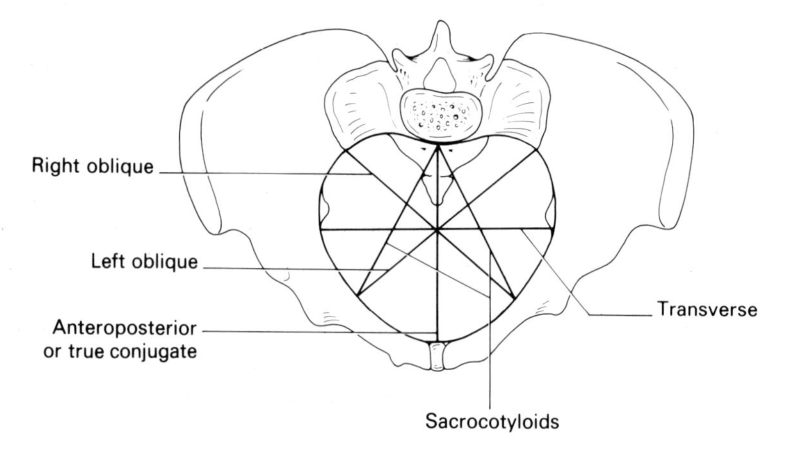

Fig. 3.48 The diameters of the pelvic inlet.

The inlet of the pelvis is therefore an oval structure with a short anteroposterior diameter and a long transverse diameter. The fetal head when engaging in the pelvis usually does so in the transverse diameter.

THE CAVITY OF THE PELVIS

The cavity extends from the inlet above to the outlet below. It is formed by the following structures:

a The posterior wall is formed by the anterior surface of the sacrum. A straight line from the promontory of the sacrum to the sacrococcygeal joint measures 11.5 cm, but if the line follows the curve the distance measures approximately 14 cm. The curve of the inner surface of the sacrum increases the anteroposterior diameter of the cavity.

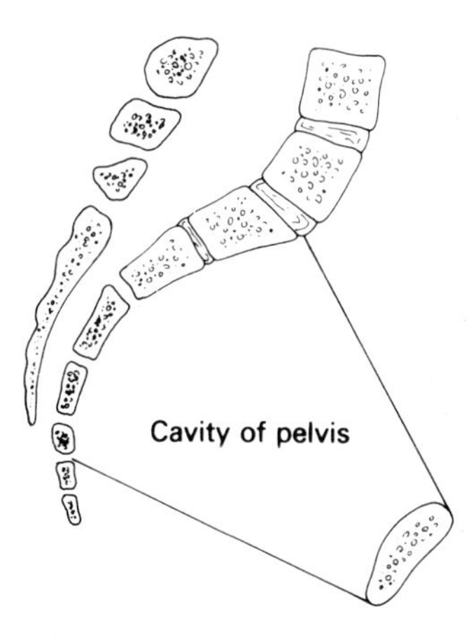

Fig. 3.49 The shape of the pelvic cavity.

b The anterior wall is formed by the inner surfaces of the symphysis pubis and superior pubic rami. It is approximately 4 cm deep.

c The side walls of the pelvic cavity are straight and formed by the inner surfaces of the iliac and ischial bones and by the ligaments filling the greater sciatic notch.

The shape of the pelvic cavity is that of a truncated cylinder (Fig. 3.49). Due to the curve of the sacrum, the upper part of the cylinder is directed downwards and backwards as far as the junction of the second and third sacral vertebrae, then downwards and, at the outlet, downwards and forwards.

The diameters of the cavity of the pelvis (Fig. 3.50). The anteroposterior diameter of the cavity is measured from the midpoint to the inner border of the symphysis pubis to the junction of the second and third sacral vertebrae. It measures approximately 12 cm.

The transverse diameter passes in the plane of the cavity between the two points farthest apart on the lateral walls, it measures approximately 12 cm.

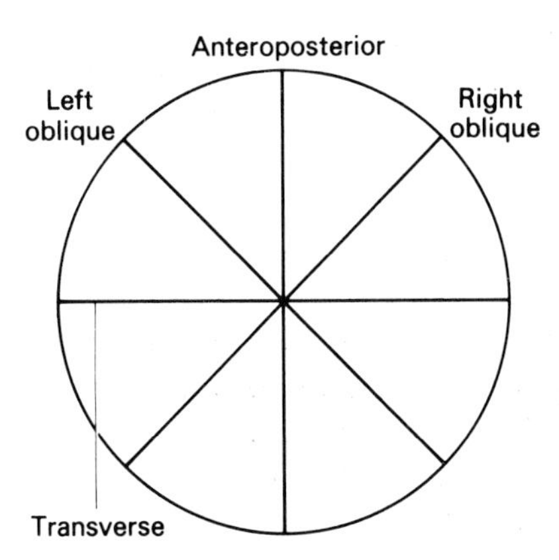

Fig. 3.50 The diameters of the pelvic cavity.

The oblique diameters pass obliquely in the plane of the cavity, parallel to the oblique diameters of the inlet. They also measure approximately 12 cm.

The cavity of the pelvis is, therefore, circular in shape, and the fetal head, having entered the pelvis in the transverse diameter undergoes internal rotation in the cavity.

THE OUTLET OF THE PELVIS

The outlet of the pelvis is divided into two parts, the anatomical outlet and the obstetrical outlet.

The anatomical outlet is formed by the structures which mark the lower border of the pelvis, i.e. the lower border of the symphysis pubis, the inferior pubic rami forming the pubic arch, the inner border of the ischial tuberosities, the sacrotuberous ligaments and the lower border of the coccyx.

The obstetrical outlet is the constricted lower portion of the pelvis and lies above the anatomical outlet. It is formed by the lower inner border of the symphysis pubis, a line passing obliquely across the ischial spines, the sacrospinous ligaments and the lower inner border of the sacrum.

The diameters of the outlet of the pelvis. The anteroposterior diameter of the outlet is measured from the lower inner border of the symphysis pubis to the inner aspect of the lower border of the sacrum. It measures approximately 13 cm.

There are two transverse diameters.

1 The interspinous diameter is the distance between the ischial spines and measures approximately 10.5 cm.

2 The intertuberous diameter is the distance between the ischial tuberosities and measures approximately 11 cm.

The oblique diameters pass obliquely in the plane of the outlet parallel to the oblique diameters of the inlet and cavity. They measure approximately 12 cm. The angle of the pubic arch is approximately 90°.

The outlet of the pelvis is therefore diamond-shaped with the longest diameter anteroposteriorly and the shortest diameter transversely (Fig. 3.51).

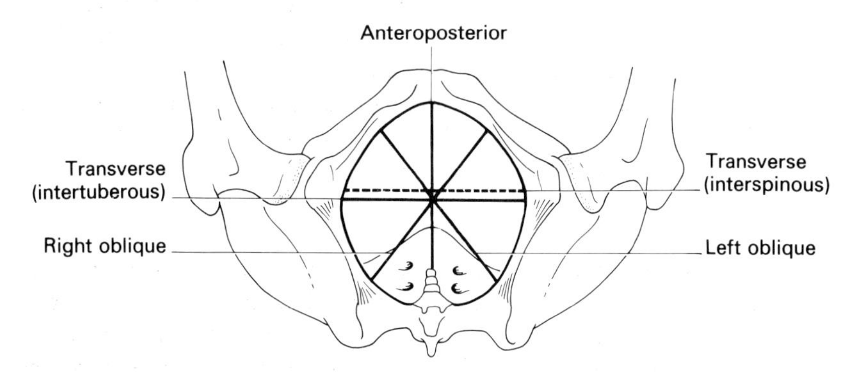

Fig. 3.51 The diameters of the pelvic outlet.

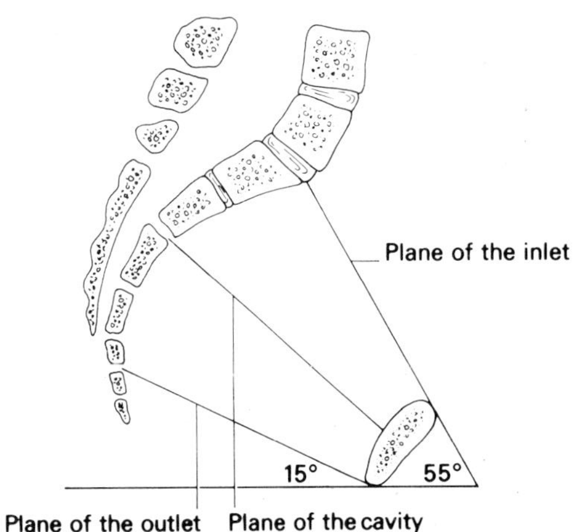

Fig. 3.52 The planes of the pelvis.

The fetal head, which entered the pelvis in the transverse diameter, underwent internal rotation in the cavity, escapes from the pelvis in the anteroposterior diameter. It is this adaption of the fetal head to the pelvic diameters which is the basis of the mechanism of labour to be described in detail later (see p. 127).

THE PELVIC PLANES

In order to determine the level of the presentation in the pelvis a number of planes or imaginary flat surfaces passing across the pelvis at different levels are described (Fig. 3.52).

The plane of the inlet. This lies across the pelvis at the level of the iliopectineal line.

The plane of the cavity. There are two planes of the cavity.

1 The plane of greatest pelvic dimensions passes across the pelvis at the level of the middle of the posterior surface of the symphysis pubis and the junction of the second and third sacral vertebrae and is circular in shape.

2 The plane of least pelvic dimensions passes through the lower border of the symphysis pubis, the ischial spines and the sacrococcygeal joint. This plane corresponds to the obstetrical outlet of the pelvis.

The plane of the outlet. This passes through the pelvis at the level of the symphysis pubis, the ischial tuberosities and the coccyx. This plane corresponds to the anatomical outlet of the pelvis.

PELVIC AXIS

This represents the direction taken by the fetal head in its passage through the pelvis. It is a curved line running parallel to the sacral curve and equidistant at all points from the pelvic walls and joining the midline points of the planes of the pelvis at the inlet, cavity and outlet. It is also known as the curve of Carus (Fig. 3.53).

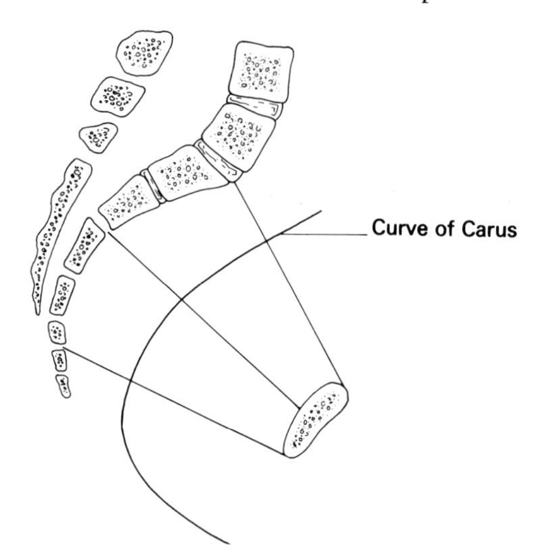

Fig. 3.53 The curve of the pelvic axis or curve of Carus.

ANGLES OF THE PELVIS

The angle of pelvic inclination. The angle between the plane of the inlet and the anterior surface of the fifth lumbar vertebra is the angle of pelvic inclination. It indicates the angle through which posterior lateral flexion of the head occurs when it becomes engaged with the occiput in a lateral position, and it should not exceed 135° (Fig. 3.54).

The sacral angle. The angle between the plane of the inlet and the anterior surface of the first sacral vertebra is the sacral angle. It usually measures 90° and indicates the dimension of the cavity in relation to the inlet (Fig. 3.54).

The inclination of the brim. The angle the plane of the inlet makes with the horizontal is termed the inclination of the brim. In the erect position the upper border of the symphysis is in the same vertical plane as the anterior superior iliac spines, and in the same horizontal plane as the coccyx (Fig. 3.54). It is approximately 55°.

The inclination of the outlet. The angle the upper border of the obstetrical outlet makes with the horizontal is the inclination of the outlet and measures 15° (Fig. 3.54).

The angle of the pubic arch. The angle between the two ischiopubic rami is the angle of the pubic arch and measures approximately 90°.

The pelvic floor

The pelvic floor is a muscular structure, which, with the perineum, forms the soft tissues which closes the outlet of the pelvis.

The structures forming the pelvic floor from within outwards are the peritoneum, extraperitoneal fat, the subperitoneal fascia, the pelvic fascia and

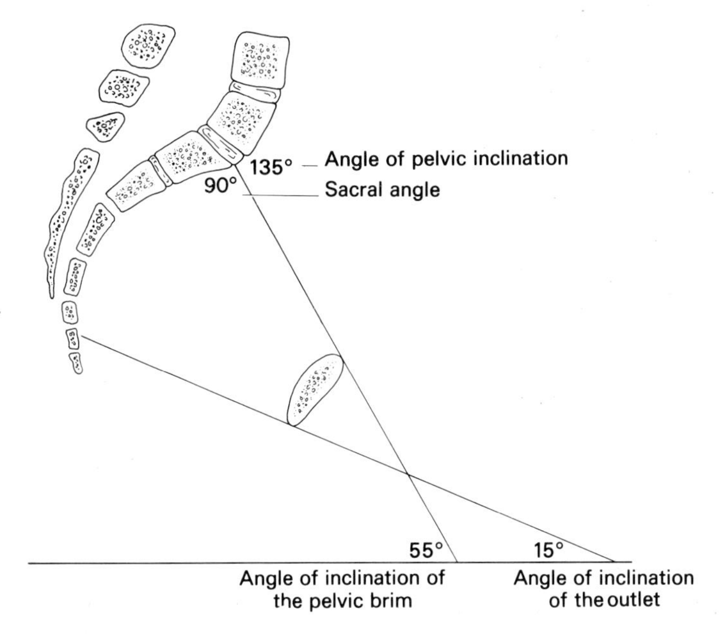

Fig. 3.54 The angles of the pelvis.

the pelvic diaphragm comprising the levatores ani and the coccygeus muscles. Of these structures the pelvic diaphragm is the most important and constitutes the pelvic floor proper.

The pelvic diaphragm

This is made up of four muscles, two levatores ani and two coccygei muscles. Together they form a muscular sheet the fibres of which interlace in different directions to form a resilient elastic, sling-shaped floor to the pelvic cavity. The upper surface is concave, the lower convex.

The levatores ani. The levator ani muscle is divided into two parts; the pubococcygeal and the iliococcygeal portions (Fig. 3.55).

The pubococcygeus arises from the posterior surface of the pubic bone and the fibres pass backwards to be inserted into the side of the coccyx. As the muscle fibres sweep backwards they pass below the bladder and on either side of the urethra, the lowest third of the vagina and the anal canal. Bands of fibres are inserted into these structures, where they blend with their instrinsic musculature. Some fibres cross from side to side to form the deep half of the perineal body, other fibres form a loop around the anal canal known as the anorectal sling. The longest fibres are inserted into the anococcygeal body and coccyx.

The iliococcygeus arises from the white line of pelvic fascia and passes

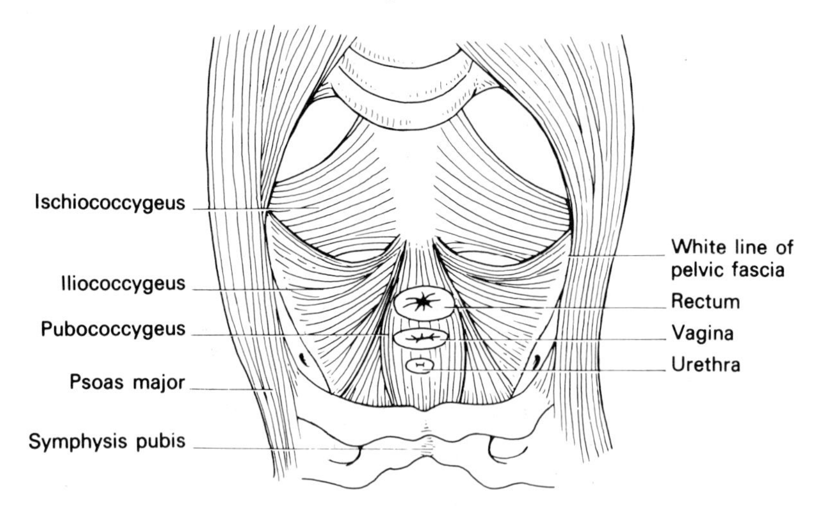

Fig. 3.55 The levatores ani and coccygeus muscles viewed from above.

downwards and inwards to be inserted into the anococcygeal body and the side of the coccyx.

The coccygeus muscle (ischiococcygeus). The ischiococcygeus is situated in front of the sacrospinous ligament. It arises from the ischial spine and passes downwards and inwards to be inserted into the side of the coccyx and lower part of the sacrum (Fig. 3.55).

FUNCTIONS

The pelvic floor provides support for the pelvic viscera, prevents their prolapse, and permits the bladder and uterus to expand and change their positions.

NERVE SUPPLY

The pelvic floor is supplied by fibres from the third and fourth sacral nerves and the pudendal nerve.

BLOOD SUPPLY

Branches of the internal iliac arteries supply the pelvic floor and venous drainage is into the corresponding veins.

THE LYMPHATICS

Drainage is into the internal iliac group.

The perineum

The perineum is the area enclosed between the lower surface of the pelvic floor above and the structures of the vulva below, extending from the symphysis pubis anteriorly to the coccyx posteriorly.

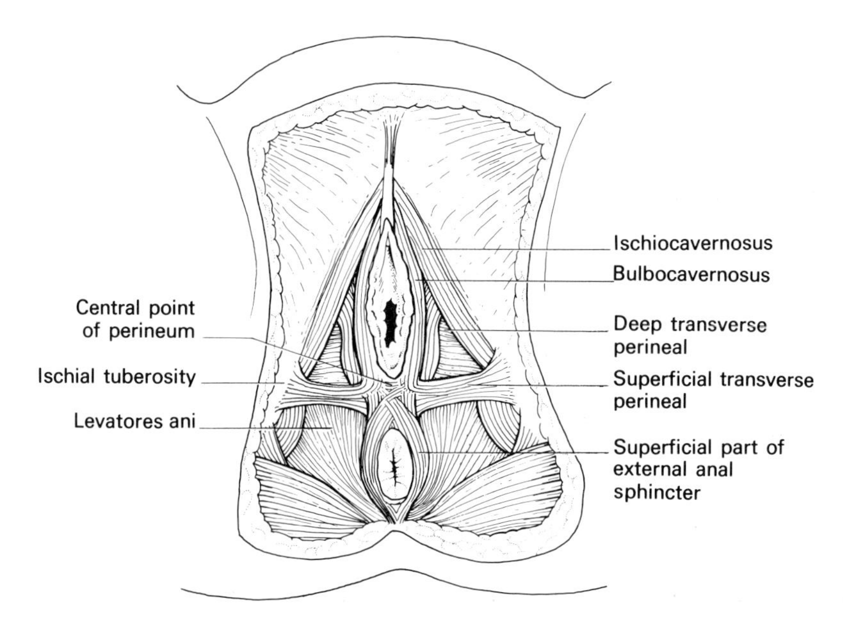

Fig. 3.56 The perineal muscles viewed from below.

The perineum is formed by two layers of muscle; the superficial perineal muscles and the urogenital diaphragm (triangular ligaments) (Fig. 3.56).

The superficial perineal muscles. These are made up of three pairs of muscles.

The transverse perinei muscles arise from the ischial tuberosities and pass medially to be inserted into the central point of the perineum. These muscles are divided into two parts, a superficial portion and a deep portion which is enclosed between layers of the triangular ligaments. The function of the transverse perinei muscles is to fix the position of the perineal body, and support the lower part of the vagina.

The bulbocavernosus muscles arise from the central point of the perineum and pass forwards around the vagina to be inserted into the corpora cavernosa of the clitoris.

The ischiocavernosus muscles have their origin at the ischial tuberosities and pass upwards along the pubic arch to be inserted into the corpora cavernosa of the clitoris.

The urogenital diaphragm. The triangular ligaments are deep fascia which invest the perineal muscles and fill the triangular spaces between the ischiocavernosus, bulbocavernosus and transverse perinei muscles.

The external sphincter of the anus surrounds the anal canal and lies below the internal sphincter. Anteriorly, it enters into the formation of the perineal body at the central point, and posteriorly some fibres are attached to the coccyx.

The membranous sphincter of the urethra is anatomically allied to the perineal muscles. The fibres arise from the pubic bone, pass above and below the urethra to be inserted into the opposite pubic bone. The sphincter lies between the layer of the triangular ligaments.

THE PERINEAL BODY

This is a fibromuscular pyramid situated between the lowest third of the vagina anteriorly, the anal canal posteriorly and the ischial tuberosities laterally.

The deep half of the perineal body consists of fibres from the levatores ani which cross over from side to side between the vagina and the anal canal. The superficial half is composed of superficial perineal muscles. The base of the perineal body is covered by skin. The central point of the perineum is the area where many of the superficial muscles converge.

The ischiorectal fossa is a deep, wedge-shaped space between the anal canal and the ischium. The fossa is filled with loose fatty tissue and allows for distension of the anal canal during defaecation. The ischiorectal fossa is of importance because it is a potential space for haematoma formation.

NERVE SUPPLY

The structures of the perineum are supplied by branches of the pudendal nerve.

BLOOD SUPPLY

The internal pudendal artery, a branch of the internal iliac artery, supplies the perineum. Venous return is by corresponding veins.

LYMPHATIC DRAINAGE

Most of the lymph vessels of the perineum pass into the medial group of superficial inguinal lymph nodes.

The pelvic floor and perineum are pierced in the midline by the urethra, vagina and anal canal.

Changes in pregnancy

Under the influence of progesterone the muscles of the pelvic floor and perineum soften and tend to sag slightly during pregnancy. The changes make pelvic assessment performed in late pregnancy less uncomfortable for the expectant mother and easier for the examiner.

Changes in labour

Owing to the fact that the pelvic floor is fixed posteriorly and has a forward slope, the fetus is directed forwards to the free space underneath the pubic arch. Pressure of the advancing fetal head causes the perineal body to flatten and the muscles to become stretched and elongated and displaced backwards in a trap door mechanism. The perineal and pelvic floor muscles may become overstretched and lacerated during delivery if preventative measures are not taken (see p. 157). There are three degrees of laceration.

First degree. The tear involves the fourchette and skin of the perineal body.

Second degree. The tear is deeper and in addition to the structures involved in a first degree laceration, the posterior wall of the vagina, the bulbocavernosus and transverse perinei muscles are involved. A deeper tear may also involve the pubococcygeus muscle.

Third degree. In addition to the structures involved in a second degree laceration the anal sphincter is torn and the tear may extend into the anterior wall of the anal canal and rectum.

Tearing of the underlying perineal tissues may occur while the external skin of the perineum remains intact. In these circumstances the posterior margin of the vagina splits away from the skin of the perineum. The injury is suspected when vaginal bleeding occurs during delivery of the head.

Changes during the puerperium

During the puerperium the relaxing influence of progesterone is no longer effective and the muscles of the pelvic floor and perineum regain their tone. If a laceration occurred or an incision was made into the muscle, healing will take place by first intention.

The fetal skull

A knowledge of the fetal skull is of great importance to the student of midwifery for it is the largest and least compressible part of the fetus to pass through the birth canal. Therefore, its shape and size are of practical importance in relation to the pelvis and the muscles of the pelvic floor and perineum, and is the reason for discussing it at this juncture as opposed to under the section relating to the fetus and neonate.

The fetal skull is divided into three parts. The vault, which is the large dome-shaped part containing the brain; the face, composed of fourteen small bones which are ossified by birth; and the base which is incompressible with the dimensions remaining unaltered by pressure.

It is the vault of the fetal skull that is of greatest importance and will now be described.

The vault of the fetal skull

The vault of the fetal skull is composed of five bones which are ossified in pre-existing membranes. The centre of ossification of each bone can be identified as a bony prominence at its midpoint.

BONES

There are two frontal bones which extend from the orbital ridge to the coronal suture. They cover the frontal lobes of the brain. The centres of ossification are called the frontal bosses.

The two parietal bones extend from the coronal suture in front to the lambdoidal suture behind. They are the largest of the bones comprising the fetal skull and cover the parietal lobes of the brain. Their centres of ossification are called the parietal eminences and a measurement between the two, the biparietal diameter. This measures approximately 9.5 cm, is the widest part of the fetal skull and forms the engaging diameter when the vertex is presenting. The biparietal diameter should be free of the ischial tuberosities before the head is allowed to extend during delivery.

The occipital bone covers the occipital lobe of the brain and the cerebellum. It lies behind the parietal bones. In the centre of the bone is a small eminence, the external occipital protuberance. There is a similarly placed bony prominence of the internal surface, the internal occipital protuberance to which a fold of dura mater is attached. The petrous portions of the two temporal bones form part of the lateral walls of the vault.

The edges of the bones do not approximate closely. They are separated by spaces known as sutures and fontanelles, formed of fibrous and membranous tissue continuous on the outer surface with the pericranium and lined on the inner surface by dura mater. Ossification of these membranous spaces occurs by degrees.

The sutures and fontanelles permit compression of the head by means of moulding, and therefore, the head can adapt to the shape and dimensions of the pelvic canal.

SUTURES

The frontal suture is a short straight suture between the frontal bones passing from the glabella to the anterior aspect of the bregma.

The coronal suture lies between the frontal and parietal bones and passes from the lateral angles of the bregma forwards. A measurement taken from the proximal points on the coronal suture across the face is the bitemporal diameter. This measures approximately 8 cm and is the narrowest part of the fetal skull.

The sagittal suture is a long straight suture between the parietal bones, passing from the posterior aspect of the bregma to the anterior aspect of the lambda.

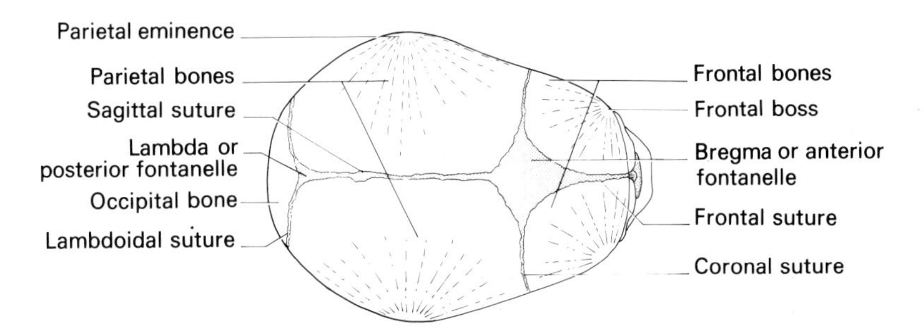

Fig. 3.57 The bones, centres of ossification, sutures and fontanelles of the fetal skull.

The lambdoidal suture lies between the parietal and occipital bones and passes forwards at an acute angle from the lateral aspects of the lambda.

The sagittal and frontal sutures allow a reduction in the width of the fetal skull from pressure on its sides, whilst the coronal and lambdoidal sutures allow a reduction in the long diameter through pressure applied anteroposteriorly (see p. 124, moulding).

FONTANELLES

There are two fontanalles of importance in obstetrics.

1 The anterior fontanelle or bregma is the larger of the two and it is situated at the junction of the frontal, coronal and sagittal sutures. It is kite-shaped and measures approximately 2.5 cm in length and 1.5 cm in width. The bregma is ossified when the baby is aged eighteen months.

2 The posterior fontanelle or lambda is situated at the junction of the sagittal and lambdoidal sutures. It is triangular and is ossified at the age of six weeks.

The sutures and fontanelles form important landmarks in identifying the presentation, position and attitude of the fetal skull in labour (see p. 148) (Fig. 3.57).

THE REGIONS OF THE FETAL SKULL

The face is the area between the mentum and the glabella. The sinciput or brow extends from glabella to the centre of the anterior fontanelle. The vertex is the area between the anterior and posterior fontanelles, bounded on either side by the parietal eminence. The occiput extends from the posterior fontanelle to the junction of the head and neck.

THE DIAMETERS OF THE FETAL SKULL

The diameters of the fetal skull are the longitudinal and the transverse diameters.

The longitudinal or anteroposterior diameters. These are of considerable clinical

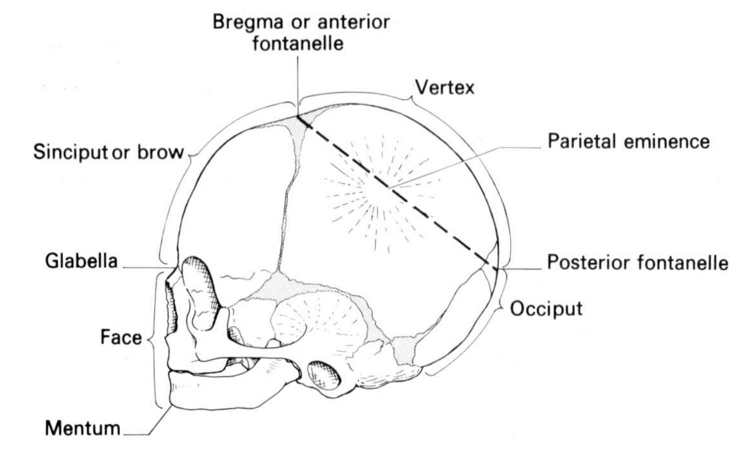

Fig. 3.58 The regions of the fetal skull.

Table 3.1 Longitudinal diameters of the fetal skull.

Attitude	*Presenting diameter (cm)*		*Presentation*
Flexion	Suboccipitobregmatic	9.5	Vertex (flexed)
Partial deflexion	Suboccipitofrontal	10.0	Vertex (partially deflexed)
Deflexion	Occipitofrontal	11.5	Vertex (deflexed)
Partial extension	Mentovertical	13.5	Brow
Extension	Submentobregmatic	9.5	Face

significance because they are the presenting diameters in relation to the pelvis, and constitute the distance the birth canal must stretch to allow passage of the head in labour. The presenting diameter varies according to the attitude of the head (Table 3.1).

a The suboccipitobregmatic diameter—from below the occipital protuberance to the centre of the bregma (Fig. 3.59).

b The suboccipitofrontal diameter—from below the occipital protuberance to the midpoint of the frontal suture. It is the maximum diameter to distend the vulva in the birth of the fully flexed vertex presentation (Fig. 3.59).

c The occipitofrontal diameter—from the occipital protuberance to the glabella. It distends the vulva in the birth of an occipitoposterior position (Fig. 3.59).

d The mentovertical diameter—from the mentum to the midpoint on the sagittal suture, i.e. highest points on the vertex. The brow presentation cannot enter the pelvis and deliver unless the pelvic diameters are increased or the fetal head less than normal size, as this diameter exceeds any diameters of the normal pelvis (Fig. 3.59).

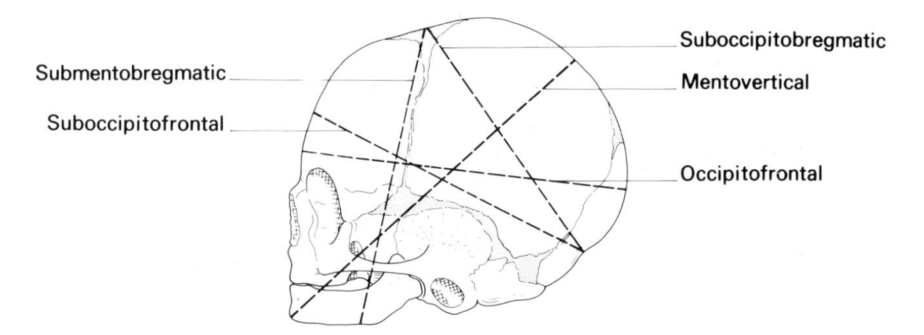

Fig. 3.59 The anteroposterior diameters of the fetal skull.

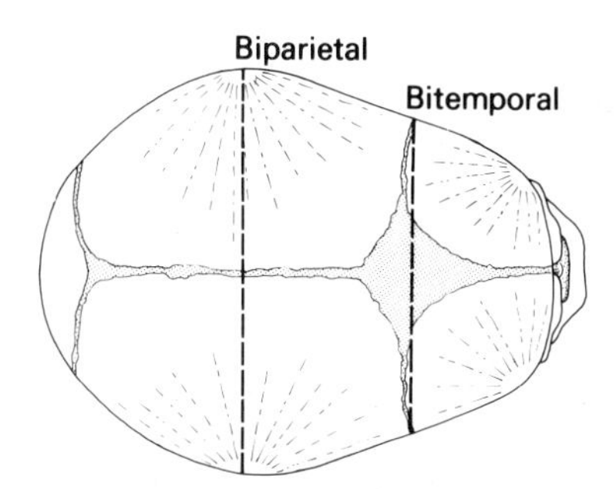

Fig. 3.60 The traverse diameters of the fetal skull.

e The submentovertical—from the junction of the chin and neck to the highest point on the vertex. It measures 11.5 cm and is the maximum diameter to distend the vulva in the birth of a face presentation.
f The submentobregmatic diameter—from the junction of the chin and neck to the centre of the bregma (Fig. 3.59).
The transverse diameters. These measure the width of the fetal skull (Fig. 3.60).
a The biparietal diameter 9.5 cm—between the parietal eminences. It is the widest part of the fetal head. When this diameter has passed through the plane of the pelvic inlet the head is engaged and when it distends the vulva at delivery the head is crowned. This indicates that the occiput has escaped under the pubic arch and the head may now be delivered by extension. The biparietal diameter is the transverse diameter that accompanies the suboccipitobregmatic, suboccipitofrontal and occipitofrontal diameters. The biparietal diameter is measured by ultrasound to assess growth of the fetal skull (see p. 317).
b The bitemporal diameter 8.5 cm—from the distal point at one end of the coronal suture across the face to the opposite end of the coronal suture. This diameter accompanies the mentovertical and submentobregmatic diameters.

HEAD CIRCUMFERENCES

There are four circumferences.

1 The suboccipitobregmatic circumference, 33 cm, the greatest circumference to pass the brim in a fully flexed vertex presentation. The greatest anteroposterior diameter is the suboccipitobregmatic, 9.5 cm, and the greatest transverse diameter the biparietal, 9.5 cm.

2 The occipitofrontal circumference, 35.5 cm, the greatest circumference in an occipitoposterior position (deflexed head). The greatest anteroposterior diameter is the occipitofrontal, 11.5 cm, and the greatest transverse diameter the biparietal, 9.5 cm.

3 The submentobregmatic circumference, 33 cm, the greatest circumference to pass the brim in a face presentation (extended head). The greatest anteroposterior diameter is the submentobregmatic, 9.5 cm, and the greatest transverse diameter the biparietal, 9.5 cm.

4 The mentovertical circumference measures 38 cm and is too large to pass the brim of the pelvis.

MOULDING

Due to incomplete ossification of the bones of the fetal skull, and the presence of the sutures and fontanelles, the fetal head is able to adapt to the shape and size of the pelvis. Pressure is applied on the head by the birth canal and the bones mould and change their shape and overlap at the sutures and fontanelles. The frontal bones slide under the anterior part of the parietal bones and the occiput under the posterior part. The posterior parietal bone slides under the anterior. Therefore, the sagittal and frontal sutures allow the diminution in width of the fetal skull, from pressure on its sides, while the coronal and lambdoidal sutures allow diminution in the long diameter through pressure applied anteroposteriorly.

The effect of moulding is to bring about a reduction in the presenting diameter and elongation of the diameter passing at a right-angle to it (Table 3.2). Therefore, although the presenting diameter is reduced, there is no reduction in the capacity within the fetal skull which would cause damage to its contents, i.e. the brain.

Moulding may be normal or abnormal. Normal moulding occurs slowly, is not excessive and is in an upwards and backwards direction (Fig. 3.61[1]). Moulding is abnormal if it takes place rapidly, is excessive or is in an upwards direction (Fig. 3.61[2,3,4]).

Excessive moulding may occur in the presence of cephalopelvic disproportion or in the immature fetus where the bones of the fetal skull are soft and more compressible.

Moulding may not be able to take place if the fetus is postmature and the bones hard and unyielding.

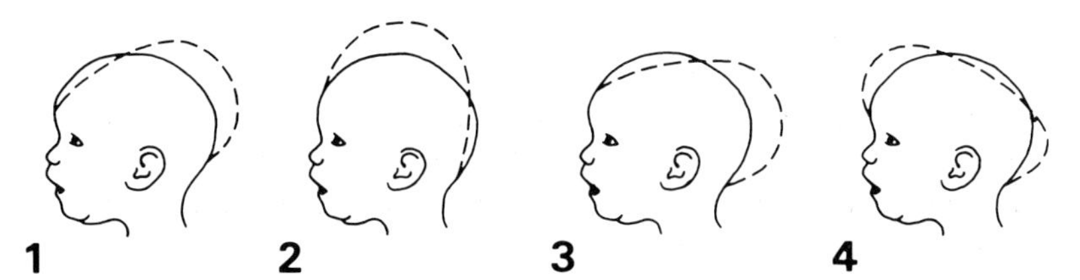

Fig. 3.61 1, normal moulding; 2, abnormal moulding (occipitoposterior position); 3, abnormal moulding (face presentation); 4, abnormal moulding (brow presentation).

Table 3.2 Effects of moulding on the longitudinal diameters of the fetal skull.

Presentation	*Presenting diameter (shortened)*	*Diameter at right-angle (lengthened)*
Vertex—flexed	Suboccipitobregmatic	Mentovertical
Vertex—deflexed	Occipitofrontal	Submentobregmatic
Face	Submentobregmatic	Occipitofrontal
Brow	Mentovertical	Suboccipitobregmatic
Breech	Suboccipitofrontal	Submentovertical

THE SCALP

The scalp consists of five layers: a layer of skin, a layer of connective tissue containing blood vessels and hair follicles, a layer of tendon and muscle, an areolar tissue layer and a layer of pericranium.

During labour, especially when the membranes are ruptured, the presenting part immediately over the os uteri is subjected to less pressure than the area which is in contact with the cervix. An oedematous swelling, known as a caput succedaneum is produced as a result of the difference between the two pressures (Fig. 3.62).

The caput succedaneum develops over the most dependent part, e.g. over the upper posterior part of the right parietal bone in a left occipitoanterior position and over the upper posterior part of the left parietal bone in a right occipitoanterior position.

It is possible to diagnose the original position of the fetus by the position of the caput succedaneum at birth.

It may be distinguished from a cephalhaematoma (see p. 346) because it is present at birth, it pits on pressure, and its infusion is into the layer of connective tissue above the pericranium and may therefore pass over the sutures. A double caput succedaneum is always unilateral and indicates a change in the attitude of the fetal head during labour, i.e. the original swelling may be found on the upper anterior part of the parietal bone when the head is deflexed, and a secondary caput succedaneum of the upper posterior part of the parietal bone when the head flexes.

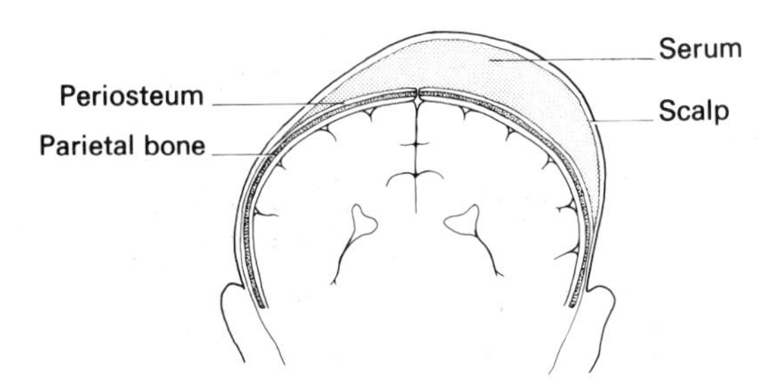

Fig. 3.62 A caput succedaneum.

The caput succedaneum will disperse within a few hours of birth without any treatment.

INTERNAL STRUCTURES

The dura mater not only covers the whole surface of the brain but forms fibrous partitions between the lobes of the brain, dividing the interior of the skull into compartments. The two most important partitions in relation to obstetrics are the falx cerebri and the tentorium cerebelli. They contain large venous sinuses which drain blood from the brain into the jugular veins of the neck.

The falx cerebri is a vertical fold of dura mater dividing the two cerebral hemispheres. The lower edge of this fold lies free and is sickle-shaped. It is attached to the inside of the skull at the root of the nose, follows the line of the frontal and sagittal sutures to the internal occipital protuberance. The venous sinus passing along its line of attachment is the superior longitudinal sinus, the inferior longitudinal sinus runs in the lower border.

The tentorium cerebelli is a horseshoe-shaped horizontal fold of dura mater which lies in the posterior part of the cranial cavity, separating the two cerebral hemispheres above from the cerebellum below. Its line of attachment is from the sphenoid bone on either side along the petrous portion of the temporal bone to the internal occipital protuberance.

The posterior part of the falx cerebri is attached to the upper surface of the tentorium cerebelli at its midline. Immediately in front of the point of junction, an arch is formed, through which the brain stem passes from the cerebral hemispheres.

The inferior longitudinal sinus ends at the junction of the falx cerebri and the tentorium cerebelli and continues as the straight sinus which passes backwards along the line of junction of the two membranes to unite with the posterior end of the superior longitudinal sinus. This point of junction, opposite the internal occipital protuberance, is known as the confluens sinium. From the confluens sinium the sinuses pass on each side along the line of attachment of the tentorium cerebelli where they are known as the lateral sinuses.

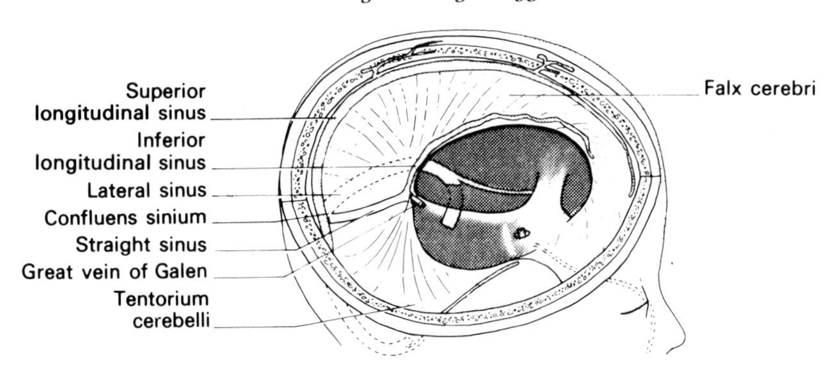

Fig. 3.63 The falx cerebri, the tentorium and the venous sinuses.

The great vein of Galen passes backwards from the surface of the brain to join the straight sinus at the point where it becomes continuous with the inferior longitudinal sinus (Fig. 3.63).

If moulding is rapid or excessive the membranes and sinuses may rupture and haemorrhage occur. Tears are more likely to occur in the tentorium cerebelli near its attachment to the falx cerebri, tentorial tear, and the great vein of Galen becomes torn at its junction with the straight sinus.

Mechanism of labour

The mechanism of labour describes the changes in the attitude and position of the fetus in its descent through the birth canal. Because these movements are necessary for the fetus to adapt to the shape and size of the mother's pelvis it is logical to describe the mechanism of labour in relation to the maternal pelvis and fetal skull although it must also be considered in association with the physiology and management of labour.

At the commencement of labour the fetus lies longitudinally in the uterus in an attitude of flexion. In the primigravida the head is normally already engaged in the pelvis; in a multigravida, owing to greater laxity of the uterine and abdominal wall muscles, flexion may be less complete and engagement does not usually take place until labour has already started.

As labour progresses the fetus descends through the birth canal and there is increased flexion. The occiput meets the resistance of the pelvic floor and internally rotates forwards through 45° (Fig. 3.64). When the occiput escapes under the pubic arch and the biparietal diameter is level with the ischial tuberosities, extension of the head takes place (Fig. 3.65). Because internal rotation of the head is not accompanied by rotation of the shoulders, a twisting of the neck occurs (Fig. 3.66). This is released (restitution) as soon as the head is born. Following restitution of the head the shoulders rotate and descend causing the occiput to externally rotate a further 45° following the direction of restitution (Fig. 3.67).

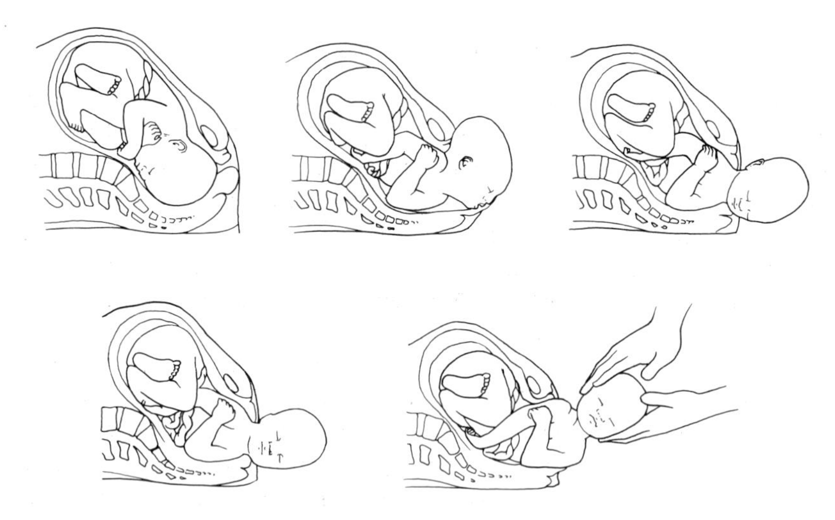

Fig. 3.64 (top left) Internal rotation.
Fig. 3.65 (top centre) Extension.
Fig. 3.66 (top right) Restitution.
Fig. 3.67 (bottom left) External rotation.
Fig. 3.68 (bottom right) Lateral flexion.

First the anterior and then the posterior shoulder and trunk are delivered in a movement of lateral flexion (Fig. 3.68). When the head is in an occipitolateral position at the commencement of labour, the long axis of the head is almost perpendicular to the plane of the inlet, the sagittal suture lies in the transverse diameter with the posterior parietal bone slightly lower than the anterior. During contractions the uterus and the long axis of the fetus move forwards and the sagittal suture moves backwards towards the middle of the inlet. The long axis of the head descends downwards and backwards parallel with the sacral curve towards the lower posterior pelvis. The forward curve of the lower sacrum prevents further backward progress and the head proceeds downwards on to the lateral and posterior parts of the pelvic floor. The shape of the pelvic floor directs the head forwards towards the posterior surface of the symphysis pubis. The sagittal suture now lies in the anteroposterior diameter of the outlet, the occiput escapes from under the pubic arch and the head is born by extension.

The body is born by a movement of lateral flexion. The interrelated factors concerned with the mechanism of labour are therefore the uterine contractions, the maternal pelvis and pelvic floor muscles, and the fetus.

The mammary glands

The breasts are modified sweat glands, which develop as fifteen to twenty cellular buds extending into the underlying dermis of the pectoral region. Although development begins before the twelfth week of fetal life only rudimentary duct development has occurred by the time of birth.

Development of the breasts occurs in relation to puberty, although some duct growth occurs before this time. Oestrogens from the ovaries cause development of the duct system, nipple and areola and are responsible for deposition of fat which is mainly responsible for the increase in size.

In females, the breasts are accessory parts of the reproductive system, being adapted to secrete milk to feed the baby. The breasts are two hemispherical swellings situated on the anterior aspect of the chest wall over the pectoralis major muscle and extending from the level of the second rib above, to the sixth rib below, and from the lateral border of the sternum to the axilla. The part of the breast tissue extending into the axilla is known as the tail of Spence.

At the most prominent part of the breast there is a projection, the nipple, on the surface of which are the openings of the lactiferous ducts (Fig. 3.69). The skin covering the nipple and the area around its base, the areola, is pigmented. Small projections, which are the sebaceous glands are seen in the outer aspect of the areola, which is approximately 2.5 cm in diameter. The nipple is about 0.5 cm long and is composed of erectile tissue covered by skin and containing smooth muscle fibres which have a sphincter-like action in controlling the flow of milk.

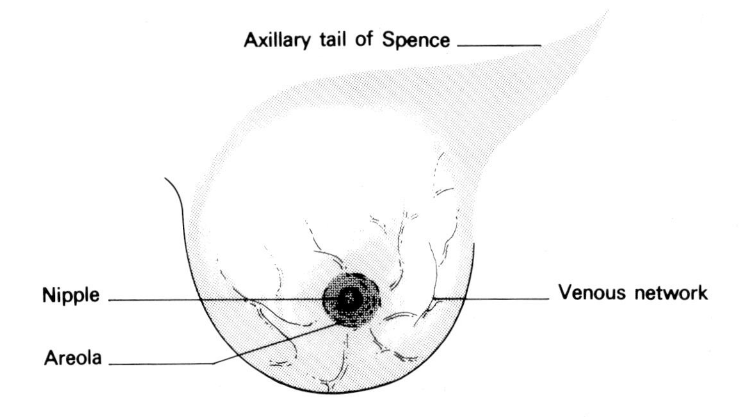

Fig. 3.69 The breast.

STRUCTURE

Because of its development from fifteen to twenty cellular buds each breast consists of fifteen to twenty segments or lobes each opening by a separate duct system on to the nipple. The lobes are separated by fibrous connective tissue partitions (Fig. 3.70). A lobe is composed of a number of lobules which terminate deep in the gland, in alveoli lined with cubical secretory cells. The lobules and alveoli are connected by small ducts which communicate with the main duct, the lactiferous duct. Each lactiferous duct dilates under the areola into a spindle-shaped ampulla, narrowing again to pass through the nipple and terminating in a minute opening at its surface. The alveoli and small ducts are surrounded by contractile cells, myoepithelial cells, which contract to eject the milk.

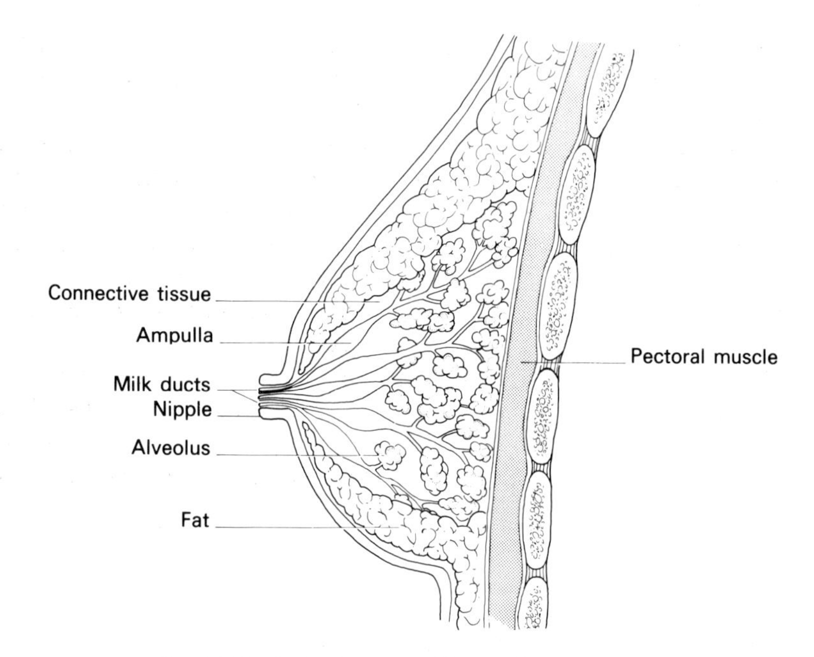

Fig. 3.70 Sagittal section of breast showing lobes.

The breasts have little natural support but are stabilised by a thick layer of fat which gives the breast its characteristic rounded appearance, and by the ligaments of Astley Cooper, fibrous processes which pass from the glandular tissue to the skin of the areola.

BLOOD SUPPLY

The breasts receive an ample blood supply from the internal and external mammary arteries and the upper intercostal artery. The veins form a network round the nipple and drain into the internal mammary and axillary veins.

NERVE SUPPLY

The nerve supply to the mammary tissue is poor, the function being controlled by hormones. Some sympathetic fibres of the cutaneous branches of the fourth, fifth and sixth thoracic nerves supply the skin.

LYMPHATIC DRAINAGE

The lymphatic vessels form a plexus beneath the areola and between the lobes and drain into the axillary glands, the glands of the anterior mediastinum and the glands of the portal fissure of the liver. The lymphatics of the two breasts communicate freely with one another.

Changes during pregnancy

Full structural development of the breasts does not take place without the stimulus of pregnancy. At the onset of pregnancy the glandular tissue, especially in a primigravida may be relatively undeveloped. Under the stimulation of oestrogens there is development of the ducts and in response to placental lactogen and the placental steroids, growth of the alveoli and secretory cells. Secretory activity begins about the third or fourth month, increases as pregnancy advances and a small amount of secretions, later colostrum, appears at the nipple. The areola becomes fuller and pigmented, the primary areola, and a mottled area of pigmentation may be seen to extend beyond the primary areola, the secondary areola.

The nipple becomes pigmented and more prominent and the sebaceous glands become enlarged and are known as the Montgomery's tubercles. There is an increased blood flow to the breasts and this causes a tingling sensation in early pregnancy and the appearance of dilated veins under the surface of the skin.

Changes in the puerperium

The physiology of lactation consists of three stages.

The production of milk. Milk production is suppressed until two to three days postpartum, the action of prolactin being inhibited by oestrogens. Following delivery of the placenta the level of oestrogens falls and the anterior lobe of the pituitary gland produces prolactin.

Milk is formed as small fatty globules in the cells of the alveoli and unite with other globules to form small droplets which are forced into the lactiferous ducts, where they unite with droplets from the other alveoli. In this way the alveoli become filled with milk. The breasts require a large blood supply from which to produce milk.

The flow of milk along the ducts. The milk present in the large ducts and ampullae forms only a very small proportion of the milk actually in the glands.

Most of the milk is contained in the alveoli and the smaller ducts. When the milk is drawn off by the baby, the myoepithelial cells contract and force more milk towards the nipple. The mechanism occurs as a result of a neurohormonal reflex in which stimulation of the nipple causes release of oxytocin from the posterior lobe of the pituitary gland (Fig. 3.71). The rise of milk pressure within the breast, the so-called 'draught' forces the milk down from the alveoli and small ducts into the larger ducts.

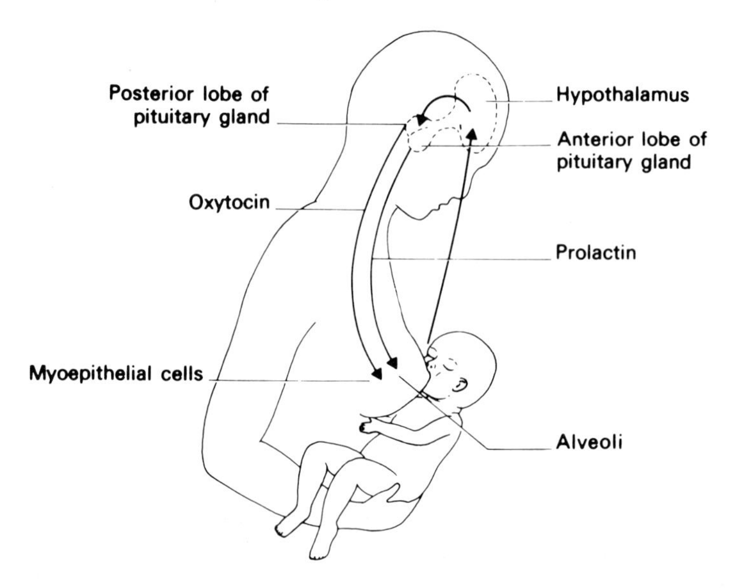

Fig. 3.71 The neurohormonal reflex.

The withdrawal of milk. The baby obtains milk from the breast by champing action with the jaws. The baby draws the nipple into its mouth, and by closing its jaws expresses the milk from the underlying ampullae. The suckling reflex causes an outflow of prolactin which stimulates further milk production in preparation for the next feed (Fig. 3.71).

INVOLUTION OF THE BREASTS

Failure to stimulate the breasts causes secretions to fail. The completeness with which the breasts return to the pre-pregnant state varies. It is thought that some functional lobules remain after lactation ceases, particularly if it has been successful and of long duration.

Table 3.3 Composition of colostrum and breast milk.

Composition	*Colostrum*		*Breast milk*
Lactose	3.5%		7.0%
Fat	2.5%		3.5%
Protein: lactalbumen, lactoglobulin	8.0%	Lactalbumen	1.0%
		Caseinogen	0.5%
Mineral salts	0.4%	Phosphorus, Calcium, Sodium, Magnesium, Potassium, Chloride	0.2%
Iron			
Vitamins A, B, C, D, E			
Water	85.6%		87.8%
Calories/30 ml	21.0		20.0
Joules/30 ml	88.2		84.0

The urinary tract

The urinary tract consists of two excretory organs, the right and left kidneys, which filter the blood circulating through them and produce urine; two collecting ducts, called ureters, which convey the urine from the kidneys to the bladder; and the bladder which acts as a reservoir for the urine until it is voided by the act of micturition, when the urine is passed to the exterior by way of the urethra (Fig. 3.72).

DEVELOPMENT

The development of the urinary tract is linked with that of the genital tract and the lower portion of the alimentary tract. At a very early stage of development, the parts which become the bladder and the urethra form with the rectum in a common cavity, called the cloaca. This cavity is later divided by a partition, called the urorectal septum, which separates the future bladder and urethra (urogenital sinus) in front from the rectum behind. The part of the cloaca which later becomes the urogenital sinus is joined by a duct, the mesonephric duct, which grows down from the mesonephros near which the gonad develops. Proximal to the junction of this duct with the cloaca a new duct, the ureteric bud, grows out towards the developing kidney, the metanephros. The ureteric bud unites with the metanephros, the ureteric bud giving rise to the ureter, pelvis, calyces and collecting tubules within the kidney, and the metanephros forming the glomerular capsules, proximal convoluted tubules, loop of Henle and distal convoluted tubules.

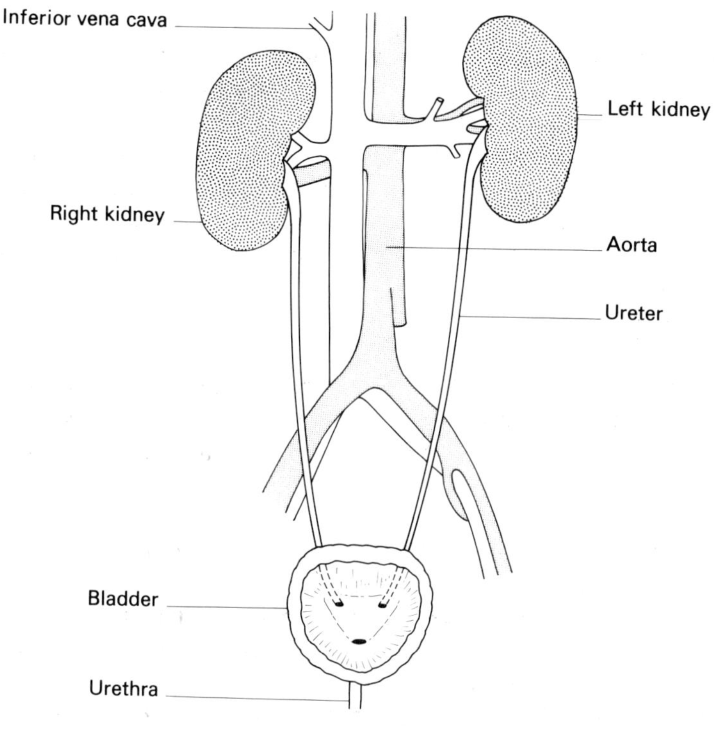

Fig. 3.72 The urinary tract.

A knowledge of the renal tract is important to the student of midwifery because of the close proximity of the bladder and urethra to the genital tract, and the effects of pregnancy on the kidneys and ureters.

The kidney

The kidney is a compound tubular gland and is one of two reddish-brown, smooth bean-shaped glands, 10 cm in length, 6 cm in width and about 3 cm thick, weighing approximately 120 g.

The kidneys lie, one on either side of the twelfth thoracic and third lumbar vertebrae, on the posterior abdominal wall behind the peritoneal cavity. The long axis of the kidney lies obliquely, the upper end being nearer the midline than the lower end. The right kidney is about 2 cm lower than the left due to the liver taking up much of the space in the upper right part of the abdominal cavity.

The anterior surface projects forwards and laterally, the posterior surface backwards and medially; the lateral border is convex and the medial is concave. The middle third of the medial border is indented, the cleft between the rounded borders being known as the hilum which transmits the ureter, renal blood and lymphatics vessels and nerves.

RELATIONS

Superiorly, the suprarenal glands cap the upper pole of each kidney. Anteriorly, the right kidney has the liver above, the hepatic flexure of the colon below, and the duodenum medially; the left kidney has the stomach and spleen, below which is the pancreas and lower still the jejunum. Posteriorly, the relations are identical on both sides apart from the lowering of the right kidney. The upper half is related to the twelfth rib and diaphragm and the lower half to the psoas major, quadratus lumbdorium and the transverse abdominus muscles.

SUPPORTS

The kidney is covered by a thick fibrous capsule and is invested by the perirenal fascia within which it is held firmly by perirenal fat. It is attached by means of the renal vessels to the abdominal aorta and inferior vena cava.

STRUCTURE

The macroscopic structure of the kidney (Fig. 3.73) is composed of three parts; the pelvis, the medulla and the cortex.

The pelvis is the funnel-shaped upper end of the ureter which opens into the cavity. It is divided into large branches, the major calyces which subdivide into smaller branches, the minor calyces.

The medulla is dark and has a striated appearance. It consists of twelve small conical masses, the pyramids. The apex of the pyramid projects into a minor calyx whilst the base extends towards the cortex of the kidney. The pyramids contain faint parallel streaks called the medullary rays which run towards the apex and are the collecting tubules which carry the urine from the cortex to the calyx, pelvis and ureter.

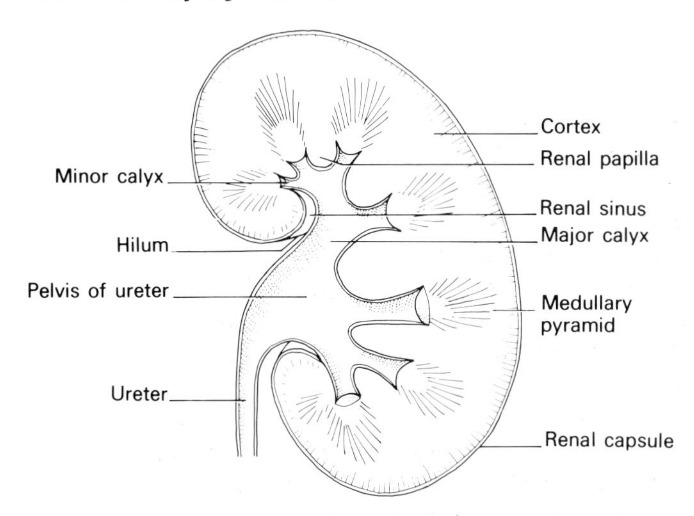

Fig. 3.73 The kidney.

The cortex is paler and has a granular appearance. It forms arches over the base of the pyramids and extends between the pyramids towards the pelvis. These projections of the cortex are known as the columns of Bertini.

The microscopic structure of the kidney is composed of the nephron which is the functional unit of the kidney. Each kidney contains about one million nephrons closely packed together in connective tissue stroma.

STRUCTURE OF THE NEPHRON

The nephron is a tubule about 3 cm in length. One end is closed and the other end opens into a collecting duct.

The closed end is a membrane formed of a single layer of flat epithelial cells reflexed back on itself which is dilated to form a cup-like structure called the glomerular (Bowman's) capsule.

The glomerular capsule is invaginated by a knot of capillary loops called a glomerulus (Fig. 3.74). An afferent arteriole carries blood to the glomerulus whilst the blood is drained from the glomerulus by an efferent arteriole. The spherical structure formed by the glomerular capsule and the glomerulus is known as a renal corpuscle or Malpighian body. Its function is filtration.

The remainder of the tubule is coiled and looped, and is surrounded by a capillary network leading from the efferent arteriole. The section near the Malpighian body has a wall of cubical cells and is called the proximal (first) convoluted tubule. This leads into the loop of Henle which extends into a medullary pyramid and back again. The tubule then forms a second coil near the Malpighian body, the distal (second) convoluted tubule, and ends by joining a collecting duct which receives many tubules and passes through a pyramid into a minor calyx (Fig. 3.75). The proximal and distal convoluted tubules and the loop of Henle concentrate the urine by selective reabsorption, and also add substances to it by secretion.

FORMATION OF URINE

Filtration under pressure. The blood pressure in the capillary loop is high because the afferent arteriole is larger than the efferent arteriole. This pressure forces water and all the other constituents of the plasma except the large protein molecules through the capillary walls and through the epithelium of the glomerular capsule into its lumen. This fluid is called the glomerular filtrate and has the composition of plasma without proteins. The two kidneys produce about 145 ml of glomerular filtrate per minute.

Selective reabsorption. This takes place in the tubule. As the glomerular filtrate passes through the proximal convoluted tubules substances useful to the body such as water, glucose, sodium and chloride ions and amino acids are reabsorbed by the cells of the tubules and passed back into the blood. The fluid passes through the loop of Henle to the distal convoluted tubule where more water may be reabsorbed depending on the fluid balance of the body. The exact

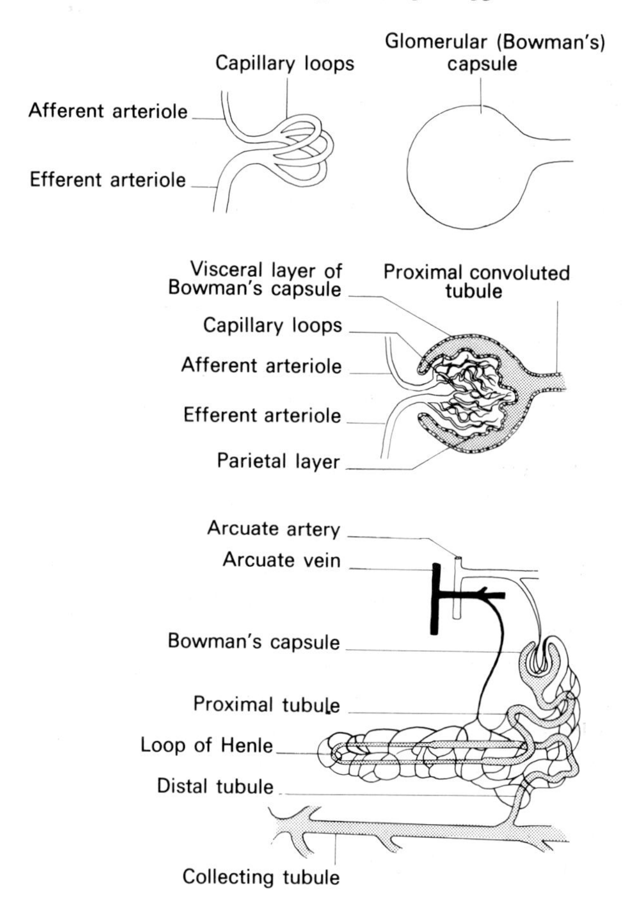

Fig. 3.74 (top) The glomerulus and glomerular capsule; (centre) Malpighian body.
Fig. 3.75 (bottom) A nephron.

amount of water reabsorbed, and therefore the volume of urine formed, is controlled by the antidiuretic hormone of the posterior lobe of the pituitary gland, which acts on the distal convoluted tubules and the collecting ducts. If the body needs to conserve water the antidiuretic hormone causes the cells to reabsorb water, and a smaller volume of concentrated urine is produced. If there is an excess of fluid the antidiuretic hormone is no longer produced and the cells do not reabsorb water, and a greater volume of dilute urine results.

Secretion. Although the tubules function mainly by selective reabsorption, they also actively secrete certain substances into the urine, for example hydrogen ions, potassium ions, creatinine and some toxins and drugs.

FUNCTIONS OF THE KIDNEYS

1 Maintain the water balance.
2 Control of sodium under the influence of aldosterone.
3 Maintain the acid base balance by eliminating acids.

The pH of fresh normal urine is between five and seven. In acidosis the kidney excretes a more acid urine and in alkalosis the urine becomes more alkaline. The cells of the kidney tubules vary the reaction of the urine according to the ions excreted into the urine.

4 Excretion of waste products.

BLOOD SUPPLY

Each kidney is supplied by a renal artery direct from the abdominal aorta. In the kidney it divides into several branches, interlobular arteries which enter the columns of Bertini and then form arcades, arcuate arteries, across the bases of the pyramids. From the arcuate arteries, branches pass into the medulla and also between the lobes, interlobular arteries, into the cortex. From the interlobular arteries an afferent arteriole goes to each glomerulus.

The blood passes through the capillary loops of the glomerulus and is carried away by the efferent arteriole which leads to a capillary network round the rest of the nephron. From this plexus the blood is drained away by vessels which eventually join up to form the renal vein.

Blood flows through the kidneys not only to nourish them, but so that they can alter its composition by removing unwanted substances according to the needs of the body. The total volume of blood in the body flows through the kidneys once every five minutes.

NERVE SUPPLY

Sympathetic fibres from the sixth thoracic to the third lumbar segments pass to the kidneys; parasympathetic fibres are derived from the vagus.

LYMPHATIC DRAINAGE

A plexus forms under the capsule of the kidney and the lymph is drained into the aortic and lumbar glands.

The ureter

The ureters convey the urine from the kidney, where it is formed, to the bladder where it is stored. The ureter begins at the medial border of the kidney by the joining of the calyces to form the funnel-shaped upper end of the ureter, the pelvis. This leads into the ureter itself which is a narrow muscular tube, 25 cm in length and 0.5 cm in diameter.

The ureter passes downwards outside the peritoneum, over the posterior abdominal wall and into the true pelvis, where it passes over the common iliac artery, at its division, into the internal and external iliac arteries. It passes down the side wall of the pelvis and medially through the pelvic fascia and ureteric canal in the transverse cervical ligaments in close relation to the isthmus. The ureter enters the bladder obliquely through the posterior wall and the posteriolateral angles of the trigone.

STRUCTURE

The ureter has four layers.

1 A lining of transitional epithelium thrown into longitudinal folds.

2 Fibrous tissue with elastic fibres.

3 Smooth muscle fibres, an inner layer of weak longitudinal fibres, a middle layer of circular fibres and an outer layer of well defined longitudinal fibres.

4 Fibrous connective tissue.

The urinary bladder

The bladder is a hollow, muscular organ which receives urine conveyed to it by the ureters from the kidney, acts as a reservoir for the urine and voids it at intervals through the urethra.

The bladder is a distensible organ and therefore its shape, size, relationships and the thickness of the wall vary at different stages of transition between the full and empty states.

The empty bladder lies within the pelvis, behind the pubic bone, anterior to the cervix and upper anterior vaginal wall, inferior to the body of the anteverted uterus and the uterovesical pouch, superior to the urethra, levatores ani muscles and the triangular ligaments, and medial to the side walls of the pelvis and transverse ligaments of the bladder (Fig. 3.76). As it fills, the bladder rises into the abdomen.

The bladder, when empty, is pyramidal in shape with its apex pointing forwards and its base backwards.

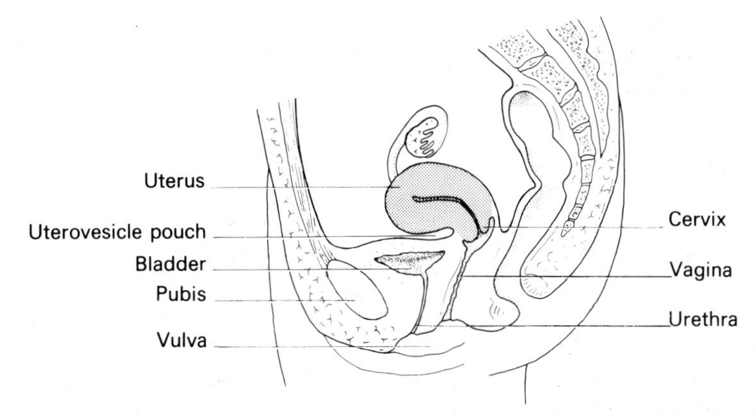

Fig. 3.76 Sagittal section of pelvic organs showing the relations of the bladder.

The bladder has a base, superior surface and two inferolateral surfaces. The superior surface is covered with the floor of the uterovesical pouch which extends from the pubic bone to the isthmus. The two inferolateral surfaces rest on the upper surface of the levatores ani muscle.

The base or trigone is triangular in shape with the base above and the apex below. The three sides of the trigone each measure about 2.5 cm in length. The ureters enter the trigone at the ureteric orifices in the upper lateral angles of the base having obliquely penetrated the bladder wall. The urethra leaves the trigone at the apex which is formed by the internal meatus and emerges from the bladder at the bladder neck (Fig. 3.77).

The capacity of the bladder is about 300 ml.

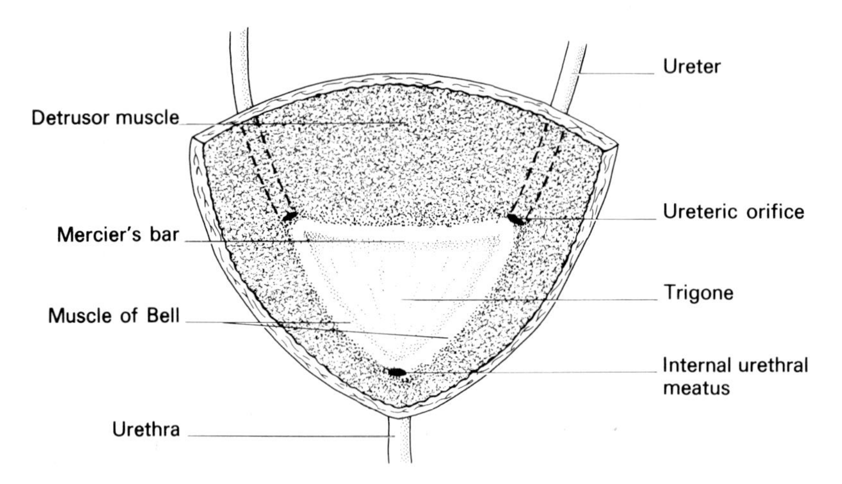

Fig. 3.77 The trigone of the bladder.

STRUCTURE

The bladder is lined by transitional epithelium which permits expansion without breaching the continuity of the lining. It is thrown into rugae and is loosely attached to the submucous and muscle layers, except over the trigone where the attachment is firmer.

The submucous layer of areolar tissue is interspersed with fine elastic fibres.

The muscular layer consists of smooth muscle fibres arranged in three ill-defined layers. The inner and outermost layers consist of longitudinal fibres and the middle layer of circular fibres. The circular fibres are thickened around the internal meatus to form the internal sphincter of the bladder. The muscle of the bladder is known as the detrusor muscle and like the muscle fibres of the myometrium possess the power of retraction. The muscles of the trigone have a special arrangement. Mercier's bar is the name given to the band of muscle fibres passing between the ureteric orifices, and the muscle of Bell is the name of the bands of muscle fibres passing from the ureteric orifices to the internal meatus. These fibres pass through the internal meatus into the urethra and play an important role in micturition.

Peritoneum covers the superior surface only, the remaining surfaces being invested in the pelvic fascia.

LIGAMENTS

There are five ligaments attached to the bladder. The urachus—from the apex of the bladder to the umbilicus; the two lateral ligaments—from the side of the bladder to the pelvic walls; and the two pubovesical—from the neck of the bladder to the pubic bone—which form part of the pubocervical ligaments.

BLOOD SUPPLY

The bladder is supplied with blood from the superior and inferior vesical arteries which are branches of the hypogastric arteries from the internal iliac arteries.

A venous plexus is situated near the ureters and the veins drain into corresponding veins.

LYMPHATIC DRAINAGE

Lymphatic drainage is into the external iliac glands.

NERVE SUPPLY

The bladder is supplied both by sympathetic and parasympathetic nerves. Stimulation of the parasympathetic nerves empties the bladder by causing the detrusor muscle to contract and the internal sphincter to relax. Stimulation of the sympathetic nerves prevents emptying by causing the internal sphincter to contract and the detrusor muscle to relax.

PHYSIOLOGY OF MICTURITION

Micturition is essentially a reflex act which has been brought under voluntary control.

The bladder fills slowly and under control of the sympathetic nerves, the internal sphincter remains closed and the detrusor muscle of the bladder wall relaxes a little to accommodate the increasing volume of urine. When the volume reaches 300 ml, the walls do not relax so readily and the pressure then rises. The increased pressure stimulates stretch receptors in the bladder wall. The impulse is relayed to the parasympathetic nerve cells which carry the impulses to the detrusor muscle causing it to contract. At the same time, the internal sphincter and the external sphincter reflexly relax so that urine is voided. However, by voluntary control of micturition, the reflex can be suppressed. The first afferent impulses, as the bladder becomes full, are interpreted by the brain, inhibitory impulses are sent from the cortex to the parasympathetic cells preventing contraction of the detrusor muscle. At the same time the internal sphincter is contracted voluntarily. When this control is removed, reflex emptying of the bladder occurs. It can be assisted by increasing the intra-abdominal pressure through simultaneous contraction of the diaphragm and anterior abdominal wall.

The urethra

The urethra is a narrow canal by which the urine is conveyed from the bladder to the exterior. The female urethra is normally 4 cm in length. It runs downwards and forwards behind the symphysis pubis, very close to the lower anterior wall of the vagina, and opens in the vestibule, behind the clitoris and in front of the vaginal orifice.

At its origin from the bladder the urethra is surrounded by thickening of the circular smooth muscle fibres of the bladder. The fibres are arranged circularly round the beginning of the urethra at the bladder neck and form the internal sphincter.

The external sphincter is composed of bands of striated muscle which surrounds the urethra just before it pierces the perineal muscles.

STRUCTURE

The wall of the urethra is thick and composed of four layers.

1 The lumen is lined with stratified squamous epithelium, except close to the bladder, where it is lined with transitional epithelium. The epithelium is thrown into small longitudinal folds.

2 Vascular connective tissue.

3 Longitudinal smooth muscle which is continuous with the longitudinal fibres of the bladder.

4 Circular smooth muscle fibres.

Several minute diverticuli or crypts open into the urethra. They run longitudinally in the wall for a short distance and communicate with the lumen of the urethra at the lowest points. The two largest, Skene's tubules, open on to the surface lateral to the urethral orifice in the vestibule.

BLOOD SUPPLY

The urethra is supplied with blood from the internal vesical and pudendal arteries and venous drainage is into corresponding veins.

LYMPHATIC DRAINAGE

The lymph drains into the internal iliac glands.

NERVE SUPPLY

The internal sphincter is supplied by sympathetic nerves and is not under voluntary control. The external sphincter is supplied by a branch of the pudendal nerve and is under voluntary control.

The effects of pregnancy

The renal blood flow increases during pregnancy from 800 to 1250 ml and the glomerular filtration from 100 to 150 ml. The kidneys may be unable to reabsorb the normal amount of glucose which passes through the glomeruli and renal glycosuria occurs.

The ureters become elongated, dilated and kinked during pregnancy. This may result in slow emptying of the ureter and renal pelvis.

Pressure of the anteverted gravid uterus causes indentation of the bladder in early pregnancy which together with polyuria causes frequency of micturition. This may also occur in late pregnancy when the fetal head enters the pelvis.

Effects of labour

The bladder becomes displaced into the lower abdomen as the fetal head descends into the pelvis. The urethra becomes elongated and the urethrovesical angle altered due to pressure of the fetal head. This may result in an inability to pass urine.

Effects of the puerperium

The increase in blood volume which occurred during pregnancy is reduced by an increase in the volume of urine produced. The ureters regain tone and return to their normal length and width. The bladder returns to being a pelvic organ.

Chapter 4
Management of Labour

Management should be taught and learnt in the clinical areas and not in the classroom or from a textbook. Therefore, in this chapter the intention is to give only an outline of the management of labour and where applicable explain the reason for a particular aspect of care to assist the student in gaining more from her clinical experience.

Management is very closely linked with physiology, and to a lesser extent with anatomy, therefore it is important for the student to have a knowledge of these subjects and to relate them to the care of the woman in labour so that she may acquire expertise from her clinical experience.

Labour may take place in hospital or in the woman's own home, but basically the management is the same. When labour commences, the woman booked for a hospital confinement is admitted to the labour ward, if booked for a home confinement she notifies the community midwife, who in turn informs the general practitioner.

Management of the first stage of labour

Admission

The reception of a woman in labour is very important and cannot be overemphasised. she must be received in a friendly and reassuring manner so as to alleviate apprehension and give her confidence in the staff who are to look after her.

The woman may have expressed a preference as to how her labour or some aspects of it should be managed, and a midwifery care plan may have been made out. This should be discussed with the woman to ascertain her current needs and where these do not conflict with a safe standard of care, her wishes should be met. It is important to leave options open and not adhere too inflexibly to the plan. For example, the woman may have stated a preference not to be given pethidine, but as labour progresses, if the midwife assesses that analgesia is necessary, the situation should be reviewed without pressure on the woman to change her mind.

Once labour has started she should not be left alone and her husband, or if he is not available some other suitable companion, should be encouraged to stay with her.

All procedures should be carefully explained and the woman's cooperation obtained. If she knows that an explanation will be given she will be more relaxed, whereas if procedures are not explained she may become apprehensive and tense, not knowing what is going to happen next. Privacy should be ensured at all times.

The midwife should be familiar with the method of preparation taught during the antenatal period so that she may encourage and assist the woman to carry out this teaching during labour.

History

The antenatal records should be studied and details of the woman's past obstetric and medical history known as well as details of the present pregnancy and relevant personal information. The management of this labour may need to be adapted to take an account of the information obtained. Enquiry is made regarding the onset of uterine contractions, whether the membranes have ruptured and if a 'show' has been noted.

Observations and recordings

The maternal and fetal conditions are observed closely during labour to detect any deviation from normal. Accurate recordings are made of all observations and any deviation from normal is reported to the doctor.

In most units, partograms are used to record maternal and fetal observations and provide a comprehensive form of record keeping that enables normal progress or any deviation from normal to be seen at a glance.

MATERNAL OBSERVATIONS

Temperature and pulse. The temperature and pulse rate are recorded on admission and thereafter the temperature is recorded at four-hourly intervals and the pulse rate at half-hourly intervals. These observations are important indicators of the woman's general condition.

Blood pressure. The blood pressure is recorded on admission and compared with the recordings made during the antenatal period. The blood pressure is then recorded at hourly intervals.

Oedema and varicosities. The legs and vulval area are inspected for varicosities and the fingers, ankles and legs for oedema.

Psychological state. The mental attitude with which a woman approaches labour has an effect on her tolerance to the discomfort and pain she experiences, and it is now also accepted that a woman's pain threshold is significantly lowered by loneliness and lack of emotional support in labour. Therefore, on admission and throughout labour the woman's mental state is observed.

FETAL OBSERVATIONS

Abdominal examination. An abdominal examination is performed on admission to establish the size of the uterus in relation to the period of gestation. There may be a discrepancy if the membranes have ruptured. The lie, presentation and position of the fetus is noted and the attitude and level of the fetal head. The fetal heart is auscultated and the rate, volume and rhythm is noted. If the membranes have ruptured the amniotic fluid is inspected for the presence of meconium. The fetal heart is monitored continuously or at fifteen-minute intervals throughout the first stage of labour.

CARE OF THE BLADDER

Because of the close proximity of the bladder to the birth canal it is an essential part of the management of labour to ensure that the bladder does not become overdistended. A full bladder may impede the descent of the fetal head or become bruised and oedematous due to the pressure of the head. An overdistended atonic bladder will reflexly reduce the strength, length and frequency of the uterine contractions and delay the progress of labour. The woman is encouraged to empty her bladder every two hours.

URINALYSIS

A specimen of urine is obtained on admission and tested for reaction, protein, ketones and glucose. Every specimen of urine is tested and the result recorded in the case record.

CARE OF THE BOWEL

The woman should be asked when she last had her bowels open and if she has any preference regarding an enema/suppositories. Some women prefer to be given an enema/suppositories even though it is not considered necessary, fearing that they may have their bowels open during the second stage of labour.

VULVAL AND PERINEAL SHAVE

It is no longer a routine to shave the vulval and perineal area, and this is another aspect of care where the woman's preference can be met. Some women may prefer to be shaved and might feel embarrassed if this is not done, but others may prefer not to be shaved.

GENERAL HYGIENE

If the membranes are intact, the woman may find a bath pleasant and relaxing. When the membranes have ruptured a shower is recommended.

Assessment of progress

ABDOMINAL EXAMINATION

Uterine contractions. The length, strength and frequency of the uterine contractions are recorded on admission and compared with the information given by the woman regarding the onset of labour. The uterine contractions become longer, stronger and more frequent as labour progresses and, therefore, they must be observed frequently to determine whether or not labour is progressing satisfactorily.

Descent of the presentation. There is progressive descent of the fetal head throughout normal labour, therefore, it is an important observation to make in assessing whether or not labour is progressing normally.

VAGINAL EXAMINATION

A vaginal examination may be performed on admission and form a baseline for subsequent examinations. The history of the labour is considered in determining whether or not adequate progress has been made.

Indications for repeating the vaginal examination during labour are:

1 When the membranes rupture to exclude prolapse of the umbilical cord if on previous examinations the presentation was not well applied to the cervix.

2 Prior to the administration of analgesia in an attempt to avoid giving drugs which have a depressant effect on the fetal respiratory centre if the second stage of labour is imminent.

Technique of vaginal examination

Prior to performing a vaginal examination it should be ensured that the bladder is empty. The examination is preceded by abdominal palpation in order that the student should gain maximum information from the procedure.

Preparation. This is an aseptic technique and therefore the hands are washed and sterile gloves worn. The use of gowns, hats and masks will vary from one unit to another.

The vulval area is swabbed using an antiseptic solution such as Savlon 1 in 100, and swabbing from front to back and from outwards in, using each swab once only. The hand to be used for the examination (usually the right) is kept clean by transferring the swabs to the other hand. The examining fingers (index and middle finger) are lubricated with an obstetric cream such as chlorhexidine 1 in 2000.

External genitalia. The external genitalia are inspected for anatomical normality, and the presence of excoriation which may indicate an infective vaginal discharge. The perineum is observed for scar tissue indicating a previous episiotomy or laceration. This tissue will not stretch as readily as undamaged tissue and therefore it may suggest the need for an episiotomy to be performed during the delivery of the baby.

Vagina. When the fingers are inserted into the vagina the tone and the elasticity is noted. If the vagina feels tight this may indicate the need for an episiotomy to prevent lacerations during delivery. Any discharge is noted because, if due to an infection, there is a risk to the fetus during delivery.

Cervix. The degree of effacement of the cervix is noted. This may have been completed before the onset of labour in which case no cervix will be felt to project into the vagina. If effacement is not complete the degree of effacement is noted, i.e. the percentage of cervix felt and the consistency.

Os uteri. During normal labour there is progressive dilatation of the os uteri. This may be slow during the latent phase of labour when progress may be determined by effacement of the cervix, but occurs more rapidly during the acceleration phase (Fig. 4.1). The dilatation of the os uteri is estimated in centimetres and the length of time taken to reach full dilatation, i.e. 10 cm, will depend on whether the woman is a primigravida or a multigravida (see p. 75).

Membranes. If the membranes are intact they may be well applied to the fetal head and difficult to feel or they may be bulging and become tense during a contraction. If the membranes are ruptured the colour of the amniotic fluid is noted for the presence of meconium (see p. 328).

Presentation. The head will be felt as a firm, smooth, rounded presentation. As the os uteri dilates and the landmarks may be more easily felt, the presentation can be confirmed and the position and attitude of the fetal head and therefore the presenting diameter, determined. The station of the fetal head in relation to the ischial spines is noted (Fig. 4.2).

Descent of the presentation is an important sign of progress in labour particularly in the latent phase when the dilatation of the os uteri is not well marked. The application of the fetal head to the cervix is noted, if well applied the danger of cord prolapse is removed and there is good stimulus to uterine contractions.

Position. It is necessary to identify the sutures and fontanelles to determine the position of the fetus. The sagittal suture is usually most easily felt and is related to a diameter of the pelvis, i.e. sagittal suture felt in the right oblique diameter of the pelvis. The line of the sagittal suture is followed and the fontanelle identified, i.e. if three sutures are felt then the posterior fontanelle is identified, if four sutures, the anterior fontanelle. The fontanelle can be related to a quadrant of the pelvis or the anterior, posterior or lateral aspects (Fig. 4.3).

Attitude of the fetal head. By identifying the fontanelles, the attitude of the fetal head and therefore its presenting diameter can be determined, i.e. if the posterior fontanelle can be felt, but not the anterior, the head is flexed and the suboccipitobregmatic diameter, 9.5 cm, is presenting. If both fontanelles

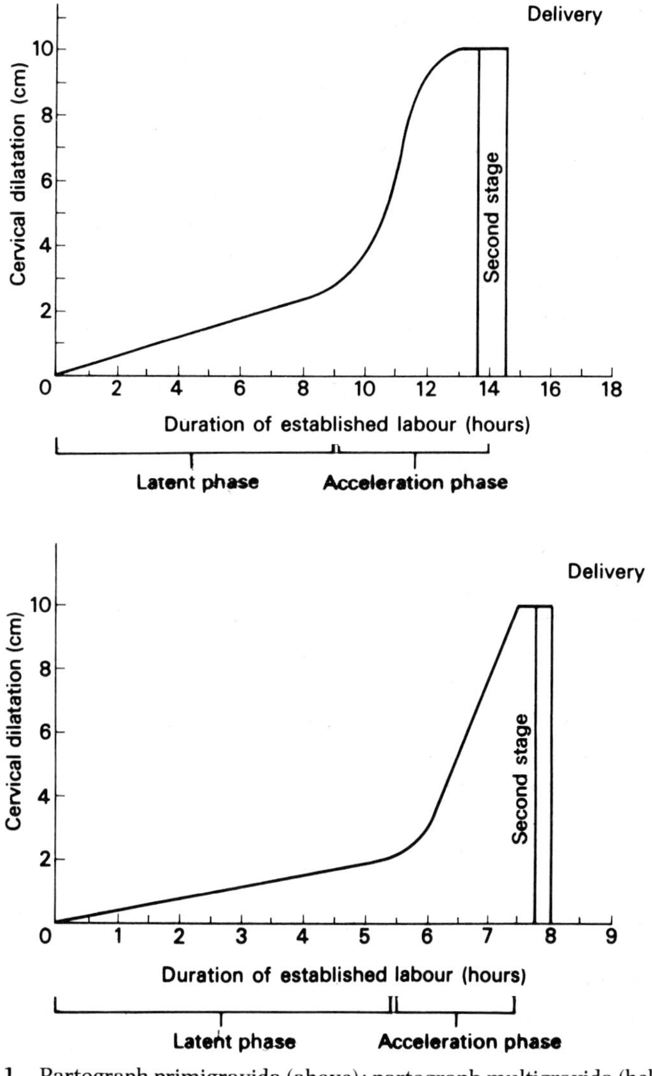

Fig. 4.1 Partograph primigravida (above); partograph multigravida (below).

are palpable, the head is partially deflexed and the suboccipitofrontal diameter, 10 cm, is presenting. If the anterior fontanelle is palpable the head is deflexed and the occipitofrontal diameter, 11.5 cm, is presenting.

The pelvis. Before completing the examination, the pelvis should be assessed. The curve of the sacrum is noted, the ischial spines are palpated and the interspinous diameter assessed. Before withdrawing the examining fingers the angle of the pubic arch is estimated. The knuckles are placed between the ischial tuberosities to assess the intertuberous diameter. Following the

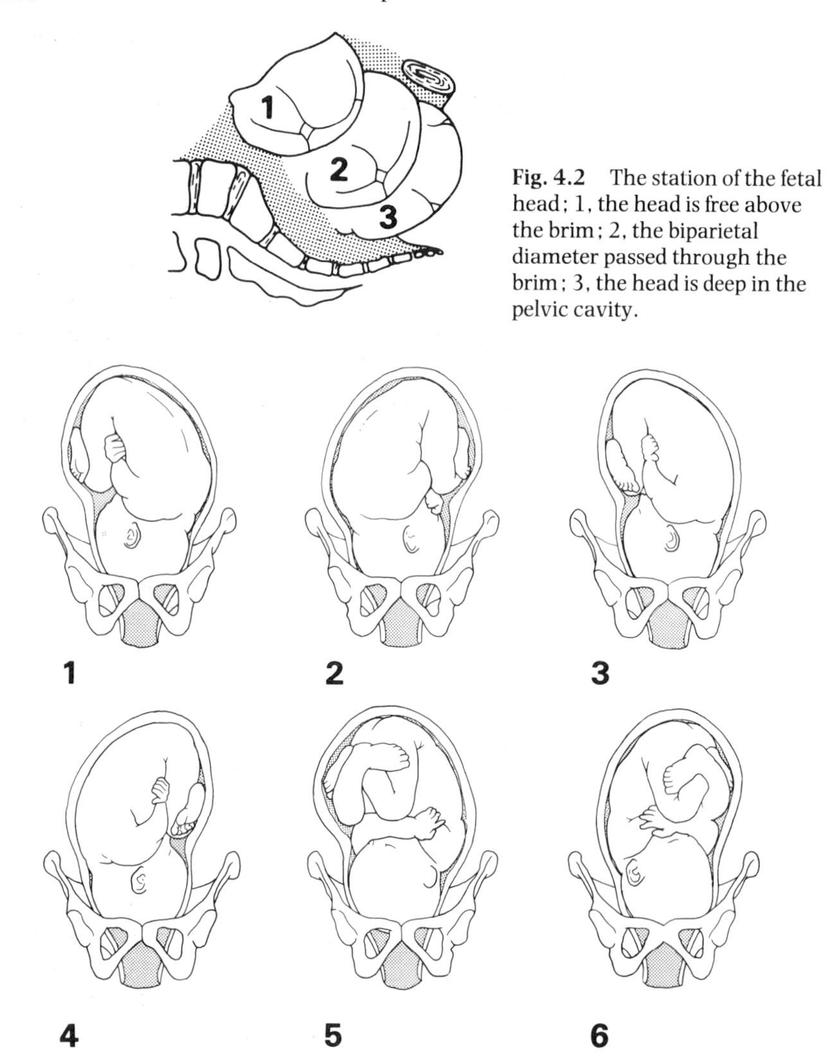

Fig. 4.2 The station of the fetal head; 1, the head is free above the brim; 2, the biparietal diameter passed through the brim; 3, the head is deep in the pelvic cavity.

Fig. 4.3 Positions of the vertex; 1, left occipitoanterior; 2, right occipitoanterior; 3, left occipitolateral; 4, right occipitolateral; 5, left occipitoposterior; 6, right occipitoposterior.

examination the woman is made comfortable and the findings discussed with her.

The midwife records the findings of the abdominal and vaginal examinations in the case records and correlates these findings with the uterine contractions in order to determine that good progress is being made.

Example:

1 Abdominal examination.

The size of the uterus is compatible with the period of gestation. Lie:

longitudinal. Presentation: cephalic, engaged. Position: left occipitoanterior. Attitude: flexed. Fetal heart 140.

2 Uterine contractions, one in three minutes lasting forty-five seconds and strong.

3 Vaginal examination.

External genitalia and vagina normal. Cervix: effaced. Os uteri: 5 cm dilated, well applied to presentation. Membranes: ruptured, clear amniotic fluid draining. Landmarks: sagittal suture felt in the right oblique diameter; posterior fontanelle in left anterior quadrant (Fig. 4.4). Conclusion: presentation, vertex at level of ischial spines; position, left occipitoanterior; attitude, flexion. Pelvis: sacrum well curved; ischial spines not prominent; angle of pubic arch 90°; intertuberous diameter four knuckles.

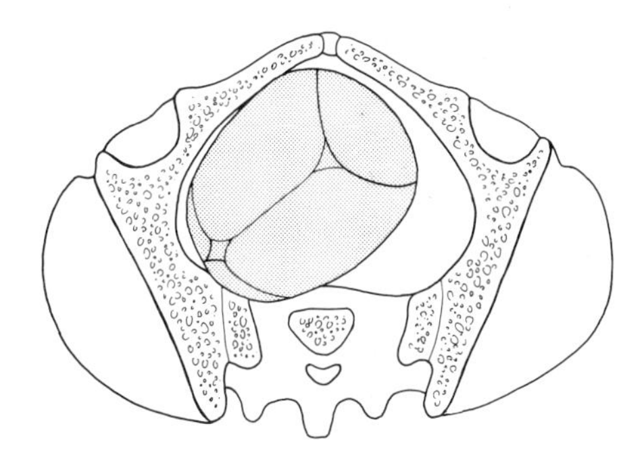

Fig. 4.4 Position of landmarks viewed from below.

Diet

The emptying time of the stomach is increased in labour and this may result in vomiting if food is taken or drugs such as pethidine are used. Therefore, there is a tendency to omit food once labour has started and allow only small quantities of water. If a general anaesthetic is required the risk of vomiting is particularly hazardous due to the danger of inhalation of vomit (see p. 292).

To counteract the acidity of the gastric contents a mixture of magnesium trisilicate (15 ml) is given at two-hourly intervals during labour. This is a precaution against acid aspiration leading to Mendelson's syndrome (see p. 292).

Position

The woman may find she is more comfortable sitting in a chair or walking about in the early stage of labour. When labour is more advanced she may be more comfortable in bed, and the position used must take into account her comfort and also fetal wellbeing. For instance, if the woman lies on her back, the uterus may compress the inferior vena cava. This may be overt when supine hypotension results or occult where there is a reduced blood flow to the uterus causing fetal hypoxia. Cord compression may occur when the woman lies on her side, if the cord lies beside the fetal head.

Drugs

Drugs used in the first stage of labour take the form of hypnotics, analgesics and tranquillisers as there may be need to induce sleep, relieve pain and allay apprehension. Drugs used must not only be safe for the woman but also for the fetus.

HYPNOTICS

In early labour the use of an hypnotic helps to ensure that the woman is well rested. Sedatives such as barbiturates are avoided because of their depressant effect on the fetal respiratory centre and because they potentiate the awareness of pain.

Hypnotics of choice include dichloralphenazone (Welldorm) 650–1300 mg, glutethimide (Doriden) 250–500 mg, nitrazepam (Mogadon) 5–10 mg, triclofos (Tricloryl) 500–1000 mg.

ANALGESICS

Pain relief should be discussed with the woman and given before she becomes distressed. The mental attitude with which a woman approaches labour has an effect on her tolerance of the discomfort she experiences and therefore the amount of analgesia she requires. The physical and emotional support she receives from a companion and the midwife looking after her will also influence the need for pain relief.

Some women express a preference not to be given analgesic drugs and may be able to cope without them, but if some pain relief becomes necessary they may find an inhalational analgesia more acceptable.

The drug used most frequently to relieve pain in labour is pethidine. It is a controlled drug and is therefore subject to controls relating to the Misuse of Drugs Act 1971. Pethidine, which was introduced in 1939, and approved by the Central Midwives Board (CMB) in 1950, is an analgesic with sedative and antispasmodic properties.

Side-effects include depression of the maternal and fetal respiratory centres which reaches a peak one hour after administration and is effective for two to three hours. It delays gastric emptying which predisposes to nausea and vomiting, and lowers the blood pressure. Pethidine interacts with some drugs and should not be administered in association with the monoamine oxidase inhibitors.

In labour pethidine may be given as an intramuscular injection by the midwife or as an intravenous injection or infusion.

The dose of pethidine ranges from 50 to 200 mg and is dependent on the size of the woman, the stage of labour and the degree of pain.

The antidote used for pethidine is naloxone hydrochloride (Narcan), a narcotic antagonist. This can be administered to the woman at the onset of the second stage of labour if pethidine has been recently given. There is also a neonatal preparation which can be given to the baby if signs of respiratory depression due to pethidine are evident at birth (see p. 345).

Pethilorphan 2 ml containing pethidine 100 mg and levallorphan 1.25 mg (a narcotic antagonist) may be used in place of pethidine, but it is less effective in relieving pain than the equivalent amount of pethidine on its own.

Inhalational analgesia. This type of analgesia can be very effective if used correctly and its successful administration depends upon attention to detail.

There are two agents approved by the ENB, these are Entonox (nitrous oxide and oxygen), and methoxyflurane (Penthrane) and air.

1 Nitrous oxide (50%) and oxygen (50%) is administered via the Entonox apparatus. It has a rapid action and is non-accumulative and must therefore be given in anticipation of the contraction. It has no depressant effect on the fetal respiratory centre. The cylinder contains premixed gases which may separate if stored at temperatures of less than 10 °C. This form of nitrous oxide was introduced in 1962 and approved by the CMB in 1970.

2 Methoxyflurane (0.35%) in air is administered via the Cardiff Inhaler. This was introduced in 1959 and approved by the CMB in 1970. It is accumulative and long-acting and causes a minimal degree of depression of the fetal respiratory centre. This apparatus requires annual inspection and certification.

The midwife must ensure that there is a valid certificate signed by a registered medical practitioner stating that the woman is fit to receive inhalational analgesia. Rules guiding and governing the midwife in her practice are included in the *Handbook of Midwives Rules* which will be discussed in Section V (see p. 495).

Regional Analgesia

The use of epidural and caudal analgesia in labour is on the increase and the midwife is involved in assisting the anaesthetist in the setting up of these methods and undertaking the 'topping-up' procedure in the maintenance of the epidural block. The CMB issued a statement in 1971 stating that the Board would raise no objection to an experienced midwife undertaking the 'topping-up' procedure in the maintenance of an epidural block provided certain safeguards are observed; this continues to apply under the rules of the United Kingdom Central Council (see Section V).

Epidural analgesia. This is the introduction of a local anaesthesia into the epidural space via the lumbar spine. Sensory nerve fibres from the uterus enter the spinal cord at the level of the eleventh and twelfth thoracic segments and from the cervix, bladder, urethra, vagina and perineal and pelvic floor muscles at the level of the second, third and fourth sacral segments.

Caudal analgesia. This is the introduction of local anaesthesia into the subdural space approached from below through the sacral hiatus (Fig. 4.5).

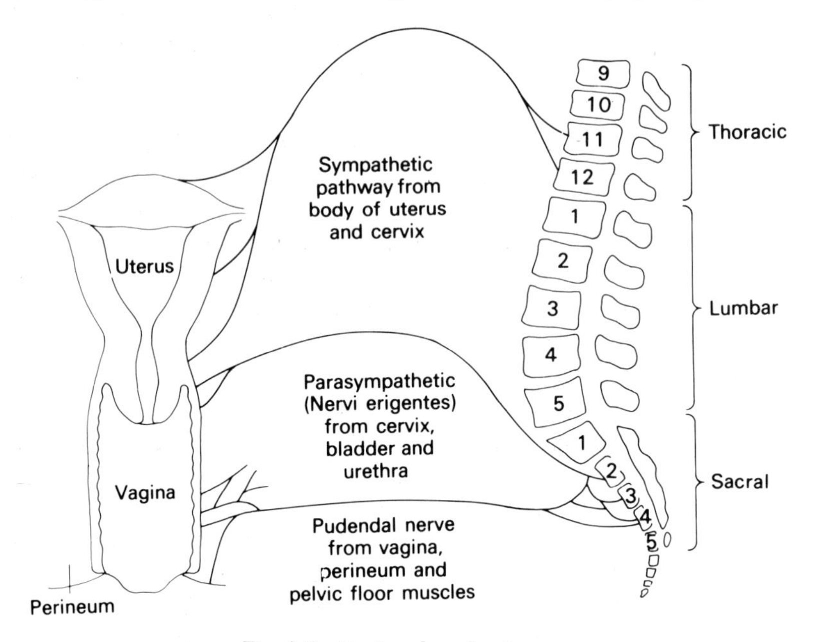

Fig. 4.5 Regional analgesia.

The technique must be carried out under strict asepsis and with the woman either sitting or in the left lateral position with the spine well flexed.

Equipment: Tuohy needle 16 gauge; Portex epidural cannular; Braunular spigot.

Drugs: Bupivocaine (Marcain) 0.375–0.25%; lignocaine (1–2%) with adrenaline 1 in 200 000.

Indications: painless childbirth without narcosis; prolonged labour; malposition of the vertex; malpresentation; abnormal uterine action; hypertension —it lowers the blood pressure; diabetes mellitus, cardiac disease.

Contraindications: diseases of the spinal cord; abnormalities of the spine; shock; skin infection of area of entry; blood dyscrasias.

Complications: hypotension; infection; headaches; retention of urine; fetal bradycardia.

Observations following procedure and after administration of first dose and 'top-up' doses are as follows:

1 Take and record blood pressure.
2 Tilt woman 5° head up with knees flexed for five minutes.

3 Take and record blood pressure every five minutes for fifteen minutes, every ten minutes for twenty minutes and then every thirty minutes until next dose.

TRANQUILLISERS

These may be used in association with pethidine and one such drug, promazine (Sparine) was approved by the CMB in 1973 as being a suitable drug to be used by midwives and may be supplied to them for use in their practice.

Promazine is a phenothiazine derivative which acts mainly on the central and peripheral autonomic nervous system. It relieves tension and anxiety without undue drowsiness and respiratory depression. It also has antiemetic properties which makes it an ideal drug to use with pethidine.

Because of its action on the peripheral autonomic system, it blocks the normal response to blood loss and severe hypotension may follow even a small haemorrhage. Fetal and maternal tachycardia may also occur in association with the use of promazine.

The dose of promazine is 25–50 mg and its duration of action is three to four hours. As this is longer than pethidine it may not be necessary to repeat the promazine as frequently as the pethidine.

Section C of the Rules of the United Kingdom Central Council includes restriction on the use of drugs by the midwife, and the Notices concerning a Midwives Code of Practice includes guidance about the drugs that may be carried and used by midwives working in the community, the use and destruction of controlled drugs and the supply of prescription only drugs to community midwives (see pp. 496, 499).

Midwives working in hospital are also restricted by the relevant Rules and Notices, but are required to either have all drugs prescribed, or a written authorisation from a doctor to use certain drugs. In addition, the employing authority will have policies regarding drugs that must be known to the midwife.

Management of the second stage of labour

As the first stage of labour nears its end, it is advisable to transfer the woman to a delivery room to avoid moving her in the second stage of labour when she is wanting to push. Many units now have dual purpose rooms which avoids the need to move the woman for delivery. The time of the onset of the second stage is noted and the length of the first stage recorded.

The onset of the second stage of labour may be confirmed by vaginal examination or noted by external signs, i.e. the woman has an uncontrollable urge to push, the perineum is bulging, the anus dilated and the fetal head may be visible at the vulva.

POSITION

The woman will find it easier to push if she is well supported by pillows in an upright position. The woman may prefer an alternative position such as squatting or kneeling, or a Birthing Chair may be used.

INSTRUCTIONS

The amount of instruction and help needed during the second stage of labour varies considerably. If the woman has attended classes and is well supported by her husband, little more than encouragement is required. But if she has either received no preparation or is not managing, then the midwife has an important part to play in ensuring that this stage of labour is not prolonged due to poor maternal effort. Instructions should be given clearly and quietly, usually between contractions, when the woman is better able to concentrate. It is important to ensure that the woman is holding her breath and maintaining a long steady push. Two or three sustained efforts are more effective than five or six short jerky ones. This can be obtained by utilising the height of the contraction rather than its beginning or ending when the power is minimal, pushing achieves little and is not conserving the woman's energy. The woman must be given time to respond to instructions and should not be expected to react immediately, i.e. when she is required to stop pushing and to pant, she should be warned that this stage is imminent and told what is required of her in advance.

The delivery should be conducted in a quiet, calm atmosphere, with only one person at a time giving advice to the woman.

OBSERVATIONS AND RECORDINGS

Maternal. The woman's general condition is noted and the pulse and blood pressure recorded at fifteen-minute intervals. The effort of pushing may cause the pulse rate and blood pressure to rise slightly.

Fetal. The fetal heart is auscultated following each contraction and the amniotic fluid observed for meconium. Placental circulation stops when the uterine pressure is 100–120 mmHg, therefore the fetus tends to become hypoxic during the second stage of labour. This is the time of maximum risk to the fetus and therefore close observation is required.

Assessment of progress. This is determined by noting the advancement of the fetal head. There should be progressive descent which will occur more rapidly in the multigravida.

GENERAL CARE

The woman will appreciate sips of iced water and her face sponged with cold water between contractions.

ANALGESIA

If an analgesic is required during this stage of labour the use of inhalational analgesia is ideal. The woman may find it helpful to use the apparatus before and as the contraction is increasing in intensity, and then discard it when she is ready to push.

Preparation for delivery

Time should be allowed for the midwife to prepare herself, the equipment and the woman for delivery. If this is hurried the preparations are going to be inadequate and the woman made anxious. If a sterile pack is used the outer cover is opened prior to the midwife preparing herself, and the inside cover opened and the contents set out ready for use once the midwife has put on sterile gloves.

Caps and masks, if used, will already be worn and following washing and drying her hands on a sterile towel, the midwife will put on a sterile gown and gloves.

The vulval and perineal areas are prepared using the same technique used prior to performing a vaginal examination (see p. 147) and the woman and bed draped with sterile towels.

Conduct of the delivery

The delivery may be conducted with the woman in the dorsal or left lateral position, if the latter, an assistant is required to support the right leg. Alternatively, the kneeling or squatting position may be adopted.

The delivery of the head is controlled by pressure on the posterior aspect of the parietal bones to maintain flexion. As soon as the biparietal diameter is distending the vulva the head is crowned, i.e. the occiput has escaped under the pubic arch and the woman, who has been encouraged to push during the contractions, is now asked to pant, and the head is born slowly by extension. As soon as the head is born, the baby's eyes are wiped clear of debris with sterile swabs, one for each eye, and swabbed from within out. Supporting the head, the midwife feels for the umbilical cord round the baby's neck. If the cord is felt and it is loose, it is looped over the baby's head. If it is tight, then it is clamped in two places and cut.

Following restitution and external rotation, the anterior shoulder is delivered by applying traction in a downward direction on the baby's head. As the anterior shoulder is released, an intramuscular injection of Syntometrine (1 ml) is given. The posterior shoulder and trunk are delivered by taking the baby up over the mother's abdomen in a movement of lateral flexion and following the curve of the birth canal. The traction being applied on the baby's head can be relieved as soon as the shoulders are born. Still supporting the head, a finger is placed under each axilla. This must not be done until the shoulders are completely free of the birth canal otherwise lacerations may occur due to increase of the bisacromial diameter.

The time of the delivery is noted and the length of the second stage of labour is recorded.

If not already done, the cord is clamped and cut. A mucus extractor may be used to clear the baby's nasopharynx and he is dried and warmly wrapped, before being placed in the mother's arms.

Episiotomy

During the second stage of labour it may become apparent that an episiotomy is necessary to avoid delay in the delivery of the fetal head, or to prevent overstretching or laceration of the perineal and pelvic floor muscles.

The term episiotomy was first introduced by Carl Braun in 1857, and refers to a surgical incision of the perineum to increase the size of the vulval outlet.

In 1967, the CMB stated that 'unless medical aid is immediately available the operation should be performed by the midwife after infiltration of the perineum with a local anaesthetic when time permits.'

INDICATIONS FOR EPISIOTOMY

1 Delay in delivery of the fetal head due to a rigid perineum.
2 To prevent overstretching and laceration of the perineum.
3 Prior to delivery in the presence of a malposition or malpresentation when a larger fetal diameter is presenting.
4 Prior to delivery of a premature infant to reduce the risk of intracranial damage.
5 Prior to a forceps delivery.

TYPES OF INCISION

Mediolateral episiotomy. The incision begins in the midline and extends backwards to a point midway between the anus and the ischial tuberosity. This method, which avoids damage to the anal sphincter and the Bartholin's glands is recommended for use by the midwife.

Median episiotomy. The incision divides the perineum in the midline. It is not recommended because of the risk of any further tear involving the anal sphincter.

J-shaped episiotomy. A curved incision that starts in the midline and curves to avoid the anus.

The three incisions are demonstrated in Fig. 4.6.

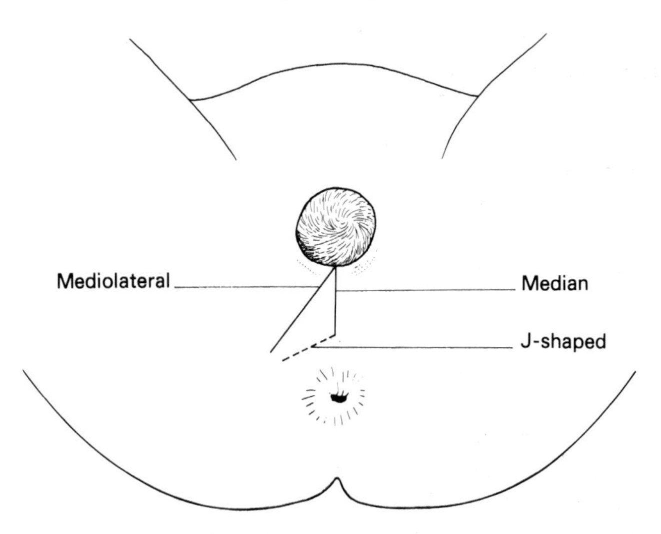

Fig. 4.6 Episiotomy.

TECHNIQUE OF PERINEAL INFILTRATION

Lignocaine (0.5%) is used to anaesthetise the perineal area, 10 ml containing 50 mg of the active agent is used. Lignocaine hydrochloride is a stable solution which is effectively absorbed and has a rapid action. It is diffused into the tissues, so only a small amount needs to be used, and it gives pain relief for thirty to forty minutes and is then rapidly diminished. Lignocaine is less effective following episiotomy, as it is rapidly absorbed due to increased vascularity. The middle and index fingers are inserted into the vagina to protect the fetal head. The needle is inserted into the midpoint of the fourchette and approximately 1 ml of lignocaine is injected under the skin. The needle is advanced slowly and the remaining lignocaine is injected along the line of the proposed incision.

TECHNIQUE OF EPISIOTOMY

The incision is made using blunt-ended episiotomy scissors. One blade is inserted into the vagina and passed flat along the fingers. The scissors are then turned so that the sharp edges are against the tissues, and a single cut is made. This should be performed as the contraction is beginning to avoid sudden delivery of the head as the pressure is released.

The length of the incision is approximately 4 cm, but varies according to the indication. It should be long enough to overcome the problem, otherwise extension tearing will occur.

The episiotomy incision should be repaired as soon as possible after delivery and before the effects of the lignocaine wear off.

Management of the third stage of labour

This is the stage of labour when the mother is most at risk and great vigilance is therefore required. The mother remains or is placed in the dorsal position with the knees flexed and the hips slightly extended. A receiver is placed close to the vulva, the cord is straightened, and the clamped end is placed in the receiver.

A sterile towel is draped over the abdomen and the midwife places her left hand on the fundus of the uterus to await a contraction.

Drugs

The drugs used to manage the third stage of labour are administered during the delivery of the baby.

Syntometrine. First introduced in 1961, it contains ergometrine (0.5 mg) and 5 units of an oxytocin in 1 ml and is the drug used most frequently. Ergometrine is an alkaloid of ergot and was first used in obstetrics in 1932 by Professor Chassar Moir. It produces a continuous uterine contraction of about two hours' duration. Oxytocin causes intermittent uterine contractions.

Syntometrine is given as an intramuscular injection with the birth of the anterior shoulder. The oxytocin component will cause a strong uterine contraction within two to three minutes of its administration. The delivery of the placenta and membranes may be timed to coincide with this first contraction. The ergometrine component acts within five to seven minutes and, therefore, the placenta and membranes should be delivered before it takes effect otherwise there is the risk of the placenta being retained.

Syntometrine shortens the length of the third stage of labour, reduces the average blood loss and the risk of postpartum haemorrhage.

An intramuscular injection of ergometrine (0.5 mg) may be used instead of Syntometrine and is given at crowning of the head.

Methods of delivery of the placenta and membranes

Controlled cord traction is used to actively manage the third stage of labour. The delivery is timed to coincide with the first contraction. The left hand is then placed on the abdomen just above the symphysis pubis. The thumb and index finger are separated, and the hand placed over the anterior aspect of the uterus at the junction of the upper and lower uterine segments with the palm towards the mother. This hand is used to control the uterus and to push it upwards towards the umbilicus. At the same time the right hand will be used to exert gentle traction on the cord first in a downwards and then, when the placenta appears at the vulva, in an upwards direction following the curve of the birth canal. As the placenta is delivering, the left hand is removed from the abdomen, and both hands used to receive the placenta. It is delivered slowly to allow the membranes to separate without tearing.

The other methods of managing the third stage of labour which are rarely used include maternal effort and fundal pressure. They necessitate awaiting the signs of placental separation and descent which considerably lengthens the third stage of labour.

SIGNS OF PLACENTAL SEPARATION AND DESCENT

Sign of separation. There is a show of blood.

Signs of descent. The uterus becomes small, hard and rounded; the uterus rises on the abdominal cavity and becomes ballottable; the umbilical cord lengthens.

MATERNAL EFFORT

It is not essential to give an oxytocic drug before using this method. The signs of placental separation and descent are noted and the mother is asked to push with the contraction. As she no longer has the urge to push, and her abdominal wall muscles are now rather lax, the mother may find it difficult to expel the placenta. This method is only used if the cord has become detached from the placenta and controlled cord traction can no longer be used.

FUNDAL PRESSURE

An oxytocic drug is administered and the signs of placental separation and descent are noted. When the uterus is contracting, the fundus is used as a piston to expel the separated placenta. This method causes considerable discomfort to the mother and the downward pressure places strain on the ligaments supporting the uterus and for these reasons it is not recommended.

The time the placenta and membranes are delivered is noted and the length of the third stage of labour determined.

Immediate postnatal care

The midwife ensures that the uterus is well contracted and the blood loss is not excessive. The perineum, vulva and vagina are inspected for lacerations or extension of episiotomy wound. The vulva and perineum are gently cleansed using an antiseptic solution, dried and covered with a sterile pad. The soiled linen is removed and the mother is made comfortable.

The temperature, pulse and blood pressure are recorded. A slight rise in these vital signs may be noted as a result of the effort used during the second stage of labour.

If an episiotomy has been performed or a laceration sustained the doctor is notified so that it can be repaired as soon as possible.

A blanket bath is given and the mother dressed in a clean gown or nightdress. She is then given a cup of tea and, if she is hungry, a light meal may be provided.

The mother is encouraged to pass urine. The bladder has a tendency to fill rapidly after delivery due to release of urine trapped in the ureters as a result of pressure from the fetal head.

An important part of the midwife's role is to facilitate and help to establish a loving bond between the parents and their baby. How this is achieved will be influenced by their wishes, for example, some mothers may wish to have the baby delivered onto their abdomen and to put the baby to the breast immediately, but others may prefer the delivery to be completed and then hold and feed their baby. If the mother does not wish to breast feed she should be given the opportunity to offer the baby a bottle feed.

The parents should be given time alone with their baby to begin the process of attachment that forms the basis of a close, loving relationship. They may want to inspect the baby to make sure all the fingers and toes are complete, and generally reassure themselves that the baby is alright.

Not all mothers respond to their baby immediately, and an allowance should be made for a variety of responses and each situation handled individually. The midwife can set an example by talking to the baby and encouraging the mother to do the same, but the mother should not be forced into making a response, as this may come quite naturally later when she has recovered from labour. However, should a mother show complete lack of interest in her baby, this should be noted and reported to the postnatal ward sister so that she can observe the mother's subsequent response.

Inspection of the placenta and membranes

As soon as possible after the completion of labour the placenta and membranes are inspected for completion and normality. A careful examination will reveal any absence of placental tissue or membranes, areas of infarction and blood clot. The insertion of the cord is noted and the number of umbilical vessels. The diameter of the placenta and the length of the cord are measured and the placenta is weighed. The blood loss is measured and an estimated total loss is calculated taking into account the staining of the drapes and bed linen. The details are recorded in the case notes and any abnormality reported to the doctor.

Full details of the labour are recorded in the case notes and a Birth Notification is completed and sent to the District Medical Officer within thirty-six hours of delivery, and the Birth Register is also completed.

Approximately one hour after delivery the mother and baby are transferred to the postnatal ward.

Immediate care of baby (see p. 334).

Chapter 5
Management of the Puerperium

The puerperium is the period immediately following labour during which the involution of the uterus and other organs takes place and lactation is established. This usually lasts for six weeks but may be longer.

The postnatal period is the early part of the puerperium and is defined as a period of not less than ten days nor more than twenty-eight days after the end of labour during which the continued attendance of the midwife is requisite.

The puerperium is a time of physiological and psychological adjustment for the mother and the care given during this period is aimed at helping her to cope with these changes. The midwife's role during the lying-in period is very important and has many aspects. She gives nursing care, makes observations of the mother's condition and keeps records of these observations. She teaches the mother to care for the baby and herself, supervises the mother to ensure she is maintaining a good standard of care, and gives advice on a wide range of subjects including family planning. Therefore, the role of the midwife is one of nurse, observer, teacher, supervisor and adviser.

The woman delivered in hospital may return home within a few days of delivery to the care of the community midwife and general practitioner, or remain in hospital for a full-stay when her care is undertaken by the hospital midwives and doctors.

The mother is admitted to the ward, with her baby, about one hour following delivery. On admission to the ward the midwife will ensure the uterus is well contracted and the lochia is not excessive. If the mother was unable to pass urine following delivery, a bedpan is offered.

Observations and recordings

TEMPERATURE AND PULSE

The temperature and pulse are taken twice daily for the first few days following delivery and then daily until discharge. Any rise in temperature or pulse rate should be reported. These observations should not be taken while the mother is breast feeding as an increase occurs at that time.

BLOOD PRESSURE

The blood pressure is recorded on admission to the ward and prior to discharge.

MICTURITION

The mother should be encouraged to pass urine as soon as possible following delivery. The urinary output may be recorded for twenty-four hours following delivery to ensure an adequate amount of urine is being passed. The abdomen should be palpated to ensure the bladder is being emptied and is not palpable above the symphysis pubis. A diuresis will occur within a few days of delivery and the woman will pass urine more frequently.

BOWELS

Due to lack of dietary intake during labour and the administration of an enema or suppositories, the mother may not have a bowel movement for a day or two following delivery. A mild aperient such as Senokot may be given on the evening of the second day following delivery and suppositories such as Beogex on the third day if there has been no bowel action.

STATE OF THE UTERUS

The tone and position of the uterus is noted; it should be well-contracted and in a central position. The rate of involution of the uterus can be estimated by measuring the height of the fundus above the symphysis pubis (see p. 79).

LOCHIA

The colour, amount, odour and constituents of the lochia are observed and is a useful indication that involution is or is not progressing normally (see p. 79).

PERINEUM

The perineum is inspected daily and any bruising, oedema or discomfort is noted. If a perineal wound is present the cleanliness and healing is noted.

LEGS

The legs are examined daily to exclude oedema and tenderness. Leg movements are encouraged as part of postnatal exercises and early ambulation is practised to improve the circulation and to reduce the risk of phlebothrombosis with the complication of pulmonary embolism.

HAEMOGLOBIN

A specimen of blood is obtained for haemoglobin estimation. If taken within the first five days following delivery the level may be lower than if taken later. This is due to the fact that the physiological readjustments in the blood following pregnancy have not taken place and the effect of the reduction in the plasma and the number of red blood cells is not evident. The mother is encouraged to continue to take iron tablets until six weeks following delivery.

MENTAL STATE

Due to the changes taking place in the puerperium a period of mental instability may become apparent. This may take the form of the mother being depressed and tearful about four to five days after the birth of her baby. This lasts for only a short period and is not a cause for concern.

Because of the danger of more serious forms of depression the mother is closely observed for early signs of onset (see p. 302). Therefore, her general behaviour, sleeping and eating habits are noted.

General care

CARE OF THE VULVAL AND PERINEAL AREAS

The vulval and perineal areas must be kept clean to prevent the risk of ascending infection to the vulnerable uterus and to aid healing of the perineal wound.

If the mother is confined to bed, vulval toilet must be performed, if she is up and about she is advised to change her pads frequently and to use the bidet following each visit to the toilet.

Baths may be encouraged to aid cleanliness and healing of a perineal wound. If non-absorbable sutures have been used for the repair these are removed on the fifth day.

POSTNATAL EXERCISES

These exercises are designed to improve the circulation and the tone of the pelvic floor and abdominal wall muscles. Leg exercises are encouraged on the first day when the mother spends the majority of time in bed, but on the following days when she is mobile more active exercises are introduced.

Postnatal exercises should be effective but easy to do and not too numerous as they are then more likely to be continued when the mother is no longer being supervised. She should be encouraged to continue these exercises until the postnatal examination.

SLEEP AND REST

During the early postnatal period the mother is encouraged to rest for a period each day. A sedative or hypnotic may be required to ensure an undisturbed night's sleep especially immediately following delivery when although tired, the mother is often too excited to sleep. Subsequently the nights may be disturbed by the need to feed the baby and therefore a rest during the day helps to prevent overtiredness.

DIET

Dietary advice as given during the prenatal period is reiterated. This is especially important if the mother is breast feeding. Also the fat deposited in the subcutaneous tissues during pregnancy needs to be shed. If breast feeding, this will happen gradually over a period of time; however if the mother elects to bottle feed she may need to take more active measures.

BREAST CARE

Whether or not the mother wishes to breast feed her baby, the breasts need to be well supported. If breast feeding, the support should be firm but not too tight otherwise the alveoli may become damaged.

If the baby has been put to the breast in the labour ward, it may be several hours before it is ready to suckle again; if not, the mother may like to put the baby to the breast following admission to the postnatal ward.

The midwife should discuss with the mother her preference regarding demand or timed feeding, night feeds and the care of her breasts. Demand feeding is putting the baby to the breast when it demands to be fed and letting it suckle as long as it wishes. Timed feeding involves feeding the baby at approximately four-hourly intervals and restricting the time at each breast to three minutes on the first day and then gradually increasing the time each day until the baby suckles for ten minutes at each breast from the fourth day. Some mothers need the reassurance of this method and their wishes should be respected, but they should also be advised that babies are individuals and some may require less time and others more time to satisfy their needs, and that this may vary from one feed to the next.

The mother is given help and advice to fix the baby at the breast to ensure that not only the nipple but the surrounding areola is included. This is important to prevent soreness of the nipples and because the ampullae, where the milk is being stored, lies under the areola. A hungry, active baby with a well developed rooting reflex will need little or no assistance to fix at the breast and, therefore, demand feeding can lead to fewer frustrations than attempting to fix a sleepy baby at the breast because it is four hours since the last feed, or a baby who has tired itself by crying because it awoke before the feed was due.

The mother should be encouraged to be flexible in relation to feed times without allowing it to totally disrupt the life of the family.

Before feeding, the mother should remove any traces of cream from the nipple area and following feeding ensure the area is well dried. The washing of the breasts before and after feeding is encouraged by some midwives and discouraged by others. If the mother's general hygiene is good it should not be necessary and may in fact lead to soreness by removing the natural skin oils. The midwife should inspect the nipple area before and after the feed to ensure that there is no soreness.

INHIBITION OF LACTATION

If the mother elects not to breast feed her baby then lactation must be inhibited, if breast feeding has been discontinued it must be suppressed.

There are three ways in which milk production can be inhibited or suppressed.

1 The natural method avoids the use of drugs. The mother is encouraged to wear a firm brassiere or binder and to avoid stimulating the breasts in any way. Milk production ceases because, due to lack of stimulus, prolactin is not produced. The breasts become engorged with blood and the pressure causes compression of the alveoli and the acini cells. Because of engorgement, the breasts are painful and a mild analgesic may be required for a few days. The method is very effective and avoids the use of oestrogens which increase the risk of embolism particularly in the high risks groups, i.e. over twenty-five years of age, obesity and following operative delivery especially if a general anaesthetic was administered.

2 Drugs containing oestrogens may be used to suppress the effect of prolactin. These include:

a An intramuscular injection of hexoestrol dipropionate 15 mg given as soon as possible following delivery and may be repeated twice at eight-hourly intervals.

b Stilboestrol 5–10 mg orally three times a day for five days or longer if necessary.

c Quinestrol (Estrovis) 4 mg given orally within six hours of delivery to inhibit lactation and to suppress lactation 4 mg is given and repeated forty-eight hours later.

3 Bromocriptine is an alkaloid of ergot and a dopamine receptor antagonist which acts on the prolactin secreting cells in the anterior lobe of the pituitary gland. The dosage is 2.5 mg twice daily.

Bottle feeding (see p. 340).

Education, supervision and advice

It is an important part of the midwife's role to teach the mother to care for her baby and herself and to supervise the care and give advice.

Teaching regarding personal care includes breast care, postnatal exercises and care of the vulval and perineal areas.

The mother is taught how to change the baby's nappy, to carry out daily toilet including care of the cord, how to bath the baby and how to make up artificial feeds and sterilise feeding utensils.

The mother should be encouraged to respond to her own instincts in caring for her baby and to treat it as an individual. She should be guided by, but not adhere too rigidly to baby care practices.

EARLY TRANSFER/DISCHARGE

If arrangements have been made for an early transfer the mother and baby may leave hospital on or after the third day, and the care is continued by the community midwife and general practitioner. The midwife will make daily visits at least until the tenth day, and then visits on approximately the tenth, fourteenth and twenty-eighth day when the health visitor takes over, although an initial visit by the health visitor may have been made on the eleventh day.

Advice regarding family planning is given and the mother referred to her general practitioner, the local family planning clinic or the clinic run in association with the postnatal clinic (see p. 416).

When the health visitor calls to see the mother she will give her information regarding the nearest child heath centre and assist with any problems that have arisen since discharge.

POSTNATAL EXAMINATION

The mother is encouraged to attend a postnatal examination approximately six weeks after the birth of the baby. At this time the process of involution should be completed. The blood pressure is recorded, the urine tested, the haemoglobin is estimated and the mother is weighed.

The breasts are examined to ensure there are no masses. If the mother is breast feeding the breasts should feel soft, although full of milk. if the mother is not breast feeding there usually should no longer be any secretions and the breasts will be soft.

The abdomen is examined to ensure the uterus is not palpable and to assess the tone of the abdominal wall muscles.

The perineum is inspected with particular regard to the satisfactory healing of an episiotomy or tear.

A speculum is passed the cervix visualised. This should be healthy with no erosion and the os closed. A cervical smear may also be taken at this time.

A vaginal examination is performed and the size and position of the uterus is noted and the tone of the vagina and pelvic floor is observed. The mother is questioned about recommencement of menstruation.

Contraception is discussed and if arrangements have not already been made, advice is now given (see p. 417).

If the examination reveals no abnormalities the mother is discharged.

SECTION II

ABNORMAL PREGNANCY, LABOUR AND PUERPERIUM

Chapter 6
Abnormal Pregnancy

Bleeding in early pregnancy

Vaginal bleeding in early pregnancy is a symptom which frequently leads women to seek advice, and may be due to one of the following causes: implantation bleeding; decidual bleeding; abortion; hydatidiform mole; ectopic pregnancy; cervical pathology—erosion, polyp and rarely carcinoma; vaginitis; bleeding from the non-pregnant horn of a bicornurate uterus.

Implantation bleeding

As the cells of the trophoblast digest the endometrial cells during implantation of the blastocyst they also erode through the walls of the arterioles. Bleeding occurs and occasionally blood escapes from the uterine cavity and is lost *per vaginum*. This blood loss, known as implantation bleeding, is very slight and occurs a few days before the menstrual period would be expected. It is of clinical significance because it may be confused with the last menstrual period if the woman normally has only scanty loss, and therefore a careful menstrual history must be obtained to avoid miscalculation.

Decidual bleeding

Menstruation is suppressed during pregnancy, but in a few women there is an occasional slight blood loss from the decidua during the first ten weeks of pregnancy before the conceptus is enlarged to fill the uterine cavity and the decidua capsularis becomes fused with the decidua vera.

Abortion

Abortion or miscarriage is the expulsion from the uterus of the products of conception before the fetus is viable. Abortion may be spontaneous or induced (Fig. 6.1).

Spontaneous abortion

The precise cause of spontaneous abortion is often unknown. It is estimated that about 10–15% of all pregnancies end in abortion, although the figure may be higher as it is probable that many fertilised ova are lost before pregnancy is recognised.

MATERNAL CAUSES: GENERAL

Chronic maternal disease. There is a higher incidence of abortion if the woman has diabetes mellitus or chronic nephritis.
Infections. Syphilis, although uncommon in pregnancy, may be the cause of a late abortion. Viral infections such as rubella and influenza especially when accompanied by a high temperature can also be a cause.
Hormonal deficiency. Progesterone deficiency, which can be demonstrated by ferning of cervical mucus, may be associated with abortion.
Nutritional deficiency. Severe nutritional deficiency may result in abortion.

MATERNAL CAUSES: LOCAL

Incompetent cervix. The internal os is dilated and there is funnelling of the cervical canal. The cervix fails to support the growing fetus and a late abortion, usually between sixteen to twenty weeks gestation results. This may be a congenital defect, or the result of injury to the cervix at a previous delivery or surgical dilatation.
Congenital abnormality of the uterus. A congenital abnormality, such as a septate or double uterus, may be the cause of an abortion.
Retroversion of the gravid uterus. This may be a cause of abortion, if it becomes incarcerated in the pelvis.

ABNORMALITY OF THE CONCEPTUS

Many abortions are due to faulty development of the embryo and the earlier the abortion occurs the more likely it is to be due to this cause.

Abortion is commonest in the second and third months of pregnancy and is more liable to occur at the time menstrual bleeding would have appeared had pregnancy not supervened.

The signs of impending abortion are uterine bleeding which precedes the pain; pain in the back and lower abdomen; dilatation of the cervix. These signs form the basis of clinical classification of abortion as follows and as shown in Fig. 6.1.

THREATENED ABORTION

The uterine size is usually compatible with the period of gestation. There is vaginal bleeding followed by lower abdominal pain, but no products of conception are expelled and the cervix is not dilated. Therefore, there is a chance that the pregnancy will continue.
Management. Bed rest, with or without sedation until the bleeding stops is the recommended treatment. If the threatened abortion is associated with progesterone deficiency, hydroxyprogesterone caproate (Primolut Depot)

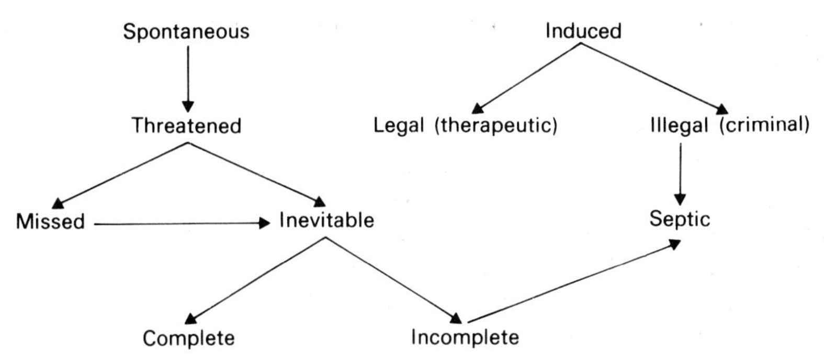

Fig. 6.1. Classification of abortion.

500 mg daily by intramuscular injection may be given until the bleeding has stopped. Maintenance treatment with 250 mg or 500 mg every three days for three doses and then weekly during the first half of pregnancy may be used.

Threatened abortion may lead to placental insufficiency and therefore the fetus should be monitored with extra care, and the pregnancy should not be allowed to become prolonged.

INEVITABLE ABORTION

If the management of the threatened abortion is unsuccessful bleeding becomes more profuse and may contain products of conception, uterine contractions occur and the cervix dilates. The abortion is then described as inevitable and may be complete or incomplete.

COMPLETE ABORTION

The products of conception are expelled intact and consequently no treatment is required.

INCOMPLETE ABORTION

If any part of the products of conception is retained in the uterus the abortion is incomplete. This is more liable to occur between the third and fifth months when the immature placenta is firmly adherent to the decidua basalis causing retention of whole or part of the placenta.

As long as products of conception are retained in the uterus the woman is liable to bleed and there is an increased risk of infection.

Management. The woman is given ergometrine (0.5 mg) or oxytocin (5–10 units) intramuscularly prior to transfer to hospital. If the haemorrhage is severe the emergency obstetric unit is called and the woman resuscitated, if necessary given a blood transfusion, before being transferred to hospital. In hospital, evacuation of retained products of conception is performed as soon as the woman's condition permits.

MISSED ABORTION (carneous mole)
Haemorrhage occurs between the decidua and the chorion causing death of the ovum. Degenerative changes occur and the moles are named according to the type of degeneration.

a Blood mole; blood clots surround the ovum.

b Carneous mole; the blood clot becomes organised and assumes a fleshy appearance.

c Stony mole or lithopaedion; calcium salts have been deposited.

The formation of the mole is marked by external bleeding, suggesting a threatened abortion. The red loss changes to brown and the woman may have a constant or intermittent brown discharge. The uterus does not enlarge, pregnancy tests become negative after two to three weeks and there is a cessation of some of the signs and symptoms of pregnancy, such as breast changes, nausea and vomiting.

If left, the uterus may retain the mole for many weeks, or even months but spontaneous abortion will eventually occur. There is little danger of serious haemorrhage or infection but the risk of defibrination syndrome must be considered.

If the mole is not expelled spontaneously within a month, medical induction is undertaken.

HABITUAL ABORTION
Some women abort repeatedly and the term habitual or recurrent abortion is used when three or more abortions have occurred consecutively.

A careful history is taken in an attempt to determine the cause. If the abortions have occurred early in the pregnancy then a chromosomal abnormality of the conceptus is suspected and may be confirmed by chromosomal studies on the aborted material. A family history may reveal a recurring abnormality and genetic studies on the parents should be undertaken.

If the abortions occurred after the sixteenth week of pregnancy incompetent cervix is suspected. There may be a history of termination of pregnancy, or trauma during a previous delivery. The diagnosis is confirmed if a Number 6 Hegar's dilator can be inserted into the cervix at midcycle.

If the history reveals that the abortions occur progressively later in the pregnancy then an abnormal uterus is suspected. It is thought that the uterine horns become larger with each pregnancy and therefore can accommodate a larger fetus.

In a subsequent pregnancy early referral is important. If vaginal cytology reveals progesterone deficiency, hydroxyprogesterone caproate may be administered (see p. 172).

If the cause is an incompetent cervix a Shirodkar suture is inserted; a purse string suture of nylon tape or braided wire is inserted around the cervical canal. If labour supervenes, the suture should be removed. The suture is removed at the onset of labour or the thirty-eighth week, whichever is sooner.

Induced abortion

LEGAL (THERAPEUTIC) ABORTION

The Abortion Act 1967, which came into effect in April 1968, stated that a termination of pregnancy could be performed with the woman's consent, if two medical practitioners are of the opinion that:

a The continuance of the pregnancy would have involved risk to the life of the pregnant woman greater than if the pregnancy were terminated.

b The continuation of the pregnancy would have involved risk of injury to the physical or mental health of the woman greater than if the pregnancy were terminated.

c The continuance of the pregnancy would have involved risk of injury to the physical or mental health of the existing child(ren) of the family of the pregnant woman greater than if the pregnancy were terminated.

d There was a substantial risk that if the child had been born it would have suffered from such physical or mental abnormalities as to be seriously handicapped.

The termination of pregnancy must be performed in an approved institution and notification sent to the Chief Medical Officer of the Department of Health and Social Security within seven days.

There is no 100% safe way of terminating pregnancy but the longer the period of gestation the higher the risk of complications. Ideally, the termination should be performed before the tenth week of pregnancy and using vacuum aspiration. Even then there is a 5% complication rate including haemorrhage, infection and trauma, i.e. cervical laceration and perforated uterus. Long-term sequelae include sterility, chronic pelvic infection and premature labour during subsequent pregnancies.

Prostaglandins E_2 and $F_{2\alpha}$ have been used for termination of mid-trimester pregnancy since 1970. One of two methods can be applied.

1 Intra-amniotic injection. Prostaglandin E_2 (10 mg) or prostaglandin $F_{2\alpha}$ (25 mg) is instilled into the uterus by the transabdominal route.

2 Extra-amniotic route. A 14 French gauge Foley catheter is inserted through the cervix so that the inflated balloon lies within the internal os. Prostaglandin is slowly instilled into the extra-amniotic space.

There was an increase in the mortality rate following legal abortion from ten in 1964–66, the last triennium before the Abortion Act was introduced, to eighteen in 1967–69, the triennium during which the Act became effective, and to thirty-seven in 1970–72, the first three year period of the Act. The subsequent decrease in the mortality rate to fourteen in 1973–75 and eight in 1976–78 indicates not only the use of safer methods of inducing abortion but also an increase in the availability of the service and in the awareness of the risk of late termination of pregnancy.

ILLEGAL (CRIMINAL) ABORTION

An abortion procured by an unauthorised person, including the woman herself, is an offence punishable by law. The risks associated with this procedure are very high and include haemorrhage, infection and trauma. These complications may result in death or morbidity such as salpingitis and sterility.

The reduction in the mortality rate following illegal abortion from ninety-eight in 1964–66, the last triennium before the Abortion Act was introduced to seventy-four in 1967–69, the triennium during which the Act became effective, and thirty-eight in 1970–72 is indicative of the effectiveness of the Act in preventing women from resorting to illegal means to obtain a termination of pregnancy. The continuing decrease to ten in 1973–75 and four in 1976–78 is probably due to the wider availability of the service.

SEPTIC ABORTION

An abortion complicated by sepsis is one of the risks associated with illegal abortion and retained products of conception as occurs in an incomplete abortion. Although deaths following illegal abortion have decreased dramatically since 1966, two of the four recorded deaths in 1976–78 were due to septicaemia. Sepsis was also the cause of death in four of the eight women who died following legal abortion.

The Report of the Confidential Enquiries into Maternal Deaths in England and Wales 1976–78 reveals the following information relevant to abortion:

Deaths from all categories of abortion were considerably reduced in 1976–78 compared with the previous triennium.

There were fourteen deaths from abortion in 1976–78 compared with twenty-nine in 1973–75.

There were four deaths from illegal abortion in 1976–78 compared with ten in 1973–75.

There were eight deaths from legal abortion in 1976–78 compared with fourteen in 1973–75. In both triennia there were six deaths in the second trimester of pregnancy.

There were two deaths from spontaneous abortion in 1976–78 compared with five in 1973–75.

Abortion is the fifth cause of maternal mortality having been the major cause in 1970–72 (eighty-one deaths) and the third cause in 1973–75 (twenty-nine deaths).

Hydatidiform (vesicular) mole

A disease of the chorion characterised by cystic degeneration of the chorionic villi and associated with a variable degree of invasion. Hydatidiform mole occurs in 1 in 2000 pregnancies. It occurs in the first twelve weeks of pregnancy and involves all the chorionic villi. The embryo dies and is absorbed. Rarely, the disease occurs after the twelfth week, when the placenta is formed. Only part of the chorion undergoes cystic degeneration and the fetus may continue to develop. The chorionic villi become distended with fluid and are converted into vesicles. The mesodermal core is oedematous and non-vascular and is covered by cytotrophoblast and syncitiotrophoblast. Due to the presence of the syncitiotrophoblast the villi are capable of invading the uterine wall causing haemorrhage and even perforation of the uterus.

CLINICAL FEATURES

The uterus is usually large for the period of gestation and it feels soft and doughy. Ballottement cannot be elicited, fetal parts and movements are not felt and the fetal heart is not heard. The woman complains of feeling unwell and may vomit excessively. Signs of pre-eclampsia may be observed at a period of pregnancy at which it would not be expected. Rapid onset of severe anaemia may occur. There is blood loss *per vaginum* which may be slight or severe and may be mixed with mucus or fluid from ruptured cysts or contain vesicles. The ovaries may be enlarged due to the presence of theca-lutein cysts.

DIAGNOSIS

Due to the proliferation of chorionic tissue, human chorionic gonadotrophin is found in excessive amounts in the urine (1500–100 000 iu/litre of urine), and remains consistently high. The diagnosis of hydatidiform mole can be confirmed by ultrasound.

MANAGEMENT

As soon as the diagnosis is confirmed, the mole is evacuated. The method is dependent on the size of the mole and the period of gestation.

If the mole is small and the pregnancy has not advanced beyond the first trimester a suction curette is used; but if the mole is large, medical induction using oxytocin or prostaglandins is preferred. Hysterotomy is rarely required.

If the woman is over forty years of age or has completed her family a hysterectomy may be indicated because of the risk of the complication of chorion epithelioma.

FOLLOW-UP CARE

The woman is kept under observation for at least a year. Curettage is usually repeated to ensure no remnants of the mole remain and human chorionic gonadotrophin assays are performed every two weeks until a negative result is obtained, and then monthly for a further year.

The woman is advised to avoid a further pregnancy for one to two years, but oral contraception should not be used until human chorionic gonadotrophin has disappeared from the urine.

Ectopic pregnancy

The fertilised ovum is arrested and develops outside the uterus. The commonest site is the outer third of the Fallopian tube, giving rise to a tubal pregnancy. Other sites include the isthmus and interstitial part of the tube, the cornua, ovary or the abdominal cavity.

The incidence of ectopic pregnancy is about 1 in 500 pregnancies.

CAUSES

The causes of ectopic pregnancy are not fully understood but the following are the predisposing causes.

Tubal pathology. As a result of infection the Fallopian tube becomes partially obstructed and the cilia destroyed.

Contraception. There appears to be an increased incidence of ectopic pregnancy in association with low dose progesterone oral contraceptives and intrauterine devices.

The outcome of an ectopic pregnancy is determined by the site of implantation of the ovum and the action of the chorionic villi. In the commonest type of ectopic pregnancy (tubal pregnancy), the fertilised ovum grows, distends and stretches the thin-walled tube; the chorionic villi penetrate the mucous membrane. While the ovum is embedding in the tube the uterus is undergoing the normal changes of early pregnancy.

Owing to the inability of the Fallopian tube to accommodate the developing ovum the pregnancy terminates in one of two ways.

1 Tubal abortion. The ovum may be expelled from the fimbriated end of the Fallopian tube into the peritoneal cavity. Usually death of the ovum has occurred due to bleeding around the ovum. Rarely a secondary abdominal pregnancy occurs when the ovum is alive at the time of expulsion.

2 Rupture of the Fallopian tube. If the attachment of the chorionic villi to the tube is firm the ovum continues to develop within the tube and when the pregnancy has advanced to the fifth to seventh week, rupture of the tube occurs.

DIAGNOSIS

Early signs and symptoms are similar to those of threatened abortion but in the case of ectopic pregnancy, pain usually presents before the bleeding. The pain may be referred to one or other iliac fossa and sometimes to the shoulder. There may be a slight 'prune juice' discharge as the decidua is shed and the woman may give a history of faintness or giddiness.

The initial symptoms may be overlooked because they are only slight. In a few cases the onset is sudden and catastrophic, there is severe lower abdominal pain due to blood in the peritoneal cavity, vaginal bleeding and shock.

MANAGEMENT

Arrangements for immediate surgery are made and this is one occasion when resuscitation should not precede but should be coincident with operation. If the diagnosis is in doubt a laparoscopy is performed to confirm the diagnosis and this is followed by laparotomy and removal of the affected tube, or in some cases, part of the tube to allow reconstruction at a later date.

SECONDARY ABDOMINAL PREGNANCY

This is a rare outcome of ectopic pregnancy and may progress undetected for some time. The fetus develops in the abdominal cavity and the chorionic villi become attached to the abdominal organs.

A laparotomy is performed prior to term and the baby removed. If there is no bleeding the placenta is left *in situ* and will eventually be absorbed. If bleeding occurs extensive surgery may be necessary to arrest haemorrhage.

There were twenty-one deaths reported as directly attributable to ectopic pregnancy in the period 1976–78 making this the fourth most important cause of maternal mortality.

Bleeding from other causes

CERVICAL PATHOLOGY

Cervical erosion and polyp are not treated until after pregnancy. With carcinoma of the cervix, the pregnancy is allowed to progress until the fetus is viable when a Caesarean section and hysterectomy is performed.

VAGINITIS (see p. 231).

BLEEDING FROM THE NON-PREGNANT HORN OF A BICORNUATE UTERUS

No treatment is required.

Antepartum haemorrhage

Haemorrhage occurring from or into the genital tract after the twenty-eighth week of pregnancy and before the birth of the baby, is known as antepartum haemorrhage. The term intrapartum haemorrhage is used if the bleeding occurs following the onset of labour.

CLASSIFICATION

The two main causes of antepartum haemorrhage are classified according to the situation of the placenta.

Placental abruption (accidental haemorrhage). Premature separation of the normally situated placenta.

Placenta praevia (*unavoidable or inevitable harmorrhage*). Separation of the abnormally situated placenta.
Extraplacental causes. Incidental haemorrhage, e.g. cervical erosion, polypi, or rarely carcinoma.
Antepartum haemorrhage of unknown origin. In a large number of cases the cause of the bleeding is not found, but the placenta is the most likely source in view of the perinatal mortality associated with this group.

Late threatened abortion is more likely to have pathology related to antepartum haemorrhage than to causes associated with bleeding in early pregnancy.

Other causes of bleeding which do not come within the definition of antepartum haemorrhage but may confuse the diagnosis and, therefore, must be excluded are haematuria, bleeding from haemorrhoids or ruptured vulval varicosities.

If the bleeding is due to separation of the placenta this is associated with disruption of the blood supply to, and therefore the function of that part of the placenta.

Placental abruption

Bleeding from the separation of a normally situated placenta may be revealed, concealed or combined (Fig. 6.2).
Revealed (when vaginal bleeding is present). The placenta separates at its edge and the blood tracks down between the membranes and the decidua vera and passes through the cervix into the vagina.
Concealed. The blood is retained behind the placenta and there is no external bleeding. The blood may infiltrate between the uterine muscle fibres and the uterine wall is infiltrated with extravasated blood and oedema fluid. This is described as a Couvelaire uterus. Shock in these cases may be severe and is the result of blood loss, sudden distension of the uterus and tissue damage.
Combined. The bleeding is initially concealed and then becomes revealed as further placental separation occurs.

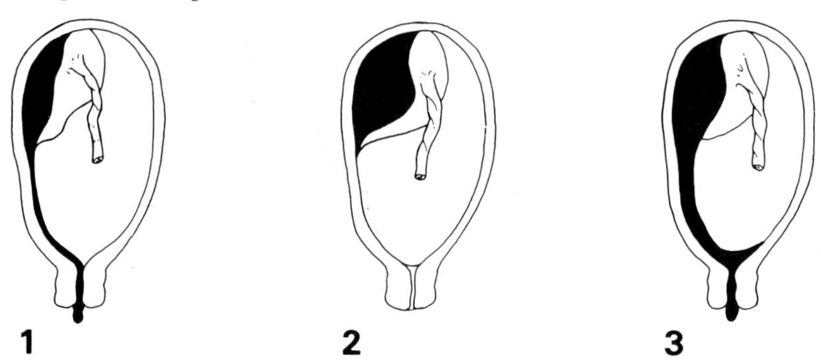

Fig. 6.2 Placental abruption; 1, revealed; 2, concealed; 3, combined.

AETIOLOGY

The cause of separation of the normally situated placenta must be some change in the uteroplacental area. It is most commonly associated with hypertension. In this condition the spasm of the spiral arteries leads to ischaemia distal to the spasm. When the spasm relaxes and the vessels again become engorged with blood, rupture occurs. Extravasation of blood occurs at the uteroplacental site with separation of the placenta from the uterine wall. It may occur following trauma, e.g. amniocentesis or by a direct blow to the abdomen, or after undue pressure on the uterus during external cephalic version, or it may occur when the tension in the uterus is suddenly decreased, as after rupture of the membranes in polyhydramnios.

Placenta praevia

Bleeding from the placenta that is situated partially or wholly in the lower uterine segment is unavoidable or inevitable because it occurs due to partial separation of the placenta following the inevitable stretching of this part of the uterus during pregnancy. Placenta praevia may be of a minor or major degree according to the relation of the placenta to the internal os. Four degrees of placenta praevia are described (Fig. 6.3).

First degree. The lower margin of the placenta dips into the lower uterine segment but the major portion of the placenta is situated in the upper uterine segment.

Second degree. The edge of the placenta reaches the margin of the internal os but does not cover it.

Third degree. The placenta covers the internal os when it is closed.

Fourth degree. The centre of the placenta lies over the internal os (central placental praevia).

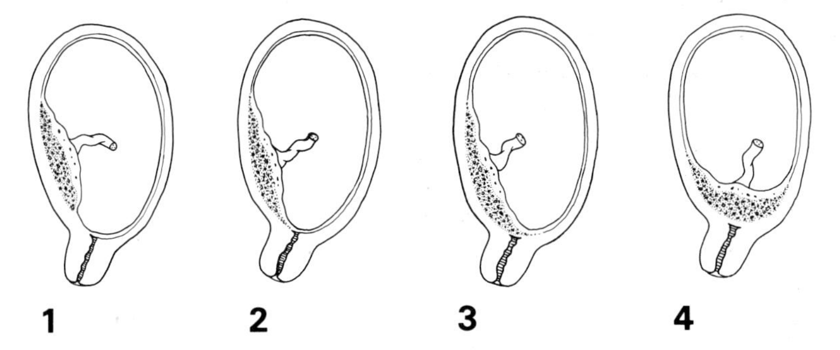

Fig. 6.3 Placenta praevia; 1, first degree; 2, second degree; 3, third degree; 4, fourth degree.

AETIOLOGY

The cause of placenta praevia is not known but it occurs more commonly in multigravidae than in primigravidae. The risk to the fetus is not as great as in placental abruption, although the risks to the mother are comparable.

Signs, symptoms and differential diagnosis

As the woman will present with antepartum haemorrhage as opposed to placenta praevia or placental abruption, it seems logical to consider the signs and symptoms as they present and to suggest how a differential diagnosis may be made.

BLEEDING

Placenta praevia. The bleeding presents without warning sometimes when the woman is asleep. It is painless, without obvious cause and may be recurrent. This is because the lower uterine segment gradually increases in size, with the result that the inelastic placenta separates and bleeding takes place. The bleeding may stop spontaneously, but as the lower uterine segment continues to stretch more of the placenta separates and bleeding recurs. The initial bleeding is usually slight and is referred to as a warning bleed, but subsequent severe haemorrhage may occur. The main source of the bleeding is the maternal blood sinuses at the placental site and therefore if intermittent or continuous slight losses of blood occur, the woman may become anaemic.
Placental abruption. The vaginal bleeding is usually of sudden onset and may be associated with some factor such as hypertension. It is accompanied by pain. In some cases the pain may be very severe and there may be no vaginal bleeding but shock is present and may be profound. All gradations of severity occur and depend mainly on the amount of blood concealed in the uterus. Combined bleeding is suspected if the degree of shock is out of proportion to the amount of external bleeding.

Abdominal examination

Placenta praevia. The more advanced the pregnancy when the bleeding occurs the more significant are the clinical signs on abdominal examination. For example, a placenta praevia, with perhaps the exception of the first degree, will prevent the head from engaging in the pelvis and, if the uterus is roomy as may be the case in multigravidae, a malpresentation or a transverse lie may occur. These findings are of little significance before the thirty-sixth week of pregnancy but may be of considerable clinical significance after that time. The index of suspicion is increased if the size of the uterus corresponds to the period of gestation, the uterus is not tender and its contents are easily palpable and the fetal heart is heard.

Placental abruption. The findings on abdominal examination vary considerably and depend on the amount of blood concealed in the uterus. The size of the uterus may correspond with the period of gestation or may be increased due to accumulation of blood in the uterus. The uterus may be tender and tense over a localised area or woody hard and painful. The fetal parts may not be palpable but if they are, the lie and presentation are usually normal. The fetal heart may be easily heard and of normal rate, there may be signs of fetal distress or in severe cases the fetal heart may not be heard.

Other causes of abdominal pain which present in pregnancy and may confuse the diagnosis are red degeneration of fibroids, twisted ovarian cyst or haematoma of the rectus sheath.

Management

If the woman is at home when the bleeding occurs she is visited by the general practitioner or community midwife before being transferred to hospital by ambulance if the blood loss is only slight and her condition is satisfactory. But if the blood loss is heavy or her condition is poor, the Emergency Obstetric Unit is summoned and the woman resuscitated, if necessary, before transfer to hospital.

On admission to hospital the woman's condition is assessed, the temperature, pulse and blood pressure are recorded. The pulse is the most valuable guide to the general condition as the blood pressure may be raised in association with pre-eclampsia, or may be maintained due to peripheral circulatory failure.

Treatment is first directed to improvement of the general condition. Opiates are contraindicated as they make diagnosis more difficult. They may, however, be needed where there is very severe pain, as in a concealed haemorrhage, when morphine (15 mg) may be given. Blood is taken for haemoglobin estimation, grouping (if this is not known), and cross-matching, fibrinogen estimations, and clotting time. The Kleihauer test is also performed to determine whether or not there has been a feto-maternal haemorrhage. If the test is positive it confirms placental separation and identifies cases where there has been disruption of placental function. A careful history is taken as to the onset of the bleeding and a gentle abdominal examination is performed. These, together with the assessment of the general condition, may give an indication of the cause of the bleeding. In addition the Doptone may be used to identify the placental souffle in an attempt to localise the placenta.

A vaginal examination must not be performed but a speculum examination may be carried out to exclude bleeding due to incidental causes.

Treatment is initiated according to the severity of the condition, the maternal condition, the fetal condition and the period of gestation.

Conservative management

If the haemorrhage is slight in degree, the maternal and fetal conditions are satisfactory and the period of gestation is less than thirty-eight completed weeks, conservative management is instituted.

The woman remains in bed until two days after the bleeding has ceased and hypertension, if present, is treated. The maternal and fetal conditions are monitored by recording the maternal pulse rate and blood pressure and the fetal heart.

PLACENTAL FUNCTION

Because placental separation leads to disruption of placental function and puts the fetus in jeopardy, tests, such as estimation of total oestrogens, are performed to assess the placental function and fetal wellbeing (see p. 322–4).

PLACENTAL LOCALISATION

Localisation of the placenta is carried out to exclude or confirm placenta praevia and if present, the degree. Various methods have been used to localise the placenta but the two most commonly used methods are:

1 Ultrasonic scan, a two-dimensional B-scan apparatus, is used and localises the placenta with 95% accuracy. This technique can be used for the purpose of placental localisation from the twenty-sixth week onwards. This method has the advantage over other methods in that it not only demonstrates whether the placenta is in the upper or lower uterine segment but on which wall and to which side. There is no radiation hazard and no special preparation is required.

2 Radioactive isotopes, using technetium or indium and a scintillation counter may be used to identify a pool of maternal blood from which to infer the placental site.

Conservative management is continued until the end of the thirty-eighth week of pregnancy. There are two reasons for the choice of this period of gestation. Firstly, the woman may go into labour at any time and, if there is a major degree of placenta praevia, uncontrollable bleeding may put the woman and fetus at risk. Secondly, the risks to fetus increase as term approachs. Maturity studies are undertaken to ensure fetal maturity before pregnancy is terminated.

A vaginal examination is performed in an operating theatre prepared for a Caesarean section. If previous investigations have suggested the placenta is not praevia, an anaesthetic may not be given prior to the examination but an anaesthetist is present. If a degree of placenta praevia has been demonstrated the examination is performed under anaesthesia so that an immediate Caesarean section can be performed if the examination confirms the diagnosis.

In the case of a first degree anterior placenta praevia it may not be necessary for a Caesarean section to be performed unless bleeding occurs. When the placenta is on the anterior wall there will be no pressure from the fetal head during labour as it will be directed in a backwards direction.

If the examination excludes a placenta praevia, the membranes are ruptured to induce labour.

Active management

If labour has commenced, or if the bleeding is severe and/or cannot be controlled, so that either the maternal or the fetal condition is deteriorating, active management is indicated. Firstly, the woman is resuscitated using plasma, O Rhesus negative blood or Reomacrodex (a plasma expander), until blood of her own group is available.

If as may be the case in a concealed or combined placental abruption, there is a clotting defect this is corrected (see p. 186).

As soon as the woman's condition permits the pregnancy is terminated by induction of labour or Caesarean section.

A Caesarean section is only undertaken if the fetal heart rate is satisfactory and the woman is not in labour as there is then a good chance of saving the baby. But if fetal death has occurred, or if labour has commenced, the woman is examined under an anaesthetic, in an operating theatre prepared to undertake an immediate Caesarean section should the findings indicate it.

If placenta praevia is excluded the membranes are ruptured and an intravenous infusion of Syntocinon is commenced.

MATERNAL CARE DURING LABOUR

In addition to the routine care given during labour the following observations are important.

Urinary output. The risk of anuria due to acute tubular necrosis is high in the presence of a severe concealed placental abruption. Vasospasm of the renal vessels occurs resulting in renal shut-down. It is therefore of vital importance to observe the urinary output in the woman and to maintain a strict fluid balance chart. A self-retaining catheter is placed *in situ* and is released hourly. Oliguria is present if less than 30 ml of urine is produced every hour. Fluid intake is then restricted and intravenous frusemide (20 mg) is given. If this condition does not resolve spontaneously with an improvement in the woman's general condition, she should be transferred to a renal unit where peritoneal dialysis can be undertaken if required.

Pulse and blood pressure. Recording of the pulse and blood pressure are made quarter-hourly to observe the general condition.

Central venous pressure monitoring is recommended to avoid the dangers associated with over or undertransfusion, i.e. hypervolaemia or hypovolaemia.

FETAL CARE DURING LABOUR

The risk of fetal hypoxia is high and therefore, where available, a monitor should be used to monitor the fetus continuously for signs of distress, which may necessitate a Caesarean section being performed.

The second stage is usually shortened by elective forceps delivery to avoid unnecessary prolongation of labour.

Postpartum haemorrhage is a not uncommon complication of antepartum haemorrhage and must therefore be anticipated (see p. 274).

MATERNAL DANGERS/COMPLICATIONS

Antepartum haemorrhage is a serious complication of pregnancy which may, if severe, endanger the woman's life.

Blood coagulation defects. In obstetrics this is usually concerned with fibrinogen depletion which may occur in one of three ways. Firstly, excessive utilisation of fibrin in the site of haemorrhage, i.e. retroplacental clot due to placental abruption. Secondly, intravascular microcoagulation due to an imbalance of the clotting factors caused by the release of thromboplastins as the result of tissue damage. Thirdly, fibrinolysis may occur, fibrinolysins are formed and destroy the fibrin.

Hypofibrinogenaemia. If the level of blood fibrinogen is below 150 mg/decilitre the blood does not clot. This condition may be suspected if the blood does not appear to clot and can be confirmed by the Fibrindex test. In this test citrated plasma from the woman, matched against control plasma, is mixed with human thrombin and the time taken for clot formation is noted. In a normal case fibrin formation is visible in 5–12 seconds. A severe defect is present if no fibrin is formed in thirty seconds. If a severe coagulation defect is demonstrated fibrinogen should be given intravenously in a dose of 4–6 g. If this is not available double or triple strength plasma should be given. Each reconstituted unit of plasma contains approximately 1 g of fibrinogen, so 2 units of double or triple strength will give 4–6 g of fibrinogen respectively. There is an increased risk of hepatitis if double or triple strength plasma is used due to pooling of blood from many donors.

If in the Fibrindex test the clot forms but later dissolves or the bleeding is not controlled by administration of fibrinogen, fibrinolysis is suspected. In this case epsilon amino caproic acid (EACA) an antifibrinolysin may be used. An initial dose of 4–6 g is given intravenously and a maintenance dose of 1 g is repeated hourly as the drug is rapidly excreted. Fibrinolysins destroy fibrin and epsilon amino caproic acid is given to prevent this from occurring.

In rare cases where the haemorrhagic state is due to excessive utilisation of fibrin as a result of intravascular microcoagulation the administration of heparin in doses of 5000 iu six-hourly for four or five days acts by liberating the trapped fibrin.

Acute renal failure. This condition is most likely to occur as the result of severe concealed placental abruption. There are three degrees of renal ischaemic disease.

1 Acute circulatory renal insufficiency caused by severe haemorrhage with inadequate replacement. Oliguria occurs as the result of deficient blood supply to the kidney and recovery is immediate and complete if the underlying condition is adequately and promptly treated.

2 Acute tubular necrosis is a more severe form of renal failure in which the tubules are damaged. Recovery will be complete provided the electrolyte balance has been maintained.

3 Renal cortical necrosis is the most severe degree of ischaemic renal damage involving not only the tubules but also the glomeruli. Although recovery may, with good management occur, it is never complete, so that there is permanent renal damage.

Sheehan's syndrome (anterior pituitary necrosis). On rare occasions some women who survive a severe and prolonged shock due to abruptio placentae later demonstrate the signs of anterior pituitary necrosis, namely failure to lactate, amenorrhaea, genital atrophy and premature sterility.

Postpartum haemorrhage. Primary postpartum haemorrhage may occur due to a blood coagulation defect following severe concealed placental abruption, or in the case of placenta praevia where the placental site is in the lower uterine segment where retractile power is poor.

Puerperal sepsis. Following blood loss, especially where massive transfusion of donor blood has been required, the woman's resistance to infection is reduced and puerperal sepsis may occur.

Chronic anaemia. A chronic iron deficiency anaemia may remain as a permanent sequel to severe haemorrhage unless steps are taken to correct it.

Haemorrhage (antepartum and postpartum) is the second most common cause of maternal death. There were eight deaths directly due to antepartum haemorrhage in the three years 1976–78, two from placenta praevia and six from placental abruption. The total of six deaths from placental abruption has remained unchanged since 1970–72 when there was a considerable reduction from twenty-seven in 1964–66 to sixteen in 1967–69. Deaths from placenta praevia have shown a gradual decline in the same period from sixteen in 1964–66 to nine in 1967–69, six in 1970–72 and two in 1973–75.

FETAL DANGERS/COMPLICATIONS

All types of antepartum haemorrhage jeopardise the fetus. Although the mortality rate in association with placenta praevia is low, in association with abruptio placenta or bleeding of unknown origin it remains high.

Causes of fetal death

a Intrauterine hypoxia due to placental separation, hypotension as the result of haemorrhage or shock or reduced maternal placental circulation as a result of hypertension. Fetal death is said to occur if more than one-fifth of the placenta is non-functioning.

b Birth injury. Malpresentation, particularly in the case of the premature infant increases the risk of intracranial haemorrhage.

c Immaturity as the result of premature onset of labour which may be spontaneous or induced.

Extraplacental causes

These causes and their management have already been considered in association with bleeding in early pregnancy (see p. 171).

Hyperemesis gravidarum

Excessive vomiting in pregnancy is termed hyperemesis gravidarum.

Many pregnant women complain of nausea and vomiting during the first three months of pregnancy. Normally it is only slight and does not cause any ill effect. Rarely is the vomiting so pronounced that it becomes pathological. But when it is, it is then termed hyperemesis gravidarum. Severe vomiting, whatever its cause, prevents the intake of food and depletes the body of water (dehydration) and salts (electrolytes). As a result a vicious circle is set up. The glycogen reserve of the liver becomes exhausted, in consequence fat is utilised as a source of energy and ketone bodies are produced faster than they can be removed and the condition of ketosis results. Dehydration and loss of electrolytes (mainly sodium chloride) occur.

AETIOLOGY

The cause of hyperemesis is unknown but it occurs more commonly in first than in subsequent pregnancies.

CLINICAL SIGNS

These women usually give a history of morning sickness which has gradually become more frequent and severe. The insidious change from the mild to severe state has constantly to be watched for.

Weight loss. The woman soon begins to lose weight due to dehydration.

Appearance. The loss of fluid will give an appearance of emaciation with sunken eyes and hollow cheeks, the tongue becomes dry and furred.

Vital signs. The pulse rate may be raised to 100 beats/min and there may be a fall in the blood pressure. In the later stages the temperature, which previously may have been subnormal, starts to rise.

Urine. The urine becomes concentrated and may contain albumin in addition to acetone and bile, with chlorides greatly diminished or absent.
Jaundice. In severe cases the woman may become jaundiced. In the later stages the woman becomes apathetic and drowsy or confused and euphoric. Squint, diplopia and nystagmus may be observed and retinal haemorrhages occur. Neurological changes such as peripheral neuritis may occur and the woman passes into coma and death.

MANAGEMENT

If vomiting becomes persistent or severe the woman should be admitted without delay to hospital. In early cases, dietetic measures will often be effective, small carbohydrate meals being taken frequently. Constipation should be corrected.

The fluid intake and urinary output is measured and recorded. The temperature, pulse and blood pressure are recorded twice daily or four-hourly.

An antihistamine preparation such as Ancoloxin which also contains pyridoxine (vitamin B_6) may be prescribed.

If vomiting does not immediately cease, all oral feeding is stopped, the loss of fluid and chlorides are replaced and the ketosis combated by an intravenous infusion of 4.3 % glucose in 0.81 % saline 3 litres being administered in twenty-four hours. Intravenous therapy is regulated according to the twice daily studies of blood chemistry. Adequate sedation is obtained by the administration of a barbiturate, for example Sodium Gardenal or promazine (Sparine) 50 mg by injection.

Oral hygiene is an important aspect of nursing care. Only when ketosis and dehydration have been overcome and the woman has stopped vomiting, are fluids given by mouth in small frequent quantities. If tolerated, solids are gradually introduced.

Injections (100 mg) of vitamin B_1 (aneurine) and B_6 (pyridoxine hydrochloride) may be given daily.

Termination of pregnancy is rarely undertaken nowadays but may be indicated if the following signs present: jaundice; persistent albuminuria; polyneuritis and neurological signs; temperature consistently above 40 °C and a pulse rate remaining above 100/min.

There was one death associated with excessive vomiting in pregnancy reported in the years 1976–78. The woman who started vomiting at the twenty-eighth week of pregnancy, inhaled vomit and died of pneumonia.

Vomiting may occur during pregnancy as the result of intercurrent illness such as pyelonephritis or gastrointestinal disorders. Careful examination will establish the diagnosis of associated disease. It is also essential to exclude other conditions such as hydatidiform mole and cerebral tumour. There were ten deaths due to cerebral tumours during the years 1970–72.

Hypertension in pregnancy

Raised arterial blood pressure is a sign common to several diseases. The systolic pressure alone, or both the systolic and diastolic pressures may be raised.

CHANGES IN THE BLOOD PRESSURE DURING PREGNANCY

Both the systolic and diastolic pressures fall to their lowest between the sixteenth and the twenty-fourth weeks of pregnancy. The fall in the diastolic blood pressure is greater than the fall in the systolic pressure but both values tend to return to normal at term. It is important, therefore, to relate the blood pressure reading to the period of gestation.

After the thirtieth week of pregnancy approximately 10 % of all normal pregnant women can develop a profound fall in blood pressure if allowed to remain supine for more than a few minutes. This is due to a lowered venous return when the uterus compresses the inferior vena cava.

HYPERTENSION DURING PREGNANCY

Hypertension with or without oedema and proteinuria is a common clinical finding in pregnancy particularly in the last trimester and is present when the blood pressure rises to 140/90 mmHg or above on two or more occasions twenty-four hours apart. This level can only be meaningful if allowance is made for the period of gestation, the woman's normal blood pressure and her posture while the blood pressure is being recorded.

The levels 139/89 mmHg have been chosen as the upper limit of normal because a rise in perinatal mortality is seen even if higher levels are found only on a single occasion.

Hypertension is classified as primary (or essential) and secondary. The term secondary is used when the hypertension occurs as a manifestation of a known disease, e.g. chronic renal disease. The term essential is given when no obvious disease can be found. Investigations suggest it may be genetic in origin and therefore it is important to enquire into the woman's family history.

Hypertension during pregnancy also confusingly described as secondary, may be due to:

1 Pre-eclampsia and eclampsia.
2 Hypertension with no associated generalised oedema or proteinuria.
3 Essential hypertension.
4 Chronic renal disease.
5 Other rare medical conditions may occur in pregnancy, i.e. coarctation of the aorta or phaeochromocytoma.

Although, with the exception of pre-eclampsia and eclampsia which are specific diseases of pregnancy, the causes are essentially medical disorders associated with pregnancy, they are discussed in this chapter because there is often difficulty in differentiating between them and making a definitive diagnosis in clinical practice because the cause of the hypertension is often obscure.

The outcome of the pregnancy in relation to both mother and baby is related to the height of the blood pressure. Morbidity and mortality rates, mainly in relation to the fetus, are increased in the presence of hypertension. There has been a gradual decline in the maternal mortality rate from hypertensive diseases of pregnancy (see p. 198).

Pre-eclampsia

A specific disease of pregnancy occurring after the twentieth week of gestation (but very occasionally earlier in connection with hydatidiform mole) and characterised by two of the following three signs.

Oedema. Slight peripheral oedema due to fluid retention is not uncommon in pregnancy. However, if there is generalised oedema it is often an indication that the woman is developing pre-eclampsia. Occult oedema may manifest as excessive weight gain, i.e. more than 1 kg in one week in the second half of pregnancy.

Hypertension. A rise of blood pressure above 139/89 mmHg on two or more occasions twenty-four hours apart.

Proteinuria. This is a late and serious sign of the disease and is due to the presence of plasma globulins as well as albumin in the urine. Other causes of proteinuria, i.e. urinary tract infection and contamination by vaginal discharge, must be excluded by obtaining a midstream specimen of urine for culture.

AETIOLOGY

The cause of pre-eclampsia is unknown but many theories have been advanced and include:

Homeostatic disturbances. These occur due to increased plasma volume, total exchangeable sodium, extracellular volume, and cardiac output and may cause a rise in the blood pressure.

Coagulation factors. An alteration in blood coagulation factors due to fibrin deposition in capillaries, in the placenta and uterus and the maternal kidneys and lungs.

Humoral or hormonal factors. Plasma renin activity is raised in normal pregnancy but may be lower or normal in association with pre-eclampsia. Renin stimulates aldosterone secretion and, therefore, higher levels of plasma aldosterone are found in normal pregnancy. As with plasma renin activity, aldosterone levels are decreased in women with high blood pressure.

PREDISPOSING CAUSES

Primigravidae. Hypertension is twice as common (10%) in primigravidae as in multigravidae (4–5%) and is more common in the elderly primigravida.
Multiple pregnancy. Pre-eclampsia presents more commonly in association with the multiple pregnancy than in a singleton pregnancy.
Polyhydramnios. Also associated with a higher incidence of pre-eclampsia.
Diabetes mellitus. Associated with vascular lesions which involves the placenta.
Obesity. A woman who is overweight is more prone to develop pre-eclampsia.
Essential hypertension. A superimposed pre-eclampsia may occur in women who present with essential hypertension.
Previous hypertension. Between 30 and 50% of women present with hypertension in a subsequent pregnancy.
Hydatidiform mole. Pre-eclampsia may present in early pregnancy in association with hydatidiform mole.

CLINICAL COURSE OF THE DISEASE

Pre-eclampsia may remain in a mild form or improve with treatment or it may progress to become moderate or severe. Indications that the disease is deteriorating are an increase in the signs and, in severe cases, the appearance of proteins in the urine and the onset of symptoms.

SYMPTOMS

The symptoms of pre-eclampsia are related to the effects of the high blood pressure, cerebral and retinal oedema.
Frontal headaches. Due to cerebral oedema.
Epigastric pain. Caused by haemorrhages into and distension of the liver capsule.
Nausea and vomiting. May be due to oedema causing pressure on the vomiting centre or in association with the headaches and epigastric pain.
Visual disturbances. Blurring of vision, photophobia, and spots or flashes in front of the eyes due to oedema of the retina.
Oliguria. A diminished urinary output may be observed and is a serious sign.

An increase in the severity of the signs and the onset of symptoms indicate that eclampsia is imminent and they are referred to as the prodromal (warning) signs of eclampsia.

COMPLICATIONS

The complications associated with pre-eclampsia are:

Maternal

a Eclampsia; the onset of epileptiform fits, indicating involvement of the central nervous system.

b Placental abruption; due to placental damage caused by arteriolar spasm.

If the diastolic blood pressure rises above 110 mmHg damage to vital organs may result.

c Cerebral oedema and haemorrhage.

d Renal and hepatic failure.

e Cardiac failure.

Fetal

a Intrauterine malnutrition due to diminished placental perfusion leading to a decrease in the nutritive function of the placenta and causing intrauterine growth retardation.

b Intrauterine hypoxia occurs when the gaseous exchange is diminished.

c Intrauterine death may occur due to anoxia where acute placental damage occurs.

Neonatal

a Immaturity due to spontaneous or induced premature labour.

b Light-for-dates as a result of intrauterine malnutrition.

c Perinatal death.

The baby's birth weight is lower and the perinatal mortality rate higher where hypertension and proteinuria presents but there is no oedema.

MANAGEMENT

The aim of antenatal care is to identify women who are 'at risk' of developing pre-eclampsia, to manage their antenatal care accordingly, and to detect and treat the condition as early as possible should it present. All pregnant women are seen with increasing frequency as pregnancy advances and at each visit they are weighed, the urine is tested for, among other constituents, protein, the blood pressure is recorded and they are examined for oedema. If signs of pre-eclampsia present the woman is admitted to hospital. The aims of management in pre-eclampsia are to monitor the maternal condition, to improve placentral perfusion, to identify the fetal risk and determine the point at which extrauterine life offers a lesser risk and to prevent complications.

Bed rest is the most important method for treating maternal hypertension and increasing the maternal blood flow to the placenta. If rest fails to reduce the maternal blood pressure to a satisfactory level, alternative methods of control will be used.

Sedation, such as amylobarbitone sodium (100–200 mg), phenobarbitone (30–60 mg), or diazepam (5–15 mg), is frequently used in association with bed rest if bed rest alone does not reduce the blood pressure, and may be given at six to eight-hourly intervals or as night sedation only.

OBSERVATIONS

Blood pressure. This is recorded twice daily but observations may be four-hourly if the blood pressure is very high.

Fluid balance. The fluid intake and urinary output are measured and recorded. In this way any reduction in the urinary output can be observed.

Urinalysis. The urine is tested daily for the presence of protein and, if present, a midstream specimen of urine is sent to the laboratory and the amount of protein is estimated.

Oedema. The presence and amount of oedema is observed daily.

Weight. The weight is estimated on alternate days. If there is a normal weight gain it indicates fetal growth, alternatively poor weight gain, static weight or loss of weight may suggest fetal growth retardation and excessive weight gain may be associated with generalised oedema.

Abdominal examination. The abdomen is examined daily. The uterine size is estimated in association with the period of gestation and also the size of the fetus and the amount of amniotic fluid present. The fetal heart is auscultated whenever the blood pressure is recorded, i.e. twice daily or four-hourly.

Estimation of placental function and fetal wellbeing. Urinary oestrogen estimation are of value in assessing the efficiency of the placenta and the wellbeing of the fetus (see p. 320). Collections of urine are made over twenty-four hours either weekly, twice weekly, on alternate days or daily depending on the severity of the condition and the results of the tests.

Hypotensive drugs. If a combination of bed rest and sedation does not lower the blood pressure to safe levels hypotensive drugs may be used.

If the condition improves, as shown by a return to and maintenance of the normal level of blood pressure and a reduction or disappearance of the oedema, increasing activity is allowed. If this does not cause a deterioration of the condition the woman may be allowed to go home. However, once she has shown signs of pre-eclampsia it is likely that it will return and therefore she should be advised to rest and is seen at frequent intervals for the remainder of pregnancy. If any sign of pre-eclampsia recurs, she is readmitted to hospital. If the hypertension persists, but is mild, the woman must remain in hospital under medical supervision.

Indications for induction of labour

If labour has not started spontaneously before the end of the fortieth week of pregnancy, induction of labour should be performed. A combination of postmaturity and pre-eclampsia carries a high risk to the fetus.

Proteinuria is of serious prognostic significance, and therefore induction of labour should be performed if proteinuria persists.

If the hypertension increases in spite of treatment, labour should be induced in the interest of the woman.

If induction of labour is an elective procedure fetal maturity tests may be performed (see p. 317–18), but if the intrauterine environment is less favourable than the extrauterine environment, the induction of labour is performed regardless of gestational age.

Severe pre-eclampsia

If the diastolic blood pressure rises to 100 mmHg, the fetus is liable to die and the woman may soon develop eclampsia. The rise in blood pressure may be rapid, occurring over the course of a few hours. It may be accompanied by an increase in the amount of oedema, and the appearance of proteins in the urine or, if already present, an increase in amount, and the occurrence of symptoms. The term fulminating pre-eclampsia is used to describe cases of severe pre-eclampsia in which the disease progresses very rapidly.

The management of severe pre-eclampsia is as for eclampsia and will be described below.

Eclampsia

The difference between pre-eclampsia and eclampsia is one of degree. Eclampsia is a serious complication of pregnancy with a 5% maternal mortality and a 30% perinatal mortality. It occurs approximately once in every 1000 births.

Aetiology

The cause of eclampsia is not known but may be due to: anoxia of the brain because of vasospasm; cerebral oedema producing encephalopathy; cerebral dysrrythmia, abnormal tracings are seen if an electroencephalogram is performed.

Eclampsia is characterised by epileptiform convulsions, often with persisting unconsciousness. Such fits may occur during pregnancy, i.e. antepartum eclampsia, during labour, i.e. intrapartum eclampsia, and in the first few days following delivery, i.e. postpartum eclampsia. In nearly every case the signs of pre-eclampsia precede the fits but occasionally fulminating eclampsia may occur.

CONVULSIONS

Three stages are described.

Tonic stage. All extensor muscles are in spasm. Opisthotonos may be present, and due to the spasm of the respiratory muscles, the intake of oxygen is stopped and cyanosis occurs. The hypoxia deprives the fetus of oxygen and severe distress or death may result. The tonic stage lasts for approximately 30–60 seconds.

Clonic stage. The muscles alternately relax and contract, producing jerking movements of the whole body. During this phase the tongue may be bitten. The clonic stage lasts for about two minutes.

Coma. Respirations are gradually restored along with the woman's natural colour, and she sinks into a coma of variable duration.

In severe cases there are recurrent fits which may occur every few minutes and be virtually continuous, i.e. status eclampticus. The woman may die of asphyxia or from inhalation of vomit or from cerebral haemorrhage. Death may also occur later due to renal failure or necrosis of the liver.

Once an eclamptic fit has occurred there is a danger of recurrence until about forty-eight hours after delivery.

MANAGEMENT

Emergency management

a Turn the woman on her side.

b Clear the airway using suction apparatus, and insert an airway if possible.

c Prevent the woman from swallowing her tongue by application of tongue forceps. A mouth gag should be put between the teeth to prevent the tongue being bitten.

d Administer oxygen as soon as the fit is over.

e Prevent injury during clonic stage.

f Summon assistance and medical aid as soon as possible.

Subsequent management

Control of fits. The greater the number of fits the worse is the prognosis for the woman and fetus. Any stimulus may precipitate another fit so the excitability of the nervous system must be reduced by sedatives, and external stimuli, e.g. bright lights, noise, discomfort and handling must be reduced to a minimum.

Medication used for controlling the fits may include one of the following:

a Diazepam (Valium) 10 mg intravenously, followed by an infusion of 20 mg in 500 ml of 5% dextrose solution. The drip rate is titrated to induce a deep sleep.

b Hydrallazine (Apresoline) 10 mg injected intravenously over a period of fifteen minutes. The blood pressure must be monitored closely during the administration. The initial dose is usually followed by a continuous slow infusion of 50 mg of hydrallazine in a litre of 5% dextrose solution. The infusion rate is adjusted to maintain the blood pressure at about 140/90 mmHg.

Other drugs such as frusemide (Lasix) 40 mg intravenously may be used to produce a diuresis which helps to reduce the blood pressure and may help to protect the kidneys from damage due to vascular shutdown.

Control of blood pressure. The aim is to prevent cerebral haemorrhage and some of the drugs mentioned above will reduce the blood pressure as well as control the fits. Medication used for lowering the blood pressure may include hydrallazine hydrochloride (Apresoline) 20 mg given by intravenous injection as an initial dose, followed by 5 mg doses as required.

NURSING CARE

Good nursing of these cases is essential and the midwife will be responsible for observations and recordings on which so much depends in the proper management of the woman. The woman is nursed in a quiet room with subdued lighting as bright sunlight or artificial light may precipitate a fit. Anaesthetic instruments and suction and oxygen apparatus must be in the room. Prevention of hypostatic pneumonia is aided by turning the woman from side to side every two hours, and the foot of the bed is slightly raised to help any respiratory secretions to drain into the mouth.

Observations

The pulse and respiratory rates are recorded quarter-hourly and the blood pressure at half-hourly intervals.

If fits occur, the number, length and time of occurrence are noted and the doctor informed immediately so that the drug therapy can be adjusted.

A strict fluid intake and urinary output charts is maintained. The amount of fluid given is based on the urinary output of the previous day plus 1500 ml for insensible loss. An intravenous infusion is in progress to provide nourishment and for the administration of drugs, two units of 5% dextrose, solution is given to one unit of normal saline.

A self-retaining catheter is inserted and released every hour. This is to prevent the discomfort of a full bladder, which will make the woman restless and precipitate a fit, and to observe the urinary output. If less than 30 ml of urine is produced in an hour this is an indication of oliguria. All specimens of urine are tested for the presence of proteins.

The fetal heart is monitored continuously or at quarter-hourly intervals.

Obstetric treatment is directed to delivering the woman in the safest way and at the earliest opportunity. Quite often the woman goes into labour spontaneously and this is easily recognised because she becomes restless and the uterus can be felt to be contracting during the times of restlessness. If the woman does not go into labour spontaneously, labour is induced by artificial rupture of membranes followed by Syntocinon infusion as soon as the fits and blood pressure are under control. If the woman is not delivered within six hours or if after a vaginal examination prior to rupturing the membranes it is considered that she is unlikely to deliver soon, a Caesarean section is performed.

Labour is supervised closely with full attention to sedation and analgesia. Epidural analgesia, which lowers the blood pressure as well as relieves pain may be an ideal method in this situation. The strain of pushing in the second stage of labour is potentially dangerous and therefore an elective forceps delivery is performed.

Ergometrine is usually avoided because it causes constriction of blood vessels and may cause a rise in the blood pressure. If a Syntocinon infusion is in progress this can be used to control the blood loss in the third stage of labour. Ergometrine would be used in the event of postpartum haemorrhage, for here the hypotensive effects of the blood loss will offset the hypertensive effect of the ergometrine.

The baby is likely to need resuscitation, and the paediatrician should be informed of the situation and called when the delivery is imminent.

Following delivery the heavy sedation is continued for forty-eight hours and then slowly withdrawn over the course of two to three days.

Maternal mortality

There were twenty-nine deaths from pre-eclampsia and eclampsia in the triennium 1976–78, thirteen due to eclampsia and sixteen due to pre-eclampsia (Table 6.1).

Table 6.1 Cause of death in association with pre-eclampsia and eclampsia.

	Pre-eclampsia	*Eclampsia*
Cerebral haemorrhage	9	8
Cerebral oedema	0	2
Anoxic cardiac arrest	2	1
Hepatic and renal failure	1	0
Adrenal cortical haemorrhage	1	0
Disseminated intravascular coagulation	1	0
Asphyxia	0	1
Cerebral infarction	1	0
Cerebellar infarction and pituitary infarction	1	0
	16	*12

* Post mortem examination was not performed in one instance.

Perinatal mortality

The perinatal mortality rate was 46.2%.

Hypertension

When the blood pressure rises for the first time during pregnancy and there is no associated generalised oedema or proteinuria, the condition cannot be classified as pre-eclampsia for, by definition, at least two signs must be present.

When hypertension is the only sign, the woman must be classified as suffering from hypertension. If subsequently generalised oedema or proteinuria develop, then the diagnosis of pre-eclampsia can be made.

AETIOLOGY

Hypertension developing during pregnancy may be the result of causative factors in the placenta or due to mechanical effects or haemodynamic changes of the pregnancy. In the majority of cases, however, some abnormality of the vascular or renal systems is present prior to the pregnancy. However, the blood pressure may be normal before pregnancy and during the first two trimesters. As a result of the haemodynamic changes of normal pregnancy the reduced vascular reserve is unmasked and hypertension develops. This may be evidence of early cases of chronic renal disease and essential hypertension.

Essential hypertension

A diagnosis of essential hypertension in pregnancy is made if the woman is known to have had a raised blood pressure before the onset of pregnancy, or if the blood pressure is raised before the twentieth week of pregnancy. A family history of essential hypertension is often given in these cases. Apart from hypertension these women appear well, as the pathological changes associated with essential hypertension are not found at the age at which pregnancy is common.

There is no significant increase in maternal mortality when a woman with essential hypertension becomes pregnant.

The perinatal mortality is dependent on the levels of blood pressure and the presence of proteinuria. Proteinuria will present in about 12% of pregnant women with essential hypertension and the incidence of a severe degree or pre-eclampsia is about 3.5%. The risk of placental abruption is increased in the severe forms of essential hypertension.

MANAGEMENT

The management of a pregnant woman with essential hypertension is similar to that outlined for the management of pre-eclampsia. Bed rest, sedation and in severe cases, the use of hypotensive drugs is maintained until the fetus is mature or the intrauterine environment is less favourable to the fetus than the extrauterine environment.

Chronic renal disease

CHRONIC PYELONEPHRITIS

The clinical manifestations of chronic pyelonephritis may closely resemble those of early hypertension. A history of previous urinary tract infections may indicate the possibility of this diagnosis. The leucocyte excretion rate and a urinary bacillary count may confirm the diagnosis but a renal bipsy may be the only method of making a definitive diagnosis. About 4–5% of pregnant women have asymptomatic bacilluria, i.e. a bacillary count in excess of 100000 organism/ml. These women are liable to develop urinary tract infection later in the pregnancy or to manifest in later years the features of chronic renal disease.

Fetal prognosis is similar to that in essential hypertension. The main risk to the mother is recurrence of urinary tract infection with further fibrosis of the kidney. The physiological changes which occur in the urinary tract during pregnancy produce a reduced rate of urinary flow with dilatation of the upper urinary tract which predisposes to recurrence of infection. Courses of varying chemotherapy periodically throughout pregnancy are usually prescribed. The principles of management additional to those mentioned above are similar to those outlined for essential hypertension.

CHRONIC GLOMERULAR NEPHRITIS

This condition complicates pregnancy far less commonly than does chronic pyelonephritis. This diagnosis is suggested if there is a history of acute glomerular nephritis or an appreciable quantity of proteinuria without an increase in the pus cells in the urine. Creatinine clearance can be estimated to determine the glomerular filtration rate and the extent to which it is reduced will give some indication of the reduction in renal reserve. A rising blood urea gives an early indication of failing renal function.

The perinatal mortality rate is high when the diastolic blood pressure is more than 100 mmHg and the glomerular filtration rate is less than 50% of normal.

Serial urinary oestrogen recordings are performed to assess the wellbeing of the fetus and ultrasonic examination used to assess fetal growth. The results of these investigations will indicate the optimum time for induction of labour.

Other causes

COARCTATION OF THE AORTA

Constriction of the aorta near its junction with the ductus arteriosus. It occurs in certain types of congenital heart disease. Pregnancy complicating coarctation of the aorta may not increase the maternal mortality but the perinatal mortality may exceed 50%, mainly due to cardiovascular and renal complications.

The physiological manifestations of coarctation of the aorta are: decreased pulse pressure below the coarcted segment; increased arterial blood pressure proximal to the coarction; increased left ventricular activity; extensive collateral arterial circulation.

PHAEOCHROMOCYTOMA

This is a non-malignant tumour arising from chromaffin tissue which is found in some glands and organs and in the sympathetic nerves. The cells stain yellow when tested with chrome salts. Ninety per cent of phaeochromocytomas occur in the adrenal medulla. About 0.5% of hypertensive diseases are due to these tumours.

A high maternal and fetal mortality result when this condition complicates pregnancy, unless the diagnosis is established and appropriate treatment is carried out.

The tumour produces large amounts of catecholamines which cause vasospasm and hypertension. The hypertension produced by phaeochromocytomas may be paroxysmal or sustained. The elevated blood pressure may be associated with other manifestations of noradrenaline or adrenaline, e.g. severe headaches, photophobia, tachycardia, profuse sweating, nausea.

Diagnosis

Measurement of the concentration of free catecholamines (adrenaline and noradrenaline) in the urine is the most reliable means of diagnosis. The measurement of the urinary metabolites of adrenaline and noradrenaline, normetanephrine and metanephrine and 3-methoxy-4-hydroxy mandelic acid (vanillylmandelic acid—VMA) may also be used.

Management

Resection of a phaeochromocytoma in pregnant women is recommended if it presents in early pregnancy or following delivery if the diagnosis is not made until late pregnancy. If resection is not performed, medical management may include administration of phenoxybenzamine (Dibenyline) 200 mg twice daily to block the tumour secretions and reduce the blood pressure and a beta-blocking agent to reduce the hyperconductivity of the heart.

One maternal death was attributed to phaeochromocytoma of the adrenal gland during the three years 1976–78 inclusive.

Renal diseases

Diseases of the renal tract are not uncommon complications of pregnancy and potentially dangerous diseases which, if they persist and become chronic, may progress to cause hypertension and ultimate renal failure. An adequate blood supply to the kidney is essential. If for any reason it is less than usual, the kidney through the renin-angiotensin system raises the blood pressure and so helps to ensure that more blood reaches it. If the nephrons receive insufficient blood because of disease in the kidney, they secrete renin in an ineffective attempt to improve the function. Severe hypertension results. It is therefore essential to recognise those women who are at risk of developing pyelonephritis and to prevent this, and to carry out effective treatment and proper subsequent investigations and care should the disease occur.

BACTERIURIA

The presence of bacteria in the urine. The presence of more than 100000 (10^5) organisms/ml in a midstream specimen of urine is found in approximately 6% of women examined during pregnancy.

The woman may give a history of recurrent attacks of urinary infection occurring throughout childhood, and often with an exacerbation with the beginning of sexual activity and during pregnancy. The infecting organism, usually the *Escherichia coli*, invades the bladder from the urethra and, if the ureterovesical sphincter is incompetent, it may ascend to the upper urinary tract. This may produce renal scarring with narrowing of the renal cortex.

ASYMPTOMATIC BACTERIURIA

In many women the bacteriuria is asymptomatic but they are more likely to develop acute pyelonephritis in pregnancy. The incidence of acute pyelonephritis can be reduced by treating women with asymptomatic bacteriuria and screening of all pregnant women at the first visit is now part of routine antenatal care. If women with bacteriuria are not treated or if they do not respond to treatment the incidence of pyelonephritis is about 30%.

Apart from the risk of developing acute pyelonephritis there is also evidence to suggest that women with asymptomatic bacteriuria are more likely to give birth to an infant of low birth weight and, that those women who fail to respond to apppropriate treatment show a high incidence of serious abnormalities of the urinary tract.

Treatment with a single course of ampicillin (500 mg eight-hourly) or sulphadimidine (0.5 g six-hourly) for eight days is effective in the majority of cases.

PYELONEPHRITIS

Inflammation of the pelvis and nephrons of the kidney. It is a common complication of pregnancy, its frequency being approximately 2% of all pregnant women. The disease may occur at any time during pregnancy but is more likely to present at about twenty weeks gestation.

PREDISPOSING FACTORS

1 Changes in the renal pelvis and ureters during pregnancy brought about by pressure at the brim of the pelvis. The right ureter is more likely to be

involved due to the tendency of the uterus to incline to the right side. This results in dilatation of the renal pelvis and ureters, kinking of the ureters and stasis of urine.

2 Congenital abnormalities of the renal tract or some other lesions such as calculus.

3 Ureteric reflux. Urine containing bacteria can enter the ureter if there is reflux at the ureterovesical junction, and during pregnancy stasis of urinary flow makes ascending infection more likely.

4 Catheterisation. There is a connection between catheterisation and subsequent development of pyelonephritis.

CAUSATIVE ORGANISM

Escherichia coli is present in approximately 80% of cases. Other organisms include *Bacillus proteus*, *Staphylococcus albus* and *Streptococcus faecalis*.

CLINICAL FEATURES

The signs and symptoms of pyelonephritis vary according to the severity of the disease which may be acute or subacute.

Acute. The onset is sudden with severe pain referred to one, usually the right, or both loins. The temperature rises to approximately 39.5–40 °C and may be accompanied by shivering and rigors. The pulse rate is rapid. The woman feels ill and may complain of headaches and nausea and vomiting. The abdomen is tender especially over the region of the infected kidney.

Subacute. The signs and symptoms are not so characteristic. The woman complains of malaise, dull backache with pain radiating to the groins and the temperature is slightly raised to 37.2–37.8 °C.

The Urine. In severe cases the urinary output is diminished and the specific gravity is high. The urine initially contains only bacilli but soon becomes turbid, contains pus and debris; the reaction is usually acid and haematuria may be present. A midstream or suprapubic specimen of urine is found to contain in excess of 100 000 organism/ml of urine, pus cells, epithelial cells and some red blood cells and protein.

MANAGEMENT

The woman is admitted to hospital and put to bed. If the right kidney only is affected, she will obtain more relief from pain if she lies on the unaffected side.

A midstream or subrapubic specimen of urine is obtained for bacteriological investigations, including sensitivities of the causative organisms.

Ampicillin (500 mg six-hourly) or sulphadimidine (1 g initially, followed by 0.5 g six-hourly) is commenced as soon as a specimen of urine has been obtained. When the bacteriological report is available the appropriate antibacterial drug is chosen. Sulphonamides should be avoided close to term because they displace bilirubin in the fetal plasma and predispose to neonatal jaundice.

A large fluid intake will increase the urinary flow and therefore reduce the proliferation of organisms in the urinary tract. A fluid intake and urinary output chart is maintained. The temperature, pulse and respiration rate are recorded four-hourly.

General nursing care includes attention to personal and oral hygiene and tepid sponging or use of an electric fan if the temperature is very high.

A midstream or suprapubic specimen of urine is obtained at intervals for bacteriological examination to check for response to treatment and to ensure the urine remains free from bacteria and pus cells.

Infection of the renal tract is commonly associated with anaemia due in part to the presence of haematuria but also as a result of a reduction in erythropoietin necessary for the production of new red blood cells. Therefore, the haemoglobin level should be estimated frequently.

MATERNAL PROGNOSIS

In the majority of cases an immediate improvement takes place following the appropriate treatment, and within a few days the pain subsides, the temperature returns to normal, and the urine contains less pus.

The acute infection is often followed by further attacks during pregnancy and the puerperium and may recur for many years. Chronic pyelonephritis may ensue as an insidious, progressive and persistent disease in which there is gradual destruction of the renal parenchyma with resulting fibrosis, scarring and contracture and the development of hypertension.

FOLLOW-UP CARE

If recurrent or persistent pyelonephritis occurs or if organisms and pus cells are found on repeated examination of the urine, an intravenous pyelogram may be carried out after pregnancy.

If excretion of pus cells and bacilli continues, even intermittently, treatment with antibiotics or long-acting sulphonamides is continued.

There were eight deaths from pyelonephritis in the years 1970–72 and there was one other death attributed to diabetes mellitus in which diabetic coma was apparently precipitated by acute pyelonephritis. Six of the eight deaths occurred during pregnancy and two in the puerperium.

FETAL PROGNOSIS

Severe pyelonephritis with high fever may result in abortion or intrauterine death. In less severe infection there may be fetal growth retardation or premature onset of labour, so that the perinatal mortality is increased.

Multiple pregnancy

The term multiple pregnancy is used when more than one fetus is present in the uterus. The incidence of spontaneous multiple pregnancy is approximately: twins 1 in 10^2; triplets 1 in 10^4; quadruplets 1 in 10^6; quintuplets 1 in 10^8.

TYPES

Twins may be binovular or uniovular.

Binovular twins are developed from two ova developing in a single Graafian follicle, or from two follicles which may or may not be in the same ovary. This type of twins is three times as common as the uniovular type. The ova are fertilised by two spermatozoa. The infants may be of the same or different sex, and are no more alike than is usual with members of the same family. As they develop from separate ova, they have separate placentae. Sometimes the placentae may fuse but there is no anastomosis of their blood vessels. Each fetus has its own amnion and chorion (Fig. 6.4[1]).

Uniovular twins are developed from a single ovum which, after fertilisation, has undergone complete division to form two zygotes. Errors of development are more likely to occur with this type of twins, conjoined twins or some form of double monster may result. Communication between the two circulations may cause unequal development of the fetuses and sometimes death. Occasionally one fetus dies early in pregnancy and is retained *in utero* until term, becoming compressed and mummified, when it is known as fetus papyraceus. The more frequent occurrence of polyhydramnios with uniovular twins is probably related to the common placental circulation.

Uniovular twins are, except in the rare cases of mosaics, the same sex and are remarkably alike in their physical and psychological characteristics. Uniovular twins which arise as the result of very early division of the ovum

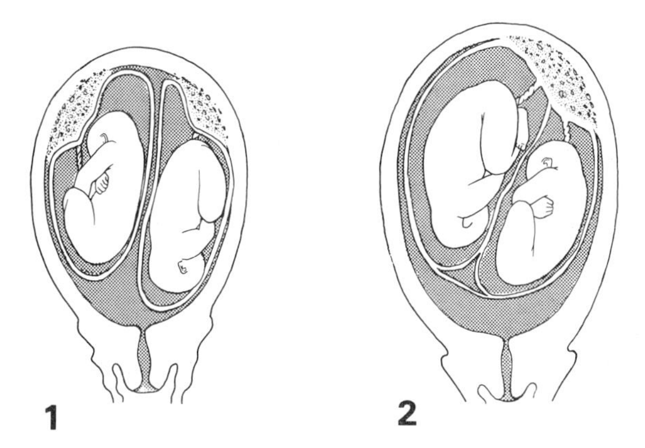

Fig. 6.4 1, binovular twins; 2, uniovular twins.

each have a chorion and an amnion; those which arise by later division have only one chorion but usually have separate amniotic sacs (Fig. 6.4[2]). Monoamniotic twins (with a single amniotic sac) are rare.

AETIOLOGY

Multiple pregnancy may be an inherited tendency, as it occurs more often in certain families. Although paternal influence is often indicated it is difficult to see how this occurs.

The frequency of twin birth is greatest between the ages of thirty-five and forty, especially when the twins are binovular, and a woman who has given birth to twins is ten times more likely to have another multiple pregnancy. Pregnancies following artificial induction of ovulation with human gonadotrophins or clomophine are not infrequently multiple especially if the dosage is not closely controlled by hormone assays. Overstimulation of the ovary may cause maturation of several ova.

Triplets may develop from a single ovum, or from two or three ova. The placenta and membranes will be arranged in the same way as in twins according to the manner in which development has taken place.

Quadruplets and quintuplets are similarly developed.

DIAGNOSIS

During pregnancy the presence of twins should be suspected if the uterus appears globular in shape and is large for the period of gestation. Other causes of the uterus being large-for-dates that must be excluded are hydatidiform mole, polyhydramnios and fibroids. On abdominal palpation three fetal poles may be felt and if the head feels small in comparison with the size of the uterus, the index of suspicion is increased. The diagnosis is made more certain by hearing two fetal hearts, recognised as two by their maximal density being at different positions, the sound being lost between them and the rates, counted at the same time by two observers over at least one minute, differing by at least ten beats. Polyhydramnios may be present and makes the diagnosis of twins by palpation and auscultation very difficult.

The diagnosis can be confirmed on ultrasonic examination or by X-ray examination after twenty-eight weeks of pregnancy. This not only confirms the diagnosis but might show evidence of abnormality such as conjoined twins, and so provide warning of difficulty with vaginal delivery.

The diagnosis of twins is sometimes missed until the birth of the first twin. If the baby's head appears small or if the uterus is unexpectedly large after the first baby is born, a multiple pregnancy is suspected and, if not already given, the Syntometrine must be withheld.

Late diagnosis of a multiple pregnancy is more likely when the labour is premature, therefore, premature onset of labour should make the attendant suspicious and more vigilant.

Effects on pregnancy

During pregnancy, the presence of twins often produces an exaggeration of the minor disorders. Thus nausea and vomiting may become excessive and hyperemesis gravidarum may occur. Pressure symptoms are also more pronounced and the tendency to oedema, varicose veins of the legs and haemorrhoids is greater. The woman often complains of tiredness and shortness of breath and she may suffer undue discomfort due to the enlarged uterus.

Polyhydramnios is more likely to occur, especially in uniovular twins and this adds to the discomfort caused by the enlarged uterus.

Pre-eclampsia occurs more commonly in association with twin pregnancy.

Antepartum haemorrhage as a result of placenta praevia is more likely to occur. The large single placenta or the two placentae produce a larger placental area which is liable to encroach into the lower uterine segment.

Anaemia due to iron and folic acid deficiency may occur due to the greater demand being made on the woman's reserves.

Malpresentations are common with twins. In about 45% of cases both fetuses present by the vertex; in about 37% one fetus presents by the vertex and one by the breech; in about 10% both present by the breech and in about 8% a transverse lie is associated with either a vertex, breech or a second transverse lie.

The prognosis for the fetus is worse in multiple than in single pregnancy. The rate of fetal growth is slower than in a single pregnancy after the twenty-eighth week. Intrauterine death affecting one or both twins may be caused by placental insufficiency associated with pre-eclampsia or antepartum haemorrhage.

MANAGEMENT OF PREGNANCY

Antenatal care should be intensified in order that anaemia, pre-eclampsia, antepartum haemorrhage and premature labour can either be prevented or detected and treated at an early stage. The woman should be seen more frequently than usual from midpregnancy onwards.

Anaemia is prevented by giving supplementary iron and folic acid daily, and frequent estimations of the haemoglobin levels.

The woman is encouraged to rest as much as possible as the effects of twins on the pregnancy may be delayed or improved by bed rest. Hospitalisation from about thirty to thirty-six weeks may be recommended.

Effects on labour

The duration of a twin pregnancy is very variable but it tends to be short. The premature onset of labour increases the risks to the fetuses.

Complications of labour, such as malpresentations placenta praevia and prolapsed cord are more common, and one twin may interfere with the descent of the other and the rare complication of locked twins may occur. The second twin may also be endangered by retraction of the uterus and premature separation of the placenta.

The overdistended uterus may not contract well and the hypotonic uterine action may lead to prolonged labour.

Primary postpartum haemorrhage may occur both due to atony of the uterus, a large placental site and if a degree of placenta praevia is present, due to lack of retractile power of the lower uterine segment.

MANAGEMENT OF LABOUR

Labour is conducted in a consultant obstetric unit with all facilities for dealing with complications should they arise. The doctor is informed of the woman's admission in labour.

Preparations should be made to receive two or more babies with the possibility that they may be premature or in need of resuscitation. The delivery trolley should contain two sets of cord clamps and some means of identifying the cords to assist in the examination of the placenta and membranes following delivery and obtaining cord blood if required.

An incubator should be available and the paediatrician and staff of the Special Care Baby Unit informed that the woman is in labour and whether or not the babies will be premature.

The first stage of labour is managed as in any other labour but attention is given to the type of analgesia used if the woman is in premature labour. Two fetal hearts are observed. Any deviation from normal is immediately reported to the obstetrician.

At the onset of the second stage of labour the obstetrician, anaesthetist and paediatrician are informed.

The delivery of both babies may be normal if they present by the vertex. The indication for a forceps delivery or breech extraction are undue delay or fetal distress. An episiotomy under local anaesthetic should be performed if indicated, e.g. to protect the premature baby's head or to prevent perineal laceration.

After the birth of the first twin the placental end of the umbilical cord must be ligated securely, because if the twins are uniovular, bleeding may exsanguinate the second twin through the anastomosed placental circulations. The cord is identified at this stage. It is after the birth of the first baby that the problems may arise and it is the second twin which is at greater risk. The lie of the second twin is ascertained by abdominal palpation and if it is transverse or oblique, external version is performed to place one pole over the dilated os. There is an advantage in converting the second twin to a breech presentation because if extraction of the second twin becomes necessary it is easier to bring down the legs of a breech than to apply forceps to a high head.

The fetal heart is auscultated and if no distress is noted the labour is allowed to progress. Uterine contractions usually recommence within a few minutes and when they do, the delivery of the second twin is usually quite rapid since the os uteri has already been fully dilated. The membranes are ruptured and the delivery is conducted in the usual way. If the uterine contractions do not recommence in about five minutes after the delivery of the first baby the forewaters should be ruptured.

An intravenous injection of ergometrine (0.5 mg) or an intramuscular injection of Syntometrine (1 ml) is given with the birth of the anterior shoulder.

COMPLICATIONS OF LABOUR

First stage

Delay due to hypotonic uterine action would be managed in the usual way but if the delay is due to one twin interfering with the descent of the other, or in rare cases in which both fetuses are lying transversely or for the very rare cases of conjoined twin a Caesarean section would be performed.

Second stage

Complications are most likely to occur in the second stage of labour.

Delay in recommencement of uterine contractions. If the uterine contractions do not return in about five minutes after the birth of the first baby the forewaters are ruptured, and a vaginal examination is performed to exclude prolapse of the cord. The delivery of the second fetus usually occurs normally without further delay.

Fetal distress. The membranes are ruptured at once and the delivery effected.

Cord prolapse. The fetus is delivered with reasonable expedition.

Premature separation of placenta. Usually both babies are born before the placenta, but rarely, with binovular twins, the placenta of the first twin separates before the delivery of the second fetus. Because of reduction in the volume of the uterus there may be separation of the placenta on which the second twin depends, so that delivery must be completed as quickly as possible.

Locked twins. This is a very rare complication, its incidence being 1 in 1000 twin labours. It is suspected when there is delay in the second stage of labour. The commonest occurrence is when the first twin presents as a breech and the second as a vertex. The chin of the aftercoming head of the first twin is caught by the forecoming chin of the second, and if disengagement is not effected quickly the delay ends fatally for the first baby. In these circumstances the aftercoming head of the first twin should be decapitated in order to free and deliver the second, the decapitated head being delivered by fundal pressure or forceps.

Primary postpartum haemorrhage. This is treated in the usual way after twin delivery (see p. 274).

The puerperium

The puerperium usually progresses normally. The lochia may be more profuse and the uterus slower to involute but this is not markedly so.

The main problem for the mother is to learn to look after two babies, and if she is a primipara she will need a lot of help and supervision. Establishing a feeding regime is important. If the mother elects to breast feed she should be shown how to feed both babies together. This can be achieved by supporting the babies on a pillow placed on either side with their head towards the centre.

A home-help may be necessary for the first few weeks to give the mother an opportunity to establish a routine for the babies while being relieved of the household chores.

The mother is eligible to claim an additional maternity grant for the second or any subsequent baby providing the infant survives for more than twelve hours.

Multiple pregnancy is a common cause of premature labour, therefore the babies may be of low birth weight (see p. 241).

In 1982 over half of all live births in a multiple pregnancy were of low birth weight as compared with 6% of singletons. Of all live-born low birth weight babies, almost 15% were in a multiple birth, but as a whole multiple births account for less than 2% of all births.

Nearly 84% of all stillbirths from multiple pregnancies were of low birth weight, while only 61% of singleton stillbirths were in this category.

Chapter 7
Medical Disorders Associated with Pregnancy

Diabetes mellitus

Diabetes mellitus is a disorder of carbohydrate metabolism, characterised by hyperglycaemia and glycosuria and resulting from inadequate production or utilisation of insulin. Without insulin the liver is unable to form and store glycogen and release it as required, and glucose accumulates in the blood. The kidney tubules are unable to reabsorb all the glucose conveyed to them by the renal vessels but continue to absorb water. Normally insulin counter-balances the influence of the diabetogenic hormone of the anterior lobe of the pituitary gland which takes part in the control of fat and protein metabolism. In the absence of insulin the liver is unable to store glycogen and converts fat to ketone bodies.

SIGNS AND SYMPTOMS OF DIABETES MELLITUS

Large quantities of urine (polyuria) containing glucose are passed. The polyuria is the result of withdrawal of tissue fluids required to counteract the rise in the osmotic pressure of the urine due to the reabsorption of water by the renal tubules. The woman complains of excessive thirst as a result of the loss of body fluids.

The glycosuria may cause pruritis vulvae. This is often associated with monilial infection of the vagina since the invading organism (*Candida albicans*) thrives in a high glucose medium.

There is an abnormal glucose tolerance test, all the normal blood glucose values are exceeded, i.e. fasting—90 mg% (5 mmol); one hour—610 mg% (9 mmol); one and a half hours—140 mg% (8 mmol); two hours—120 mg% (6.5 mmol); and two and a half hours—100 mg% (5.75 mmol).

CLINICAL CLASSIFICATION OF DIABETES MELLITUS

Clinical diabetes. There is an abnormal response to a glucose tolerance test and signs and symptoms or complications of diabetes.

Chemical diabetes. There is a diabetic response to a glucose tolerance test but no clinical signs and symptoms of diabetes.

Latent diabetes. There is a normal glucose tolerance test currently, but the woman has been known to have had a diabetic response to a glucose tolerance test in the past, i.e. during pregnancy, infection or when obese. There is an abnormal response (similar to that found in diabetes) to provocative tests, such as corticosteroids or tolbutamide.

Potential diabetes. There is a normal glucose tolerance test but a potential risk of developing diabetes because:

a An identical twin has diabetes mellitus.

b Both parents have diabetes mellitus or one parent has diabetes, and the other non-diabetic parent has either a parent, sibling or has a sibling with a diabetic child.

c The obstetric history reveals a live or stillborn baby weighing more than 4.5 kg, or a stillborn child showing hyperplasia of the pancreatic islets.

Effects of pregnancy on the diabetic state

Pregnancy has a diabetogenic effect and therefore this may lead either to the diagnosis of chemical or latent (gestational) diabetes being made, or to a worsening of an established (clinical) diabetic state during pregnancy, evidenced by an increase in the insulin requirement.

It is routine practice to screen the urine for glucose at booking and at each subsequent antenatal visit in order to detect women who have undiagnosed chemical diabetes or gestational diabetes. Investigation by glucose tolerance test is usually performed routinely on all women who fall into the group listed under the heading potential diabetes. Other women at special risk are those with:

1 A history of diabetes mellitus in a blood relative.
2 A previous baby with a birth weight in excess of 4.5 kg.
3 Glycosuria on two or more occasions during the present pregnancy.
4 A history of unexplained stillbirth.
5 A history of infertility or recurrent abortions.
6 Gross obesity.

GLYCOSURIA IN PREGNANCY

Glycosuria may present in pregnancy for one of the following reasons: clinical diabetes; chemical diabetes; gestational diabetes; lowered renal threshold (renal glycosuria).

Lowering of the renal glucose threshold is thought to be due to increased blood flow through the glomeruli. A large amount of glucose enters the glomerular filtrate and the tubules cannot reabsorb it adequately during the time the fluid is passing through. The function returns to normal after pregnancy.

Due to lowering of the renal threshold for sugar during pregnancy, urine testing is a less reliable guide in the management of diabetes mellitus. However, if urine tests are correlated with blood glucose estimations whilst the woman is in hospital the reliability of urine testing is increased.

Effects of diabetes mellitus on the pregnancy

Pre-eclampsia. There is an increased incidence of pre-eclampsia in women with diabetes mellitus and this is probably a major contributory factor in late intrauterine death and is therefore a serious complication.
Polyhydramnios. An increase in amniotic fluid is common and the incidence is increased if the control of the diabetes is poor. Polyhydramnios may also be seen in association with a congenital malformation.
Vulvovaginitis. Glycosuria predisposes to monilial infection due to the yeast-like fungus *Candida albicans.*
Infections. Women with diabetes mellitus are more prone to infection of all types which usually result in instability of the diabetic state.

EFFECTS OF DIABETES MELLITUS ON THE FETUS

In diabetes mellitus, the intrauterine environment of the fetus is abnormal and this is shown by the increase in the perinatal mortality rate. Provided the diabetes is controlled before the twenty-eighth week of the pregnancy the fetal outcome is good, but if early control is poor the subsequent care and control has little effect on the outcome.
Fetal abnormalities. There is an increased incidence of fetal malformation in diabetic pregnancy and this is further increased if the father also has diabetes mellitus.
Large fetus. This occurs as a result of high maternal blood glucose concentrations stimulating the fetus to produce insulin. Excess insulin secretion results in deposition of fat and protein.
Intrauterine death. This may occur due to placental insufficiency as the result of oedema of the placental tissue, spasm of placental blood vessels may be due to high capillary glucose acting as an irritant and the large fetus outgrowing the placental function. Pre-eclampsia would aggravate this condition. Placental insufficiency may result in the fetus being small-for-dates. Hypoglycaemia appears to have no effect on the fetus but ketoacidosis in midtrimester is associated with fetal loss. There is a greater fetomaternal gradient for glucose in diabetic pregnancy than in normal pregnancy.

Management of pregnancy

The aim of antenatal care is to establish good diabetic control by keeping the maternal blood glucose levels as near physiological as possible. The management is undertaken jointly by a physician and an obstetrician.

The woman is admitted to hospital as soon as possible for investigation of serial blood glucose levels. Urine testing is unreliable in pregnancy as a guide to plasma glucose levels and good control of diabetes demands plasma glucose estimation.

Insulin is adjusted to secure maximum control of the diabetes. In mild cases control may be by a 120–140 g carbohydrate diet only or a low carbohydrate diet plus lente (long-acting) insulin. In more severe cases soluble and isophane insulin may be combined to give good control throughout the twenty-four hours. The use of oral hypoglycaemic drugs such as chlorpropamide is not recommended because they cross the placenta and may cause hypoglycaemia in the neonate if not stopped forty-eight hours before delivery. (Insulin was discovered by Banting and Best in 1922 and introduced into the management of diabetes mellitus in 1924.)

Following discharge the woman is seen at fortnightly intervals in early pregnancy and weekly intervals in late pregnancy. She tests her urine on waking, before meals and before retiring.

Readmission to hospital would be indicated if an obstetric complication such as pre-eclampsia occurred, if she developed an infection or if the diabetic state becomes unstable and cannot be controlled as an outpatient.

There is usually an increase in insulin resistance in the midtrimester and a further increase in the third trimester. If there is an abrupt fall in insulin requirements near term it may indicate failing placental function.

Placental lactogen is an antagonist of insulin and causes an accelerated fasting syndrome which is present from the eighth week and falls rapidly after delivery returning to normal within six hours.

The pregnancy is usually allowed to progress to the end of the thirty-eighth week if the diabetes is well controlled, or if diet only is required the pregnancy may be allowed to proceed to term but not beyond. Earlier intervention would be indicated if the diabetic condition is not well controlled or an obstetric complication occurred.

Management of labour

If the diabetes has been well-controlled during pregnancy and there is no obstetric contraindication, a vaginal delivery is anticipated. Artificial rupture of membranes is performed followed by Syntocinon infusion immediately, or within six hours, if labour is not established.

The usual insulin is given during labour and an intravenous injection of glucose 50 g given every six hours. Alternatively, an intravenous infusion of 10% dextrose with added insulin may be used to give 10 g of glucose and 2 units of insulin each hour.

Continuous monitoring of the fetal heart should be made, as this is an at-risk fetus.

If labour does not progress satisfactorily or if fetal distress develops, a Caesarean section is performed.

Management of the puerperium

The insulin requirements may fall precipitately following the birth of the baby, and frequent blood glucose estimations will be needed until the level again becomes stable. Breast feeding is not contraindicated although lactation does slightly increase the difficulties of stabilisation.

Oral contraceptives precipitate diabetes and therefore are not recommended as a method of contraception.

EFFECTS OF DIABETES MELLITUS ON THE INFANT

The baby born to a woman with diabetes mellitus is more prone to develop respiratory distress syndrome than another baby of similar gestation. It may be large and plethoric if the diabetes has been poorly controlled, but despite its size may be physiologically immature. The baby is also prone to symptomatic and asymptomatic hypoglycaemia (see p. 393).

MATERNAL MORTALITY

There were three deaths attributed to diabetes mellitus in the triennium 1976–78, and all were considered to be of indirect causation.

Anaemia

Anaemia is any condition in which there is an alteration in the quality or quantity of the blood causing a decrease in the haemoglobin concentration.

Physiological anaemia

During pregnancy there is an increase in the blood volume but there is a relatively greater increase in the volume of plasma than of the red blood cells. This leads to a fall in the red cell count and haemoglobin concentration. This physiological haemodilution of pregnancy creates a physiological anaemia, so called because while there is in pregnancy an increase in haemoglobin in the body, there is less per decilitre of blood. The haemoglobin reaches its lowest level at thirty-two weeks gestation when haemodilution reaches its maximum. Haemoglobin values of less than 12 g/decilitre are abnormal before twenty-five weeks of pregnancy whereas values of less than 11 g/decilitre are abnormal after this time. The increased blood volume is maintained until term, there is then a sudden fall but the original level is not reached until about six weeks postpartum.

High absorption rates of up to 40% of dietary iron are attained in the latter half of pregnancy so that utilisation of iron supplements is facilitated. This facility is increased if the woman is anaemic.

Anaemia in pregnancy

Types. Iron deficiency; folic acid deficiency; haemoglobinopathies including sickle cell disease and thalassaemia; haemolytic, e.g. glucose 6 phosphate dehydrogenase.

Iron deficiency anaemia

This is the most common cause of anaemia in pregnancy.

CAUSES

Increased demand for iron. The normal daily requirement of 1 mg is increased to 3–4 mg a day in pregnancy. The uterus and its contents require 300 mg, the fetal iron requirements reaching a maximum during the last three months of pregnancy. The increase in red blood cells requires 300 mg and during the puerperium lactation requires 80 mg.
Daily loss. Approximately 1 mg of iron is lost each day in urine, bile and sweat.
Reduced iron intake. This may occur as the result of poor diet or excessive vomiting.
Low reserves. Regular depletion by menses may result in the woman commencing pregnancy with low iron stores. A loss of 70 ml is easily made up but a loss of more than 120 ml is difficult to replace. Frequent pregnancies, especially of the interval between the pregnancies is less than two years, reduces iron stores.
Abnormal demands. This will occur if there is a multiple pregnancy.
Blood loss. Chronic or repeated small losses of blood may occur as the result of haemorrhoids or antepartum haemorrhage.
Chronic infection. Erythropoietin released from the kidney stimulates the bone marrow to produce new red blood cells. In the presence of an infection of the urinary tract erythropoesis is reduced.

SIGNS AND SYMPTOMS

In mild cases the woman often does not complain of any symptoms but in more severe cases she may look pale although this can be an unreliable sign in pregnancy due to peripheral vasodilatation. She may complain of tiredness, breathlessness and palpitations.

A well nourished woman has good iron stores and this delays the onset of anaemia in pregnancy or other stress situations such as haemorrhage. There may be a sudden fall in the haemoglobin concentration when the iron stores are depleted. Women with poor iron stores become anaemic as a result of the demands made by the pregnancy.

DIAGNOSIS

There is a reduction in the mean corpuscular volume (MCV) to less than 80 fl. Hypochromia and a reduction in the mean corpuscular haemoglobin (MCH) to less than 27 pg occurs in the more severe degrees of iron deficiency.

Serum iron levels of less than 60 mg/decilitre and an increase in the total iron binding capacity (the ability of the cells to transport iron) which is normally 300–325 μg/decilitre indicates reduced iron stores. A bone marrow biopsy may be performed and this is normal in a woman with iron deficiency anaemia.

MANAGEMENT

The management of iron deficiency anaemia in pregnancy has mainly become preventative by daily supplements of elemental iron throughout pregnancy. A daily intake of 78 mg is sufficient to prevent the development of anaemia in the absence of an adequate diet. Dietary advice is given to all women during pregnancy and foods rich in iron such as red meat, peas, lentils, green vegetables and dairy produce are recommended.

It is important to exclude other causes of anaemia by ensuring that the woman does not have any chronic blood loss, septic foci, e.g. dental caries or infection of the urinary tract.

The haemoglobin concentration is estimated routinely at booking, at twenty-eight weeks and at thirty-four to thirty-six weeks gestation. If there is an increased demand, as in a multiple pregnancy, the haemoglobin concentration is estimated more frequently. If the haemoglobin concentration is low a full blood count is performed if this is not done routinely.

If the cause of the anaemia is iron deficiency the supplementary dose of iron is increased and is very effective in correcting the anaemia. Parenteral iron is only indicated if oral iron fails to correct the anaemia.

TYPES OF IRON

Oral. Ferrous sulphate, ferrous gluconate, ferrous succinate, or ferrous fumarate, may be given as sugar-coated tablets or contained in other forms of iron preparation.

Parenteral. Jectofer is an iron sorbitol citrate complex which is rapidly transported from the injection site. It has a small molecule and is therefore excreted rapidly through the kidneys. It is contraindicated if the woman has a history of urinary tract infections. An intramuscular injection of 100 mg is given daily.

Ferrivenin, a saccharated iron oxide is an intravenous preparation. An initial test dose of 40 mg is given followed by daily injections of 100–200 mg.

Imferon is an iron dextran complex and is used for a total dose infusion of iron. The amount of Imferon is calculated according to the degree of anaemia and the woman's body weight. The dose is diluted in 5% dextrose or normal saline. Because there is a risk of an anaphylactic reaction the intravenous infusion is run at a rate not exceeding ten drops/min for ten minutes under strict medical supervision. If this test dose is tolerated, the rate of infusion is increased to 40–60 drops/min.

Blood transfusion is rarely given because of the risk of overloading the circulation, but on the rare occasions when there is insufficient time to achieve a reasonable haemoglobin concentration before delivery a transfusion of packed cells would be used.

Parasitic infestation

Hookworm infestation is endemic in some areas of the world and this should be suspected in women from an immigrant population if persistent anaemia occurs. The infestation may persist for a long time after arrival in Britain.

Diagnosis. The ova of the hookworm are found in the stools. Treatment is to give bephenium hydroxynaphthoate (Alcopar) 5 mg on an empty stomach to be repeated if required.

Folic acid deficiency

Folic acid is required for normal maturation of red blood cells. If there is a deficiency of this substance the cells in the bone marrow become megaloblastic and the number of mature red cells in the circulation is reduced. The presence of megaloblasts in the bone marrow is the reason why this condition is also referred to as megaloblastic anaemia. The red blood cells are macrocytic and the peripheral blood picture may be similar to pernicious anaemia. The mean corpuscle haemoglobin (MCH) is raised above 90 pg although the haemoglobin concentration falls.

Serum folate levels may give abnormal results but often these are not significantly different from results in healthy pregnant women.

The anaemia may develop rapidly in late pregnancy and be accompanied by a very low haemoglobin concentration which does not respond to oral iron.

There is a higher incidence of folic acid deficiency in multigravidae, multiple pregnancy and in poorly nourished populations. The incidence varies considerably with populations being as low as 0.5% in Western countries and as high as 50% in parts of India. There is an increased folate requirement in women receiving anticonvulsants.

The daily folate need is increased from the non-pregnant requirement of 50 μg to 100–130 μg in pregnancy due to transfer of folate to the fetus.

MANAGEMENT

Folic acid is usually given prophylactically during pregnancy usually in a combined pill with iron, e.g. Slow-Fe folic containing ferrous sulphate (150 mg) and folic acid (0.5 mg). Intramuscular folvite (15 mg) may be administered if folic acid deficiency occurs. Dietary advice is given and the woman advised to eat foods rich in iron which also contain folic acid (see p. 52).

Haemoglobinopathies

Three types of haemoglobin are normally found in man HbA, HbA_2 and HbF. There are four globin chains designated alpha, beta, gamma and delta which differ in the sequence and content of their amino acids. Alpha chains are common to all three haemoglobins. The normal haemoglobin molecule of the adult (HbA) has two pairs of polypeptide chains two alpha and two beta chains. During intrauterine life alpha chains combine with gamma chains to form HbF. At term, gamma chain synthesis ceases and alpha chains combine with beta and delta chains to form HbA and HbA_2 respectively. By six months of age, HbA reaches the adult level of over 95% and HbF forms less than 1% of total haemoglobin.

Haemoglobinopathies are inherited defects of haemoglobin, resulting from impaired globin synthesis (thalassaemia) or from structural abnormalities of globin (haemoglobin variants, e.g. sickle cell disease).

The routine screening for haemoglobinopathies should be undertaken by means of haemoglobin electrophoresis in all women at risk, e.g. negroid populations in the case of haemoglobin variants, and Mediterranean, negroid and Indian populations in the case of thalassaemia.

HAEMOGLOBIN VARIANTS

Both heterozygous and homozygous forms of each variant occur. Heterozygous subjects inherit one abnormal haemoglobin chain from one parent. They are carriers and transmit the abnormal haemoglobin although they are not anaemic and show no clinical abnormality. This is known as sickle cell trait (HbAS). Homozygous subjects inherit the same abnormal chain from each parent and no normal HbA is synthesised. This is known as sickle cell disease (HbSS).

It is possible for subjects to be doubly heterozygous for a haemoglobin variant, for example, they can inherit the sickle cell gene from one parent and an HbC gene from another (HbSC).

CLINICAL MANIFESTATIONS

Sickle cell disease (HbSS)

The structural alteration in the haemoglobin molecule results in alteration in the shape of the red cells (sickling) when the oxygen tension is reduced, haemoglobins being less soluble in deoxygenated states. This gives rise to chronic haemolytic anaemia of varying severity which occurs from an early age. The sickle-shaped cells are fragile and easily destroyed and their life-span is therefore reduced. Thrombosis, due to the high viscosity of the cells, causes slowing of the circulation.

Crises are characteristic of the disease. These acute episodes occur due to intravascular sickling and cause vascular occlusion resulting in tissue infarction. These crises, which present with pain in bones, joints and abdomen often accompanied by fever, are often precipitated by changes in oxygen tension, drugs or infections, and are more common in pregnancy.

Sickle cell trait (HbAS)
This occurs in about 10% of the negroid population and only results in sickle cell crises if gross hypoxia occurs.

Sickle cell HbC disease (HbSC)
This is a mild variant of sickle cell disease with normal or near normal levels of haemoglobin. Because of the mild nature of the disease it may go undiagnosed but these women are at risk from sickling crises in pregnancy and particularly the puerperium.

MANAGEMENT

Pregnancy. Folic acid supplements are given during pregnancy but iron therapy is not given. People with sickle cell disease have a high serum iron concentration and a low iron-binding capacity, so that administered iron may be deposited in the reticule-endothelial system with haemosiderosis. Because infection precipitates crises, even mild infections are treated with antibiotic therapy. Blood transfusions may be used to reduce the incidence of complications. Regular transfusion of three to four units of blood at approximately six-weekly intervals maintains the proportion of HbA cells at 60–70% of the total. This regime not only dilutes the number of sickle cells in the circulation but reduces the number of sickle cells produced by reducing erythropoeisis.
Labour. It is essential that hypoxia, dehydration and acidosis do not occur in labour.
Puerperium. This is a very dangerous time and following delivery, magnesium sulphate may be administered. This is a calcium antagonist and because it delays formation of thrombi, acts as an anticoagulant. It is also a vasodilator. An intravenous injection of 50% magnesium sulphate (2 ml) is given slowly and repeated four-hourly for two days.

THALASSAEMIA

Thalassaemia results from an inherited defect in the synthesis of normal haemoglobin which leads to the production of red cells with deficient haemoglobin content. It most frequently occurs in Mediterranean races.

There are two main types of thalassaemia, alpha and beta and both types occur in homozygous and heterozygous forms.

Thalassaemia major is the homozygous form of thalassaemia. The alpha type is incompatible with life; the beta type responds to blood transfusion and survival is prolonged into adolescence. Thalassaemia minor is the heterozygous form of thalassaemia. It is the most common type of thalassaemia and the one most likely to present in pregnancy. The peripheral blood picture is characteristic of an iron deficiency anaemia but it is often associated with overloaded iron stores.

MANAGEMENT

Iron suppplements are not given unless iron deficiency is diagnosed by measurement of iron stores. The red cells are often hypochromic because of the failure to produce adequate amounts of haemoglobin. Extra folic acid should be given.

Haemolytic anaemia

Glucose-6-phosphate dehydrogenase is an enzyme which is essential for normal metabolism in the red blood cells. It is an inherited sex-linked gene found more commonly in males and predominantly in Eastern Mediterranean and African populations.

Acute haemolytic episodes associated with this condition are most commonly precipitated by oxidant drugs such as salicylates, sulphonamides and vitamin K.

EFFECTS OF ANAEMIA ON PREGNANCY

1. It undermines the woman's general health.
2. Lowers the resistance to ante and postpartum blood loss.
3. Predisposes to thromboembolic disease.
4. A contributory cause of maternal mortality.
5. If severe causes intrauterine hypoxia.
6. The perinatal mortality is increased in severe anaemia.

Cardiac disease in pregnancy

The physiological changes that occur in the cardiovascular system during normal pregnancy are significant in the diagnosis of heart disease during pregnancy and the management of the pregnancy complicated by heart disease (see p. 27). The incidence of heart disease is 3% of all pregnancies and with the decline of rheumatic heart disease there has been a change in the pattern of heart disease seen in pregnancy. Congenital heart disease now occurs as frequently as rheumatic heart disease because more patients are surviving surgery for congenital heart disease in infancy. This trend is likely to continue.

The main causes of heart disease in pregnancy are:

1 Rheumatic heart disease: mitral stenosis or incompetence; aortic incompetence.

2 Congenital heart disease: atrial septal defect; ventricular septal defect; patent ductus arteriosus; coarctation of the aorta; pulmonary stenosis.

The effect of pregnancy on heart disease is to expose the woman to certain risks which are related to the increased work undertaken by the heart throughout pregnancy and may precipitate heart failure. Even with adequate care and supervision, pregnancy not infrequently results in the functional capacity of the woman with heart disease degenerating by one grade.

GRADES OF FUNCTIONAL CAPACITY

Grade one. The woman has no symptoms or limitation of activity.

Grade two. There is slight limitation of activity and symptoms with strenuous activity.

Grade three. There is marked limitation of activity with dyspnoea on effort.

Grade four. The woman is unable to undertake any physical effort without dyspnoea and exhaustion.

Although the lesion present is important, the functional capacity is the most significant factor in prognosis. The medical and obstetric care and supervision, and adequate rest during the antenatal period are also important factors in prognosis, as are age, parity and social class.

The aim of antenatal care is to prevent the woman's condition from deteriorating and the complication of heart failure from occurring.

The management of pregnancy

The woman is seen at frequent intervals during the antenatal period and ideally she should be seen at each visit by both an obstetrician and a cardiologist. If this is not possible she should be thoroughly assessed as early as possible by a cardiologist who should then see her at least monthly throughout pregnancy. The frequency of antenatal visits will place an additional burden on the woman and therefore transport should be provided if necessary.

The dangers during pregnancy are cardiac decompensation and failure. Precipitating factors to these conditions are described below.

Anaemia. Because of the risks of anaemia the haemoglobin level is estimated at frequent intervals during pregnancy and prophylactic iron and folic acid are given.

Infection. The risks of infection, especially respiratory infection, are very high and the woman is admitted to hospital for rest and antibiotic therapy. Dental caries should be treated, and if dental extractions are required, penicillin should be prescribed before and afterwards to reduce the risk of bacterial endocarditis.

Bacterial endocarditis. There is a risk of the woman developing the serious and sometimes fatal complication of bacterial endocarditis if infections are not prevented or adequately treated.
Excessive weight gain. The normal weight gain of pregnancy places a strain on the heart and therefore if weight gain is excessive there is an additional strain.
Hypertension. The development of hypertension is a serious complication and if this is accompanied by oedema the heart may be unable to cope with the fluid retention and the strain of the hypertension.

Adequate rest is essential to help to counterbalance the additional strain placed on the heart during pregnancy. The woman is encouraged to rest for ten to twelve hours each night and for two hours during the day. The provision of a home-help can relieve the woman of the household chores. The decision to hospitalise the woman for bed rest is made on an individual basis but many women with heart disease benefit from a period of bed rest in the last trimester. This may not apply to the woman with functional grade one heart disease who may be managed as an outpatient. Women with functional grades three and four will spend most or all of the pregnancy in hospital. The woman's social circumstances must be taken into consideration and the social worker will need to be involved to ensure that existing children are being cared for adequately. This may involve the use of day nurseries, child-minders or even foster parents.

In addition to the normal obstetric examination undertaken at each antenatal visit the woman's pulse rate is counted and jugular venous pressure recorded. A careful examination is made for oedema including auscultation of the lungs for any evidence of pulmonary oedema. A pulse rate in excess of 100 beats/min, jugular venous pressure exceeding 2 cm, a rise in blood pressure and the presence of anything more than slight oedema are indications for admission to hospital.

Women who are classified as functional grades two, three and four may require digitalis and oral diuretics such as chlorothiazide during pregnancy especially if they show any signs of heart failure. Women with artificial heart valves, mitral valve disease or pulmonary hypertension are usually taking anticoagulants such as warfarin before they become pregnant. Because the risk of thrombosis is further increased in pregnancy the therapy is continued. At thirty-six weeks gestation subcutaneous heparin (10 000 units twelve-hourly) is substituted for warfarin and continued for forty-eight hours postpartum. There is a risk that warfarin which crosses the placenta will increase the risk of bleeding in the neonate. Heparin being of large molecular weight does not cross the placenta.

Miral stenosis is the most dangerous of cardiac conditions encountered in pregnancy because it is not possible to determine functional grading from physical activity and because the overloading and hypertrophy of the left atrium causes hypertension and the danger of pulmonary oedema.

PULMONARY OEDEMA

The development of pulmonary oedema may be sudden and unexpected with no precipitating factor, or it may occur as a result of one of the precipitating factors mentioned earlier, e.g. anaemia or infection. The onset of acute pulmonary oedema is recognised by dyspnoea accompanied by the coughing up of a frothy, often bloodstained sputum. Rhonchi and crepitations are present throughout the lung fields and signs and symptoms may worsen rapidly. Treatment consists of the immediate intravenous injection of frusemide (20 mg) accompanied by morphine sulphate (15 mg). If there is no anaemia a venesection of 500 ml should be performed, but if anaemia is present a sphygmomanometer cuff is applied at the root of all four limbs and inflated to a pressure of 50 mmHg in order to block venous return. The cuffs are temporarily deflated in rotation every fifteen minutes. If the woman is not already digitalised, digitalisation is carried out as quickly as possible. Aminophylline (500 mg) by intravenous injection may be prescribed if bronchial spasm is an element in the dyspnoea.

The subsequent management depends on the precipitating cause, if there was no precipitating cause, mitral valvotomy may be performed. This is the only form of cardiac surgery advocated in pregnancy.

CYANOTIC HEART DISEASE

Fallot's tetrology is the most common type of cyanotic heart disease in pregnancy. There is an increased incidence of fetal growth retardation and intrauterine death due to placental insufficiency.

The more severe types of cyanotic heart disease such as Eisenmenger's syndrome carry a very high risk to the pregnant woman.

The management of labour

Minimal interference is advocated during labour and induction of labour is only undertaken if there is a strict obstetric indication for so doing. Cardiac disease alone is not an indication for induction of labour in fact it is a contraindication. The aim is for an easy labour and the woman with no obstetric complication is allowed to go into spontaneous labour.

A course of penicillin is usually given prophylactically during labour and continued for the first fourteen days of the puerperium.

During labour the woman is usually most comfortable in an upright position well supported by pillows. Dyspnoea may be alleviated by the administration of oxygen.

Adequate pain relief is essential to prevent distress and this is achieved by the use of pethidine or nitrous oxide via the Entonox apparatus. Epidural analgesia should be used with caution because of the risk of hypotension. It may be used for women with mild heart disease, and some women with severe heart disease such as mitral stenosis who are at considerable risk of developing pulmonary oedema in labour may benefit by the decreased venous return caused by epidural anaethesia. However, in the women who are not at risk of developing pulmonary oedema epidural anaesthesia is contraindicated. They usually have mild or moderate mitral stenosis and are unable to increase their cardiac output to maintain their blood pressure if peripheral resistance is reduced as in the case of epidural anaesthesia. Not only may the resultant hypotension harm the woman but, since maternal placental blood flow depends on perfusion pressure, the fetus may also suffer.

The second stage of labour is usually managed by elective forceps delivery although in a mild case a short second stage may be allowed.

There is a difference of opinion regarding the routine administration of an oxytocic drug in the late second stage. Intravenous ergometrine is contraindicated because the strong uterine contraction it stimulates produces a sudden transfer of 300–500 ml of uterine blood into the circulation and this increase in the effective blood volume may precipitate pulmonary oedema. However, in some types of congenital heart disease, i.e. atrial septal defect, a postpartum haemorrhage is more hazardous than in a woman with a normal heart. Cardiac failure may follow a blood loss that would not have endangered either the woman with a normal heart or a woman with more serious heart disease but with an intact atrial septum. For this reason and because of the danger of uncontrollable postpartum haemorrhage intramuscular Syntometrine is usually prescribed. In the event of a postpartum haemorrhage it would be managed in the usual way with additional measures taken to manage the pulmonary oedema should it present.

Management of the puerperium

The puerperal management of the woman with a functional grade one heart disease differs little from the normal apart from the continuance of antibiotic therapy. Those women with a higher grade of functional disability should rest in bed for five to ten days followed by a week of graduated activity before being allowed home. Attention must be paid to passive movements to reduce the risk of thromboembolism. Provided the woman is well enough to care for her baby there is no contraindication to breast feeding, although if she is receiving anticoagulant therapy it must be remembered that active metabolites of warfarin may be excreted in breast milk. If lactation is suppressed oestrogens are best avoided because of the risk of hypertension. The puerperium is a time when particular vigilance is needed because this is the time when the woman may die (Table 7.1).

Table 7.1 Maternal deaths due to acquired cardiac disease 1976–78.

Coronary artery disease	7
Rheumatic valvular disease	3
Bacterial endocarditis	3
Other conditions including cardiomyopathies	5

Table 7.2 Maternal deaths due to congenital malformations 1976–78.

Eisenmenger's syndrome	2	One died the day after an emergency Caesarean section at the thirty-eighth week of pregnancy for a third degree placenta praevia; the other died seventeen days postpartum following induction of labour in the thirty-ninth week of her first pregnancy and a vacuum extraction under epidural anaesthesia
Ventricular septal defect	1	Died four weeks postpartum

CONTRACEPTIVE ADVICE

Although there is no evidence that pregnancy causes deterioration in the cardiac condition unless the woman has been in cardiac failure, it is not desirable for her to have repeated pregnancies. Tubal ligation may be performed if the woman and her husband are agreeable. If this is not acceptable another method of contraception must be advised. Oral contraceptives containing oestrogen are contraindicated because they are likely to cause hypertension, whilst the low dose progestogen-only pill carries a higher risk of pregnancy. Intrauterine devices are contraindicated because of the increased risk of infection.

SOCIAL ASPECTS

Careful consideration must be given to the woman's social circumstances and if these are unsatisfactory the social worker would be asked to see her. If the home conditions are unsuitable, e.g. the family may live in a flat with no lift or the building may be substandard and damp, this may involve rehousing.

The home-help services may be required to relieve the woman of household chores.

If she has other children to care for they could be placed in a day nursery or with a child-minder. Rarely is there a need for residential care, but if such a need arose it would involve a residential nursery or fostering.

MATERNAL MORTALITY

Twenty-one women died from cardiac disease associated with pregnancy during the period 1976–78, compared with twenty in 1973–75 and forty-two in 1970–72. Eighteen deaths occurred in women with acquired cardiac disease, and three with congenital malformations. These deaths were all classified as indirect maternal deaths.

Avoidable factors were considered to be present in four of the twenty-one deaths associated with cardiac disease; three with an acquired cardiac disease and one with a congenital cardiac malformation. In each case the woman alone was deemed responsible. The avoidable factors all related to failure to attend for care or to take advice during pregnancy and not where the woman had failed to take advice about avoiding pregnancy or having a termination of pregnancy.

Termination of pregnancy is rarely necessary and has no place in deteriorating heart disease as the stresses are greater than the continuance of pregnancy. If a termination of pregnancy should, however, be necessary, it must be confined to early pregnancy when the woman's cardiac state is well compensated. In this context, the 1967 Abortion Act contains the following clause, 'the continuance of the pregnancy would involve risk to the life of the pregnant woman greater than if the pregnancy were terminated'.

Respiratory diseases

Pulmonary tuberculosis

Tuberculosis is an infectious disease characterised by the presence of small nodules (tubercles) in the tissues caused by the organism *Mycobacterium tuberculosis*. Tuberculosis may affect any part of the body, but pulmonary tuberculosis is the commonest and most dangerous form.

PULMONARY TUBERCULOSIS COMPLICATING PREGNANCY

Pregnancy does not adversely influence the course of pulmonary tuberculosis provided adequate treatment and supervision are given during and after pregnancy and provided pregnancy and labour are uncomplicated.

The incidence of pulmonary tuberculosis is between 0.2 and 0.5%, but some communities have a far higher incidence.

Routine X-ray of the chest during pregnancy has been discontinued in some clinics and is now only performed if indicated, e.g. if there is a family history of the disease or in women from an immigrant community who are very susceptible to the disease.

MANAGEMENT OF PREGNANCY

If the condition has already been diagnosed and the woman is receiving treatment this is continued throughout pregnancy. Antituberculosis therapy by means of streptomycin and sodium aminosalicylate or isoniazid is not thought to have an adverse effect on the fetus although there is some evidence that streptomycin given in the first trimester of pregnancy may occasionally lead to eighth nerve damage in the fetus. The placenta acts as a successful barrier against the tubercle bacilli and the disease should not present in the neonate if the mother has received adequate and proper chemotherapy.

MANAGEMENT OF LABOUR

Prolonged labour must be avoided and the management of labour in a woman suffering from pulmonary tuberculosis is along the same lines as for the woman with cardiac disease. The second stage may be terminated by forceps delivery under pudendal block unless progressing rapidly.

MANAGEMENT OF THE PUERPERIUM

There is a risk of reactivation of the disease in the puerperium and therefore continued treatment and supervision is essential. Breast feeding is contra-indicated except in those mothers whose disease has been inactive for at least two years.

THE INFANT

In active cases the danger of infecting the baby is very high and the child must be separated from the mother. All infants of mothers suffering from tuberculosis, or if there is a case in the immediate family, must receive BCG vaccination. If the mother has active tuberculosis the infant must be isolated from her until the Mantoux test is positive, usually after six to eight weeks. In the meantime this may involve the baby being fostered.

Pulmonary sarcoidosis

This is a chronic granulomatous disease of unknown aetiology characterised by tubercle-like lesions. There is a relatively high incidence of pulmonary sarcoidosis amongst West Indian immigrants.

This condition is usually diagnosed as a result of routine chest X-ray but can present as erythema nodosum. During pregnancy the diagnosis may be confirmed by scalene node biopsy and by the presence of a negative Mantoux and a positive Kveim test.

The disease usually remains static during pregnancy. Occasionally, however, rapid deterioration can occur and steroid therapy may be necessary. There is a very slightly increased risk of fetal malformation if steroids are given in the first trimester of pregnancy.

Chronic bronchitis and emphysema

The woman with chronic bronchitis is liable to become very severely dyspnoeic during pregnancy. In spite of the dyspnoea, women with chronic bronchitis and emphysema usually tolerate pregnancy quite well, provided they have adequate rest including, if necessary, hospitalisation. If they develop a respiratory infection they must be treated in bed with a suitable antibiotic such as Ampicillin (250 mg six-hourly). In some cases the drug at half-dosage may be used prophylactically during autumn and winter.

The management of labour is similar to that for a woman with cardiac disease. Oxygen is often helpful. Drugs causing respiratory depression should be used with caution and only given if specifically prescribed. Epidural analgesia may be preferable for these women. The second stage of labour should be short and may need to be terminated electively by forceps.

Asthma

Asthma is not usually adversely affected by pregnancy. Treatment is essentially the same as treatment in the non-pregnant states although steroids should be avoided in pregnancy, especially during the first trimester of pregnancy unless the severity of symptoms indicates their use. The management of labour is similar to that advocated for women suffering from chronic bronchitis.

There were four deaths ascribed to asthma and one anaesthetic death where the patient's asthmatic condition was considered to have contributed to her death in the triennium 1976–78.

Essential hypertension

Although a medical disorder of pregnancy essential hypertension has been discussed in the previous chapter. There is often difficulty in deciding the cause of hypertension in pregnancy and making a definitive diagnosis in clinical practice because the cause of the hypertension is often obscure (see p. 199).

Chronic renal disease

Because chronic renal disease is complicated by hypertension, the two main causes of this condition, chronic pyelonephritis and chronic glomerulonephritis have been discussed in the chapter dealing with hypertension in pregnancy (see p. 199).

Epilepsy

Epilepsy is a disease of the nervous system characterised by convulsive seizures accompanied by paroxysmal cerebral dysrhythmia and followed by a period of unconsciousness.

Epilepsy as such has no adverse effect on pregnancy but fits and the controlling drugs do. The effect of pregnancy on the epilepsy is variable. The number of fits may be unchanged or increased or they may cease during pregnancy.

DIFFERENTIAL DIAGNOSIS BETWEEN EPILEPSY AND ECLAMPSIA

Clinical differentiation between epilepsy and eclampsia as a cause of convulsions may be necessary during pregnancy. The following points should be considered

1 History of fits before pregnancy.

2 Time of onset of fits. Apart from its association with hydatidiform mole eclampsia is essentially a disease of the latter half of pregnancy.

3 The number of fits. In epilepsy, apart from the rare status epilepticus, fits occur singly, in eclampsia they may occur in series.

4 The blood pressure. In epilepsy the blood pressure is unchanged but in eclampsia it is always above the non-pregnant level.

5 Proteinuria. Except for a trace which is occasionally found immediately after a convulsion, proteinuria is not a feature of epilepsy. Equally, it is rare for protein not to present in eclampsia.

6 Quantity of urine. Oliguria is usually a feature of eclampsia, whereas in epilepsy the amount of urine secreted is unchanged.

TREATMENT

The treatment of a woman with epilepsy during pregnancy is the same as if she were not pregnant. If she is already taking a drug which is controlling the fits this would be maintained during pregnancy. If medication is commenced during pregnancy phenobarbitone (30–60 mg three times a day) may be prescribed. The disadvantage of high doses of phenobarbitone is that it causes drowsiness. If this is unacceptable or it fails to control the convulsions, phenytoin (100 mg two or four times a day) may be given in addition or to replace the amount of phenobarbitone. If both fail to control the convulsions primidone may be given in dosages up to 250 mg four times a day. The optimum dose of these drugs for any particular woman is obtained by commencing her on the smallest dose and gradually increasing until the fits are controlled.

Anticonvulsant drugs may result in a folic acid deficiency anaemia, therefore the pregnant epileptic woman who is receiving such therapy should be given folic acid (5 mg twice a day). Deterioration in epilepsy during pregnancy may be related to retention of fluid and for this reason a restricted salt diet and diuretics may be prescribed.

STATUS EPILEPTICUS

The mortality of this condition in pregnancy is high and once the fits have been controlled the pregnancy is usually terminated. Paraldehyde (10 ml) is given intramuscularly using a glass syringe, followed by 5 ml half-hourly until the fits cease. When this point is reached the intervals between the injections may be prolonged.

MATERNAL MORTALITY

Three women died from epilepsy in the three years 1973–76. One died in status epilepticus following Caesarean section and this was classified as an indirect maternal death. The other two deaths were classified as fortuitous and occurred at twenty-two days and two months after delivery.

VAGINAL DISCHARGES, SEXUALLY TRANSMITTED AND VENEREAL DISEASES

Vaginal discharge may be physiological or pathological.

PHYSIOLOGICAL

An excessive white or yellow mucoid discharge often occurs during pregnancy due to an increase in the circulating oestrogens and increased vascularity of the cervix and vagina. The discharge, referred to as non-infected leucorrhoea, is non-irritant, does not cause soreness and is odourless.

PATHOLOGICAL

The discharge is usually due to an inflammatory condition causing cervicitis, vaginitis or vulvovaginitis.

There are three venereal diseases designated by Parliament, namely syphilis, gonorrhoea and chancroid or soft sore. There are, however, other sexually transmitted diseases including non-gonococcal urethritis in the male, and trichomoniasis and candidiasis in the female.

Sexually transmitted diseases

Trichomoniasis

Trichomonas vaginalis is a species of protozoon infecting the vagina and causing vaginitis with an abundant, frothy, offensive, greenish-yellow discharge and intense pruritis and burning of the vulva. The discharge may be bloodstained and may be a cause of incidental bleeding.

TREATMENT

Metronidazole (Flagyl) 200 mg may be given three times a day for a week or a 400 mg tablet may be used, two tablets in the morning and three at night for two days only. It is usually recommended to give the same course of treatment to the sexual partner and to ban intercourse for the duration of treatment. The cure rate exceeds 80%. If the first course is unsuccessful a response is often obtained by repeating the dosage. Complete failure sometimes occurs in late pregnancy, to be followed by success after delivery. Failure to respond to metronidazole may necessitate acetarsol pessaries being used. Two pessaries are inserted high in the vagina each night for two to four weeks. The fetus is not affected during its passage through the birth canal.

Candidiasis

This condition is usually caused by the fungus *Candida albicans*. The organism thrives in a glycogen and acid medium and is the cause of approximately 28% of all vaginal discharges investigated during pregnancy.

The *Candida albicans* causes a white or yellow discharge and intense itching of the vagina and vulva. The vagina is coated with a grey, whitish or yellow curd-like substance which is adherent to the epithelium, and if removed causes bleeding.

TREATMENT

Nystatin pessaries 100 000 units inserted for fourteen successive nights is usually effective. Candicidin (Candeptin) vaginal ointment (supplied with applicator) or vaginal tablets (3 mg) may be used as an alternative. One application of ointment or one tablet is used night and morning for fourteen days.

The fetus may be infected by the *Candida albicans* during its passage through the birth canal (see p. 376).

Herpes genitalis

Herpes genitalis is caused by *Herpesvirus hominis* type II. The primary infection may be severe with marked regional adenitis and systemic symptoms. The blisters, which characterise the first stage of herpes genitalis, usually break down within twenty-four hours and present as a cluster of small, round shallow ulcers. Other signs and symptoms include cervicitis, vaginal discharge and dysuria. There is no specific treatment for herpes genitalis.

The *Herpesvirus hominis* type II does not appear to cause intrauterine infection, but infection occurring in late pregnancy is a potential hazard to the baby during delivery. All babies born to mothers with herpes infection at the time of delivery should be isolated and barrier nursed.

Group-B haemolytic streptococci

The pathogenesis and epidemiology of group-B haemolytic streptococcal infection are incompletely understood. The emergence of group-B haemolytic streptococci pathogens in the newborn has focused attention on the mother. The fact that strains from mother and baby are usually identical suggests that infection is transmitted directly from the mother to child during delivery (see p. 378). There appears to be a link with complications such as premature labour and prolonged rupture of membranes. In some centres, women are screened for group-B haemolytic streptococci in late pregnancy and if found to be carriers, treated with penicillin.

Venereal diseases

Syphilis

This disease is caused by the micro-organism, *Treponema pallidum*. The term syphilis comes from Syphilus, the name of the shepherd infected with syphilis in a poem written by Fracastorius in which the disease was described for the first time (1530).

The organism requires moisture for survival, hence the commonest sites of infection are the genitalia, vulva and cervix, and the mouth. The incubation period ranges from ten to ninety days and averages from fourteen to forty-two days. There are four stages in the disease.

Primary stage. A primary sore or chancre appears at the site of inoculation. If the site of inoculation is the cervix the disease will be symptomless and may go undetected. The sore may present as a hard, painless indurated ulcer or as a fissure. Diagnosis is made by examination of the discharge under the darkground microscope. A blood test becomes positive after an interval varying from ten to ninety days. About the same time as the chancre appears or soon afterwards, the *Treponemata* penetrate into the lymph and bloodstream. The lymphatic nodes local to the chancre enlarge painlessly. The chancre heals spontaneously, except for slight induration.

Secondary stage. This appears within six to eight weeks of the primary stage. There is a generalised non-irritant rash accompanied by enlarged lymphatic glands, sore throat and general malaise. The disease if untreated enters the latent phase.

Latent phase. After the secondary phase *Treponema pallidum* tends to disappear from the bloodstream. The response in each case is individual but if the disease is untreated one of three things may occur. The disease may remain latent, except for a persistent positive serological reaction, tertiary manifestations may develop, or a spontaneous cure may occur.

Tertiary stage. The manifestations of late syphilis are rare. chronic inflammatory reactions in the central nervous and cardiovascular system occur.

DIAGNOSIS

Serological tests for syphilis are performed as a routine at the booking visit and include the Reiter Protein Complement Fixation Test and the Veneral Disease Reference Laboratory (VDRL) Slide Test. A positive serological test is not absolute proof of infection and further investigation by another serological test and by the treponemal immobilisation test is required.

TREATMENT

Benzylpenicillin 2.4 g is injected intramuscularly and repeated after two weeks. In penicillin sensitive women erythromycin 500 mg three times a day for twenty-one days is an alternative treatment. Penicillin crosses the placenta and therefore the fetus is treated at the same time.

EFFECTS ON PREGNANCY

Untreated syphilis may cause abortion, premature labour or intrauterine death. During the active stage of syphilis the *Treponema pallidum* invades the placenta from the maternal bloodstream. The organism causes inflammation with endarteritis, and soon invades the fetal bloodstream. In less severe cases the baby may appear well at birth but develop signs weeks, months or even a year later. Early signs include skin rashes, snuffles with sometimes a purulent bloodstained nasal discharge, hepatosplenomegaly and jaundice (see p. 373).

Gonorrhoea

This disease is caused by the Gram-negative diplococcus *Neisseria gonorrhoeae* and has an incubation period of two to ten days. In the female the classical symptoms consist of a white discharge which tends, after about two days to become greenish-yellow. However, at least 30% of women who are infected have no symptoms at all.

There is an increased chance of the disease being overlooked in pregnancy due to the fact that slight discharge due to the pregnancy itself or to other conditions such as candidiasis and trichomoniasis is quite common. Approximately 50% of women who have gonorrhoea also have trichomonas vaginitis.

The disease is unlikely to affect the pregnancy but during labour the baby's eyes are in danger of being infected and the diagnosis of gonococcal ophthalmia in the baby (see p. 376) may be the first indication for suspecting the presence of the infection in the mother. Therefore, full investigation of any vaginal discharge during pregnancy is indicated.

The diagnosis of gonorrhoea in females is very difficult. High vaginal swab alone is unreliable and accurate diagnosis may only be made of urethral and cervical smears and cultures. The Gonococcal Complement Fixation Test is of limited value in the diagnosis of the disease as it is not positive in the acute stage and it is only positive in a proportion of cases of long-standing.

TREATMENT

Procaine penicillin is the drug of choice and a single intramuscular injection of 2.4 g is usually sufficient. It is only necessary to have an adequate blood concentration for twenty-four hours to cure the disease in some cases. Repeat smears and cultures are taken at frequent intervals during pregnancy. In resistant cases the treatment may need to be supplemented with erythromycin, kanamycin, spectinomycin or tetracycline, although the last is contraindicated in pregnancy. Treatment is continued until smears and cultures are repeatedly negative.

The recent isolation of strains of gonococci which can produce penicillinase (β-lactamase) is causing concern as this represents a change in the survival capability of the organism. Following the introduction of penicillin in the early 1940's for the treatment of gonorrhoea there was a significant change in the clinical pattern of the disease due to the sensitivity of the organism to its action. After the initial success it was realised that, although total resistance to the drug did not occur, certain strains were much less sensitive to its action with the doses then used and an increase in the therapeutic dosage of penicillin for clinical and bacteriological cure became necessary. This tendency for a gradual increase in the relative resistance of the gonococcus has continued and has been accompanied by an increase in penicillin dosage required.

The difference between the less sensitive strains of gonococcus, which may fail to respond to the usual therapeutic penicillin regimes, and those which fail because of penicillinase production is important. Penicillin resistance is caused by an altered permeability of the cell wall to the drug; as it becomes less permeable it presents a stronger barrier to the entry of penicillin into the cell thus preventing its destructive activity. This is a gradual process which occurs over a long period of time. Penicillinase-producing strains are absolutely resistant to the action of penicillin because of their ability to produce an enzyme which destroys the drug. These properties are carried genetically and are transferred to subsequent generations of the organism.

Chapter 8
Abnormal Labour

Induction of labour

Induction of labour is a method by which an attempt is made to stimulate labour after the twenty-eighth week of pregnancy and before the onset of spontaneous labour. Induction of labour was introduced in 1756 by Thomas Denman who used artificial rupture of the forewaters for cases of contracted pelvis.

No method of induction is absolutely certain or safe and it is only justified if the risk of prolongation of pregnancy to the mother or fetus is greater than the risk of Caesarean section if it is necessary. The nearer to term the induction is performed the better the results.

INDICATIONS

Pre-eclampsia, eclampsia and essential hypertension. Hypertension is the commonest indication for premature induction of labour. The procedure may be performed because of the effects of the hypertension on the placental function and fetal wellbeing or to reduce the risk of maternal complications.

Prolonged pregnancy. The pregnancy is terminated in the interest of the fetus.

Antepartum haemorrhage. Induction of labour may be performed in the interest of the mother and fetus in the case of severe bleeding or to prevent the complication of placental insufficiency as the pregnancy nears term where a threatened abortion or antepartum haemorrhage has occurred earlier in pregnancy.

Cephalopelvic disproportion. Induction of labour is performed where there is a minor degree of disproportion between the fetal head and maternal pelvis as part of the procedure of trial of labour.

Diabetes mellitus. The risk to the fetus is increased after the thirty-sixth week of pregnancy and induction of labour is usually indicated.

Breech presentation. Induction of labour is advocated about thirty-eight weeks gestation to permit easier delivery of the aftercoming head.

Rhesus haemolytic disease. The timing of the induction depends on the severity of the disease as determined by the liquor bilirubin estimations.

Intrauterine death. The knowledge that her baby is dead is very distressing to the woman and, since this may give rise to hypofibrinogenaemia, induction of labour is justified.

Fetal abnormality. Induction of labour may be advocated in certain types of abnormality.

Polyhydramnios. Induction of labour by hindwater rupture of the membranes may be indicated in this condition.

To avoid the risk of prematurity due to an inaccurate history of the menstrual cycle and last period, investigations of fetal maturity should be undertaken before an induction of labour is planned when the indication is prolonged pregnancy.

METHODS

The methods of induction of labour used in modern obstetric practice are amniotomy (artificial rupture of membranes) and the administration of oxytocic agents, oxytocin and prostaglandins. In practice these methods are often combined.

Amniotomy

Artificial rupture of the membranes is a quick and efficient method of inducing labour. The forewaters are usually ruptured or both the forewaters and hindwaters, although occasionally only the hindwaters are ruptured.

TECHNIQUE

The procedure and the reason for it are carefully explained to the woman.

Artificial rupture of membranes is an aseptic procedure and should, therefore, be performed in a labour room.

Prior to the procedure, the vulval and perineal areas may be shaved and the woman may be given suppositories or an enema. An abdominal palpation is performed to check the lie, presentation and position of the fetus and the level of the presentation. The fetal heart is auscultated.

After emptying her bladder, the woman is placed in the lithotomy position and, following swabbing the vulva with antiseptic solution, draped with sterile towels. The operator, wearing a mask and sterile gown and gloves, makes a vaginal examination to confirm the presentation of the fetus and the state of the cervix. A finger is passed through the cervical canal, and the membranes are separated from the lower uterine segment. Low rupture of the membranes is performed by the use of Kocher's forceps or Goodwin's amniotomy forceps. Once the membranes are ruptured as much amniotic fluid as possible is drained.

CONTRAINDICATIONS

This method of induction of labour is not recommended if there is polyhydramnios, because the sudden reduction in the volume of the uterus may cause placental separation due to retraction of the placental site. Where the fetus is dead, the risk of infection is very high and therefore amniotomy is contraindicated.

DANGERS

There is a risk of prolapse of the umbilical cord if the presentation is not engaged in the pelvis.

Vaginal bleeding may occur if there is an undiagnosed placenta or vasa praevia.

Amniotic fluid embolism may occur, either at the time of amniotomy or some hours later.

The risk of infection is increased once the membranes are ruptured but is minimal if the induction–delivery interval does not exceed twenty-four hours.

Hindwater rupture of membranes is seldom used now as it carries the risk of damaging the placenta. A Drew-Smythe catheter is introduced through the cervix and passed round the head outside the membranes. The hindwaters are tapped by means of a stilette within the catheter. The amount of amniotic fluid drained can be controlled and it is therefore the method used if there is polyhydramnios. Amniotomy may be followed immediately or within a few hours by a Syntocinon infusion if labour is not established.

MANAGEMENT

The fetal heart is auscultated immediately following the amniotomy, then quarterly-hourly for an hour and then at half-hourly to hourly intervals. The amniotic fluid is examined for meconium at frequent intervals. When uterine contractions commence the labour is managed in the usual way.

Oxytocic agents

OXYTOCIN

Oxytocin ('Syntocinon') is the drug most frequently used to induce labour and is given as an intravenous infusion. It may be administered by using two units of 500 ml of 5% Dextrose, one containing 5 units of Syntocinon the other used as a control. The plain solution is used to set up the infusion and the solution containing the Syntocinon is connected to this. The drip rate is gradually increased until the desired uterine response is obtained but not exceeding forty drops/min. The drip rate is adjusted according to the response and the infusion can be switched over to the control solution if the contractions are too strong or too frequent when the drip rate is at a minimum. In this way the vein can be kept open and the infusion reverted back to the Syntocinon if it is required. The infusion rate can be counted and adjusted manually by an observer or automatically by a drip rate counter attached to the infusion.

Cardiff Infusion Unit

This equipment automatically administers Syntocinon by gradually increasing the dose and by means of measuring the frequency and response of the uterus, regulating the dose of oxytocin administered. A concentration of 10 units of Syntocinon in 500 ml of 5% Dextrose solution is used. The dose rate can be adjusted manually by means of a control knob used to set the dose rate or automatically when the dose rate is automatically increased. When the maximum dose of 32 micro units/min is reached the dose rate motor is automatically switched off and the dose continues at a consistent rate. The equipment's control section enables the rate of increase in dose rate to be linked to the strength and frequency of uterine contractions. Because the pump accurately meters small quantities of fluid, more concentrated solutions are used and less fluid is infused. This is particularly important for women suffering from pre-eclampsia. The equipment contains alert condition warnings so that if, for example, the uterine contractions are too strong the pump switches off and an audible alert will sound.

PROSTAGLANDINS

In the latter weeks of pregnancy the levels of prostaglandins rise and this, in association with the falling levels of progesterone, is thought to be responsible for the cervical changes ('ripening') that precede labour.

Prostaglandins stimulate smooth muscle to contract and therefore preparations of prostaglandins E_2 and F_2 are being used increasingly to ripen the cervix and induce labour.

Method

Prostaglandins may be administered vaginally, intravenously and orally.

Vaginal Prostaglandins—Prostaglandin pessaries or gel containing 2.5 mg prostaglandin E_2 (Prostin) inserted into the posterior fornix of the vagina may be used to ripen the cervix prior to amniotomy. The dose and timing of the treatment will depend on the state of the cervix. In a primigravida with an unfavourable cervix 5 mg may be inserted on the evening before or morning of induction. In a multigravida the usual dose is 2.5 mg inserted on the morning of induction. The treatment may induce labour.

PROSTAGLANDIN INFUSION

Prostaglandin E_2 and $F_{2\alpha}$ may be administered by intravenous infusion for induction of labour. This method is proving to be more effective than Syntocinon when the period of gestation is less than thirty-six weeks. Side-effects, including nausea, vomiting and diarrhoea, limit the acceptability of this method.

ORAL PROSTAGLANDINS

Oral prostaglandins in the form of Prostin E_2 may be given as an alternative to prostaglandin infusion. One tablet containing 0.5 mg is given hourly until delivery. When uterine contractions are established the tablet is given or omitted according to uterine activity. Again, the side-effects limit the acceptability of this method, and more recently the tablets have been used vaginally.

MANAGEMENT

Close supervision is essential in the management of labour induced by use of oxytocin.

Observations of the maternal pulse and blood pressure are made at half-hourly intervals and the temperature recorded four-hourly. The fetal heart is monitored continuously if this facility is available otherwise, at fifteen-minute intervals. The amniotic fluid is inspected frequently for signs of meconium.

The uterine response to the oxytocin is continuously monitored if the Cardiff Infusion Unit is used or at half-hourly intervals if this method is not in use. The strength, length and frequency of the contractions are observed and the resting tone of the uterus between contractions. The infusion rate is adjusted accordingly and the concentration of the solution and infusion rate is recorded.

Assessment of the progress in labour is based on the uterine response, descent of the presentation as determined on abdominal palpation and vaginal examination, and the degree of effacement and dilatation of the cervix and os uteri.

Because induction is an abnormal procedure and may be undertaken because of a complication of pregnancy, the psychological support of the woman is very important. The addition of equipment for administering the Syntocinon and monitoring the fetus may increase the woman's anxiety and the support of an understanding and sympathetic midwife, and if possible the presence of her husband, goes a long way to help the woman to accept the procedure.

Premature labour

Premature labour is the onset of labour before thirty-seven completed weeks of pregnancy. This is an important complication of labour because one-third of all low birth weight babies are immature and this is a major cause of perinatal mortality.

Causes

Premature labour may occur spontaneously or be induced because of a complication of pregnancy.

SPONTANEOUS

In 50–75% of all labours which commence prematurely, the cause is unknown and there is evidence that this may occur in subsequent pregnancies. Multiple pregnancy accounts for about 12% of premature labours of spontaneous onset.

INDUCED

Approximately 13% of all premature labours are induced and in about 55% of these cases the reason is maternal hypertension, mainly as the result of pre-eclampsia. Other reasons include placenta praevia and placental abruption, diabetes mellitus, Rhesus haemolytic disease and polyhydramnios.

Management

PREGNANCY

The management is aimed at preventing the onset of premature labour or the need for premature induction and, should it occur, preventing labour from progressing to delivery of the baby.

Good antenatal care is designed to detect early signs of pre-eclampsia and to treat the condition in its early stages. In this way the complications of pre-eclampsia and the indications for inducing labour prematurely can be reduced. The modern management of Rhesus incompatibility should continue to reduce the incidence of Rhesus haemolytic disease. Early diagnosis and management of multiple pregnancy will help to reduce the incidence of spontaneous onset of premature labour.

LABOUR

Attempts may be made to suppress uterine activity by use of the beta sympathomimetic drugs, salbutamol and ritodrine.

1 Salbutomol. This drug may be given by intravenous infusion or orally.

Intravenous infusion. An initial dose of 0.04 mg/minute is given increasing by 0.04 mg/minute every ten minutes until uterine contractions are suppressed. This dose is maintained for six hours and then decreased gradually over the next six hours.

Oral. A maintenance dose of oral salbutamol 8 mg every eight hours is commenced following completion of the intravenous regime and is continued for up to seven days.

2 Ritodrine hydrochloride is a uterine relaxant for use in the management of uncomplicated premature labour. It may be given in one of the following ways.

Intravenous infusion. An initial dose of 0.05 mg/min is gradually increased according to the response by 0.05 mg/min every ten minutes until the desired response is obtained or the maternal heart rate reaches 135 beats/min. The effective dose usually lies between 0.15 mg and 0.35 mg/min. The infusion should be continued for twelve to forty-eight hours after the uterine contractions have ceased.

Intramuscular injection. An injection of 10 mg is given every three to eight hours according to response. The usual frequency is four-hourly and the injections continued for twenty-four to forty-eight hours.

Oral. A maintenance dose of 10 mg every two to six hours is used and the dosage is increased or decreased according to response up to a maximum of 120 mg in any twenty-four hours. The medication is continued as long as it is desirable to prolong pregnancy.

Prostaglandin metabolism is an important determinant of the timing of the onset of spontaneous labour and its duration. Theories being put forward suggest an antiprostaglandin could prove to be important in reducing the incidence of premature labour but evidence suggests they may have dangerous effects on the fetus.

Management of premature labour

The management of uncomplicated premature labour differs little from that of labour commencing at term, although certain points need to be emphasised. In addition the labour may be complicated by the presence of an obstetric complication such as pre-eclampsia.

The obstetrician is informed of the woman's admission and the paediatrician and staff of the Special Care Baby Unit are notified that there is a woman in premature labour. Continuous monitoring of the fetal heart should be undertaken if the facilities are available as this is an 'at risk' fetus.

The use of respiratory depressant drugs in the first stage of labour should be kept to a minimum because of the risk of asphyxia of the baby at birth. Epidural anaesthesia or nitrous oxide and oxygen may be more suitable methods unless contraindicated.

The second stage of labour may be conducted in one of two ways. A short second stage with elective episiotomy to protect the soft fetal head may be permitted or an elective forceps delivery may be performed. A paediatrician should be present at delivery to undertake resuscitation of the baby should it be required.

Following delivery the baby is transferred to the Special Care Baby Unit (see p. 351).

Abnormal uterine action

It is important for the student to understand the physiology and management of normal labour before considering abnormal labour because the latter is an extension of the former rather than a separate entity. Many of the causes of abnormal uterine action are a reversal of the normal process, e.g. polarity, a feature of normal uterine action, describes the opposite and contrasting functions of the upper and lower uterine segments. The contractions in the upper uterine segment are stronger and more sustained than in the lower uterine segment and retraction occurs in the upper uterine segment, whereas relaxation occurs in the lower uterine segment. Loss or reversal of polarity may be a feature of abnormal uterine action. Therefore, unless the student understands polarity she will never understand loss or reversal of polarity.

The student is therefore recommended to read again the section on normal uterine action (see p. 72) before proceeding to read this section.

The introduction of partographs and the active management of labour has prevented many of the problems associated with abnormal uterine action and prolonged labour. However, delay in cervical dilatation due to inefficient uterine activity continues to occur and the midwife must be aware of these, as failure to recognise an abnormality in uterine action can lead to unnecessary prolongation of labour.

Types of abnormal uterine action

1 HYPOTONIC UTERINE ACTION

The uterine action is weak and the upper uterine segment does not contract strongly enough to efface the cervix and dilate the os uteri. The tone of the contractions is usually less than 25 mmHg. The uterus relaxes between contractions which are not only weak but infrequent and of short duration. There is minimal interference with the uteroplacental blood flow and the fetus is in no immediate danger.

Primary hypotonic uterine action. The uterine contractions are weak from the onset of labour.

The cause of primary hypotonic uterine action is unknown but it may be associated with muscular development and nerve innervation or hormonal factors. It is rarely seen in a multigravida.

Secondary hypotonic uterine action. The uterine contractions are of normal strength, length and frequency at first becoming weak, short and infrequent.

Secondary hypotonic uterine action may occur as the result of cephalopelvic disproportion which may be due to a contracted pelvis or malposition or malpresentation of the fetus. Overdistension of the uterus due to a large fetus, multiple pregnancy or polyhydramnios may affect the contractile power of the uterus. An overdistended, atonic bladder will reflexly affect uterine contractions. Uterine activity usually increases in efficiency with parity but with each pregnancy, muscle fibres are replaced by fibrous tissue and eventual uterine action becomes less effective.

2 HYPERTONIC UTERINE ACTION

The uterine action is excessive and may be of normal or abnormal distribution.

Precipitate labour. There is normal polarity and, in the absence of cephalopelvic disproportion, labour progresses rapidly and is completed within two hours. This type of uterine action is found more commonly in parous women. Once a woman has had a precipitate labour subsequent labours are liable to be even shorter.

A very rapid labour can be very alarming for the woman who may deliver in the ambulance on the way to hospital or at home before the midwife arrives. There is an increased risk of lacerations of the cervix and perineum due to rapid delivery. Primary postpartum haemorrhage, retained placenta or inverted uterus may occur due to sudden relaxation of the uterus following the birth of the baby. Fetal hypoxia may occur due to the strong uterine contractions or cerebral injury due to late engagement of the fetal head and rapid moulding and decompression.

Bandl's ring. This abnormality occurs as the result of an obstructed labour due to cephalopelvic disproportion. The uterus continues to contract and retract in an attempt to overcome the obstruction. The upper uterine segment becomes progressively shorter and thicker; the lower uterine segment becomes progressively longer and thinner, and the line of demarcation between the two segments, the retraction ring, becomes more marked. Eventually the retraction ring can be seen and felt through the abdominal wall and is known as Bandl's ring. If labour is allowed to continue the ridge rises progressively due to continued shortening of the upper uterine segment. The uterine contractions become stronger and longer and the interval between the contractions shortens until eventually the uterus is contracting continuously.

Because there has been excessive thinning out of the lower uterine segment there is the danger of uterine rupture. This type of uterine action only occurs in multiparous women, the response of the primigravid uterus would be to stop contracting, resulting in secondary hypotonic uterine action.

Tonic contraction. The whole of the uterus is in a state of sustained and powerful contraction and has moulded itself to the fetus. This is a manifestation of obstructed labour.

Incoordinate uterine action. This type of uterine action occurs when the polarity of the uterus is lost or reversed and there is loss of the pacemaker of the uterus leading to failure of synchronisation between the two lateral halves of the uterus. Spasmodic contractions occur in various parts of the uterus. The tone of the uterus is high but because of the lack of coordination the contractions are ineffective at dilating the os uteri. The resting tone is also high and this leads to the woman experiencing pain in between the contractions and to continued interference with the placental blood flow. The woman complains of colicky pains exceeding the length of the palpable contraction, unlike normal uterine action when the observer can palpate the contraction before and after the woman herself is aware of it.

The cause of incoordinate uterine action is unknown but malpresentation and malposition of the fetus and cephalopelvic disproportion may be underlying causes.

Constriction ring. This is a localised form of incoordinate uterine action where there is spasm of part of the uterus. The most usual site is at the junction of the upper and lower uterine segments. The constriction ring encircles the fetus around a depression in the fetal outline, usually the neck, and prevents further descent from taking place. The lower uterine segment is not excessively thinned out so there is no danger of uterine rupture.

Hypertonic uterine action interferes to a greater or lesser extent with uteroplacental blood flow which stops when the uterine pressure is 100–120 mmHg, therefore, the risk to the fetus is high. This risk is increased in the presence of incoordinate uterine action, when not only is there interference to the uteroplacental blood flow during a contraction, but, because the resting tone of the uterus is high, the blood flow does not return to normal between contractions. This rapidly leads to intrauterine hypoxia which will eventually progress to anoxia and fetal death.

3 CERVICAL DYSTOCIA

This is a rare condition in which there are normal uterine contractions but the cervix fails to dilate. This may occur as a result of a developmental abnormality or due to fibrosis and scarring.

With the exception of hypertonic uterine action, which leads to precipitate labour in the absence of disproportion, all the other types of abnormal uterine action lead to prolongation of labour and their management will be considered in that section (see p. 270).

Abnormal pelves

Radiological studies have shown that there are four basic types of pelvis, although in clinical practice very few pelves fit the criteria exactly. The four main types of pelvis are gynaecoid, android, anthropoid and platypelloid.

The size is the most important factor relating to the pelvis because if the pelvic dimensions are large enough the fetal head will have no mechanical difficulty in its passage through the pelvis. The shape of the pelvis is of secondary importance because only if the pelvic diameters are small in relation to those of the fetal head passing through it will mechanical difficulty occur.

Contracted pelvis

This term is used to describe a bony pelvis having one or more of its diameters reduced by a centimetre or more, and may apply to any of the four main types of pelvis.

GYNAECOID PELVIS

This pelvis has been described elsewhere (see p. 105) and the student is advised to read again the section describing the gynaecoid pelvis in order to be able to compare the variations in pelvic shape and how these may affect the outcome of labour.

Justominor pelvis. This is the small gynaecoid pelvis. All the diameters are equally reduced, therefore, although this is a contracted pelvis, the basic shape of the gynaecoid pelvis is retained. This type of pelvis is found in women of small stature, petite with small hands and feet.

The outcome of labour depends on the size of the fetus. If the fetus is small then labour will progress normally but if the fetus is of average or above average size cephalopelvic disproportion will occur.

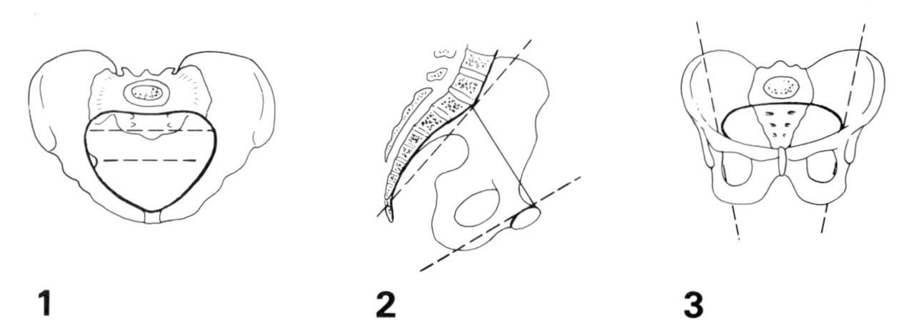

Fig. 8.1 The android pelvis; 1, inlet; 2, cavity; 3, outlet.

ANDROID PELVIS

This is the male type of pelvis (Fig. 8.1).

Inlet. The inlet is heart-shaped. The iliopectineal lines and superior pubic rami are straight forming a sharply angulated, narrow fore-pelvis. The widest transverse diameter is nearer the sacral promontory than it is in a gynaecoid pelvis, thus the posterior section of the pelvis is shallow. The narrow fore-pelvis predisposes to occipitoposterior position of the occiput, the wider posterior aspect of the fetal head is accommodated in the more spacious posterior aspect of the pelvis. Because the widest diameter of the inlet is nearer the sacral promontory, the head is directed more posteriorly and this may result in the biparietal diameter becoming caught in the sacrocotyloid diameter and the possibility of a secondary brow or face presentation (see pp. 259–261).

Cavity. The sacrum is straight and the side walls converge resulting in a deep funnel-shaped cavity which, unlike the spacious, round cavity of the gynaecoid pelvis, does not encourage the fetal head to rotate. The sacrosciatic notch is long and narrow and the sacrospinous and sacrotuberous ligaments are correspondingly shorter.

Outlet. The subpubic arch is narrowed to an angle of less than 90° as a result of which the fetal head is directed posteriorly onto the pelvic floor with an increased risk of severe tearing. The ischial spines are prominent and, if the occiput has not rotated, the head may become arrested transversely (see p. 251).

ANTHROPOID PELVIS

This type of pelvis is long and narrow, the transverse diameters are reduced throughout and the anteroposterior diameters exceed the transverse diameter. The sacrum is long and shallow and frequently contains six vertebrae. Laterally the sacrosciatic notch is wide and the sacrospinous and sacrotuberous ligaments are correspondingly longer (Fig. 8.2). At the outlet the subpubic angle tends to be narrow. The head engages with the occiput posterior because of the roomy posterior section, it does not undergo internal rotation and the baby is born face to pubes.

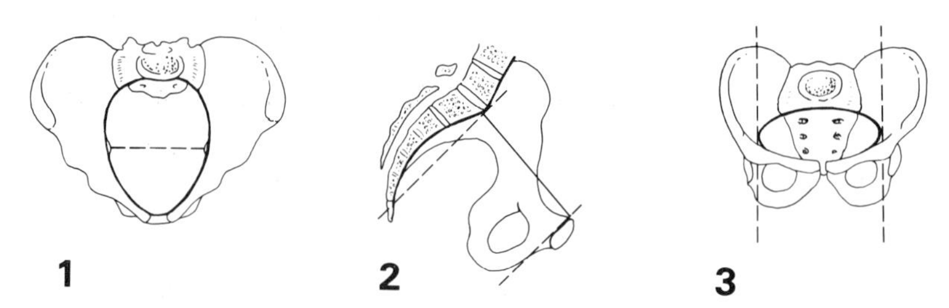

Fig. 8.2 The anthropoid pelvis; 1, inlet; 2, cavity; 3, outlet.

PLATYPELLOID PELVIS

This is known as the flat pelvis. The anteroposterior diameters are reduced and the transverse diameters are increased throughout (Fig. 8.3). At the outlet the subpubic angle is wide. The head enters the brim by a process known as asynclitism. The head is tilted sideways so that one parietal bone, more commonly the anterior, descends first. When the anterior parietal eminence has descended past the symphysis, the posterior parietal eminence is forced past the sacral promontory by tilting of the head towards the anterior shoulder. If the biparietal diameter becomes fixed in the midline of the brim the head may become extended to a secondary brow or face presentation (see pp. 259–261).

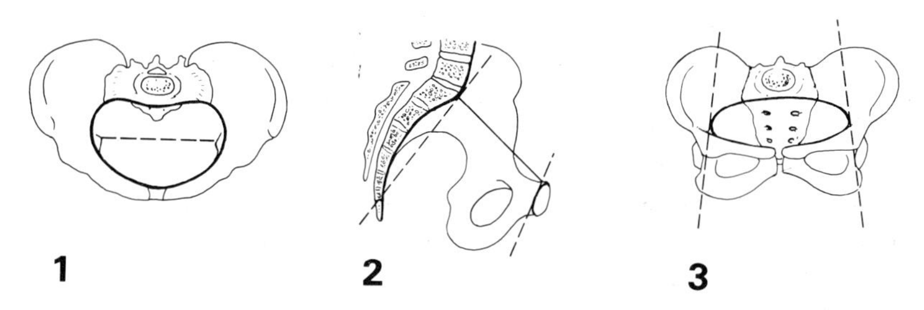

Fig. 8.3 The platypelloid pelvis; 1, inlet; 2, cavity; 3, outlet.

DEVELOPMENTAL ABNORMALITIES

Naegele's pelvis. This is a rare abnormality of the pelvis where there is defective development of the sacral ala on one side of the pelvis and the ilium is fused to the main part of the sacrum.

Robert's pelvis. There is bilateral absence of the sacral alae. This is an exceedingly rare abnormality.

PELVIC DISEASE OR INJURY

In addition to the developmental abnormalities the pelvic size and shape may be altered by disease or injury.

The rachitic pelvis. Rickets causes softening of the pelvic bones and rachitic deformity in early life.

Osteomalacia. A disease that occurs in Africa and Asia, and can cause severe distortion of the pelvis.

Fractured pelvis. Failure of the pelvis to unite following fracture may cause distortion of the pelvis.

ABNORMALITIES OF SPINE, HIP JOINTS AND LOWER LIMBS

The shape and inclination of the pelvis may be affected by kyphosis, spondylolisthesis, congenital dislocation of the hip and abnormalities of the lower limbs. Therefore, it is important not only to consider the woman's stature but also her gait.

Malposition of the occiput

Definition. A vertex presentation in which the occiput is directed towards the posterior aspect of the pelvis and the sinciput towards the anterior aspect of the pelvis. The incidence is about 10%. The cause of malposition of the occiput is unknown but it is associated with abnormal types of pelves such as android and platypelloid.

DIAGNOSIS

Occipitoposterior position can be diagnosed by abdominal and vaginal examination.

Abdominal examination. On inspection the abdomen may appear flat because the fetal back is directed towards the posterior aspect of the uterus. There may be a depression between the pubis and the umbilicus, the space usually occupied by the anterior shoulder of the fetus.

On palpation the fetal back is felt as a ridge in the lateral aspect of the uterus; the limbs are felt under the anterior wall of the uterus on both sides of the midline and the anterior shoulder is felt on the same side of the midline as the back. The fetal head is usually deflexed and the occiput and sinciput may be felt at the same level. The head may not be engaged in the pelvic brim in a primigravida at term.

On auscultation the fetal heart sounds are heard best either in the midline through the anterior wall of the fetal chest or far out in the flank on the same side as the back.

Vaginal examination. In labour a vaginal examination will reveal the head high in the pelvis. As labour progresses and the head descends and the os uteri dilates the landmarks can be identified. The sagittal suture will be felt in the right or left oblique or anteroposterior diameter of the pelvis, the anterior fontanelle will be felt if the head is deflexed and this will be directed towards the anterior aspect of the pelvis (Fig. 8.4).

OUTCOME OF LABOUR

Long anterior rotation

In the majority of cases the head flexes and long internal rotation of the occiput through 135° takes place.

Mechanism. Descent takes place with flexion of the head. The occiput meets the resistance of the pelvic floor. Long internal rotation of the occiput through 135° to the anterior is accompanied by internal rotation of the shoulders through 90°. The occiput escapes under the pubic arch and the head is born by extension. Restitution and external rotations of the occiput is accompanied by internal rotation of the shoulders through a further 45°. The anterior shoulder escapes under the pubic arch, the posterior sweeps the pelvic floor and the body is born by lateral flexion.

Short posterior rotation

The sinciput meets the resistance of the pelvic floor anterior to the mid-point and rotates forwards through 45°, the occiput rotates backwards and the baby delivers face to pubes.

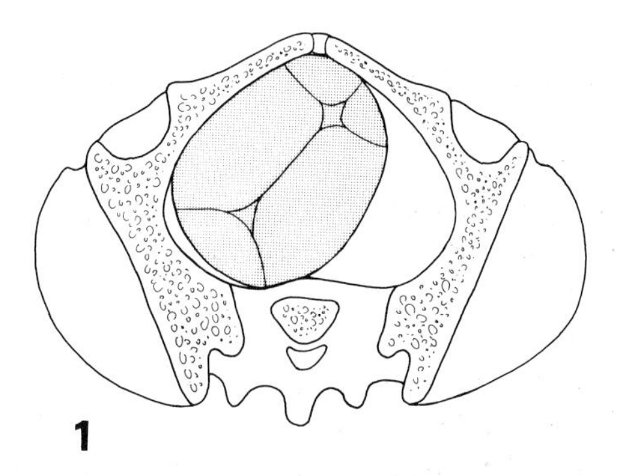

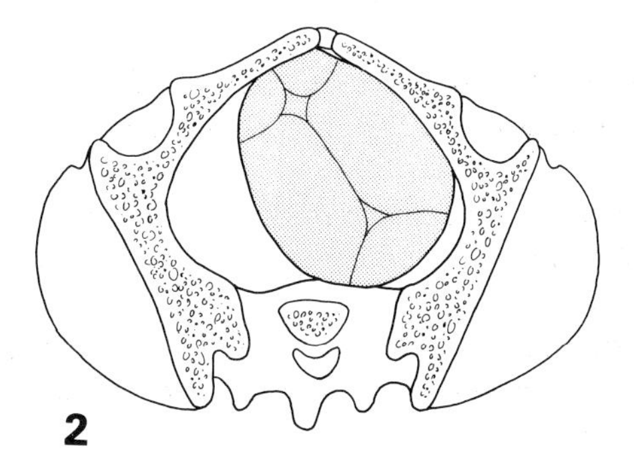

Fig. 8.4 1, right occipitoposterior position; 2, left occipitoposterior position; viewed from below.

Persistent occipitoposterior

The occiput is directly posterior with the sagittal suture in the anteroposterior diameter of the pelvis. As the head descends the occiput remains posterior and delivers as an unreduced occipitoposterior.

Deep transverse arrest

The occiput rotates forwards through 45° instead of 135°, the sagittal suture lies in the transverse diameter and the occiput to one side of the pelvis. Further descent is unable to take place and the head is arrested at the level of the ischial spines. This situation, which occurs in the second stage of labour, is due to one of three factors. The head fails to flex and rotation cannot proceed, failure of the head to flex is due to ineffective uterine contractions. The presenting diameter of the deflexed head is the occipitofrontal measuring approximately 11.5 cm which is greater than the interspinous diameter which may be reduced due to prominent ischial spines. One or more of these factors may be at fault.

Secondary brow or face presentation

Occasionally, instead of flexion of the head occurring at the pelvic brim, extension takes place and a secondary brow or face presentation occurs (see pp. 259–61).

PROGNOSIS

In the majority of cases labour progresses normally, but in a small percentage, labour is prolonged with increased risk to mother and fetus (see p. 271).

Malpresentations of the fetus

A malpresentation is any presentation other than the vertex and includes breech, face, brow and shoulder presentations.

The cause of malpresentation is unknown but it is associated with premature onset of labour, multiple pregnancy, conditions permitting movement *in utero* in late pregnancy, polyhydramnios and multiparity, factors preventing the head from entering the pelvis, contracted pelvis, hydrocephaly and placenta praevia, and uterine abnormalities such as bicornuate uterus.

Breech presentation

There are three types of breech presentation, the flexed or complete breech with both legs fully flexed at both hip and knee (Fig. 8.5), extended or frank breech with both legs fully flexed at the hip and fully extended at the knee (Fig. 8.6), and footling breech where the legs are fully flexed at the knee but partially extended at the hip. The extended breech is the commonest type, especially in primigravidae. The incidence of breech presentation at the onset of labour is about 3% but varies from unit to unit according to the policy for managing breech presentation during pregnancy (see p. 253).

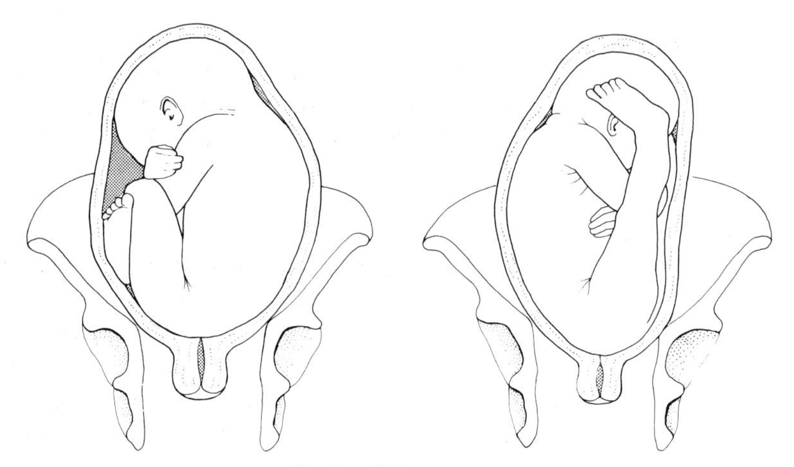

Fig. 8.5 (left) Flexed breech.
Fig. 8.6 (right) Extended breech.

DIAGNOSIS

Abdominal examination. When the breech is presenting, examination of the lower pole of the uterus fails to demonstrate the presence of the hard fetal skull. The fetal head can be felt as a hard, mobile pole in the fundus. The woman often complains of pain in this area due to pressure of the head against the diaphragm. The mobility of the head may not be very pronounced if the legs are extended and splinting the head, and for this reason undiagnosed breech presentation is more likely to occur in an extended breech. The point of maximal density of the fetal heart is slightly above the level of the umbilicus.

Positions of the breech

The four positions of the breech are left and right sacroanterior and left and right sacroposterior.

Vaginal examination. If the diagnosis is uncertain following abdominal examination a vaginal examination will often confirm the suspicion. The soft breech can be felt through the lateral fornices.

If the diagnosis is still in doubt X-ray examination or an ultrasonic scan can be used to confirm the diagnosis. These examinations not only confirm the presentation but the type of breech presentation, the size of the fetus and excludes or diagnoses hydrocephaly.

ANTENATAL MANAGEMENT

There are various schools of thought on how a breech presentation should be managed during pregnancy. In some cases an attempt is made to convert the breech to a cephalic presentation after the thirty-fourth week of pregnancy unless there is a contraindication. External cephalic version is not indicated before this time because due to the size of the fetus a spontaneous version is likely to take place.

However, in some other cases no attempt is made to correct the breech presentation and, if spontaneous version does not take place, an elective Caesarean section is performed or, if there are no contraindications a vaginal breech delivery is planned.

EXTERNAL CEPHALIC VERSION

Contraindications. External cephalic version is contraindicated in pre-eclampsia and hypertension because of the risk of placental abruption; also following antepartum harmorrhage; when there is a multiple pregnancy; in cases of hydrocephaly and in the presence of a uterine scar. If an elective Caesarean section is planned, a version is not necessary, and if there is a hydrocephalic fetus the management of the second stage of labour is easier if the breech is presenting.

Procedure

The manoeuvre is explained to the woman and her cooperation sought, as she should be as relaxed as possible. The bladder is emptied. If the breech is in the pelvis it is disengaged by raising the foot of the couch. The position of the fetus is ascertained and the fetal heart is auscultated. It is essential to maintain the fetus in an attitude of flexion and to achieve this, one hand is placed on the occiput and the chin pressed into the chest. The other hand is placed on the breech and the two hands, working together, gently manoeuvre the fetus round until the head lies over the brim. The head is then pushed into the brim. At the conclusion of the version the fetal heart is auscultated, it is always a little slow after version but should return to normal within a minute or two. If the fetal heart is very slow or absent, the fetus is turned back to a breech presentation. This complication suggests a short cord or cord entanglement. The vulva is inspected for evidence of placental separation or rupture of membranes. Fetal distress, antepartum haemorrhage or ruptured membranes would necessitate the woman being admitted to hospital for observation.

Dangers

External cephalic version is not without risk. The fetal mortality rate is 0.6% but this must be compared with the mortality rate for breech delivery which is 2% in the most experienced hands. The manoeuvre may cause partial detachment of the placenta, early rupture of the membranes or premature onset of labour.

Failure to turn the fetus, especially in a primigravida, is followed by re-examination of the pelvis and fetus by X-ray. A decision as to the mode of delivery would depend on the findings of the X-ray and other factors such as age and parity of the woman. If there is any other complicating factor, such as elderly primigravidity, a Caesarean section may be planned. Careful selection reduces the risks associated with a breech delivery.

MANAGEMENT OF LABOUR

A breech delivery must take place in a major obstetric unit with experienced obstetricians and all facilities for operative intervention should this become necessary. Perinatal mortality rates as high as 30% have been reported when breech delivery is conducted by inexperienced personnel in unsuitable units.

Induction of labour at the end of the thirty-eighth week of pregnancy is sometimes advocated to prevent the fetus from becoming too large and the fetal head too ossified.

First stage of labour

The management of the first stage of labour differs little from the management of this stage when the vertex presents. If the membranes were not ruptured artificially to induce labour they may rupture early in labour, as the poor fit of the presenting part means that the forewaters are subjected to the full force of the contractions. As soon as the membranes rupture a vaginal examination must be performed to exclude prolapse of the umbilical cord. This is more likely to occur when there is a flexed breech. Meconium-staining of the amniotic fluid is not uncommon in a breech presentation due to compression of the buttocks and, in the absence of other signs, is not a sign of fetal distress. Continuous monitoring of the fetal heart should be undertaken where possible, and the maternal condition and progress of labour carefully observed so that any deviation from normal can be detected.

Second stage of labour

The woman may feel the urge to push before the os uteri is fully dilated because the narrow breech can pass through the dilating os. Therefore, a vaginal examination must always be performed to confirm full dilatation of the os uteri before the woman is allowed to push. The obstetrician should be informed of the onset of the second stage, and in addition an anaesthetist is present at the delivery in case operative intervention under general anaesthesia is required. A paediatrician is also in attendance as the baby is likely to require resuscitation. Spontaneous breech delivery will occur in a large percentage of cases whether the legs are extended or not, especially in parous women. The second stage should be allowed to continue with minimal interference so long as progress is being made and in the absence of fetal distress.

MECHANISM OF LABOUR

The bitrochanteric diameter (10 cm) enters the pelvis in the right or left oblique diameter. The movements are:

1 Descent occurs with compaction due to increased flexion of the limbs.

2 The anterior buttock meets the resistance of the pelvic floor and undergoes internal rotation through 45° to the anterior. The bitrochanteric diameter is then in the anteroposterior diameter of the outlet.

3 With lateral flexion of the trunk the anterior buttock escapes under the pubic arch, the posterior buttock sweeps the pelvic floor and the body is born. The shoulders are entering the brim at this stage in the same oblique diameter as the bitrochanteric diameter. The bisacromial diameter of the shoulders measures approximately 11 cm.

4 The buttocks undergo restitution and external rotation. This is accompanied by internal rotation of the shoulders bringing the bisacromial diameter into the anteroposterior diameter of the outlet. The anterior shoulder escapes under the pubic arch, the posterior shoulder sweeps the pelvic floor and the shoulders are delivered.

5 The head enters the pelvis in the transverse diameter and internal rotation of the occiput through 90° to the anterior is accompanied by forward rotation

of the back. The occiput escapes under the pubic arch and the mentum, face sinciput and vertex sweep the pelvic floor and the head is born.

TYPES OF BREECH DELIVERY

There are three types of breech delivery; spontaneous and assisted breech delivery and breech extraction.

Spontaneous breech delivery

This type of breech delivery occurs with minimal interference. The woman is placed in the lithotomy position when the posterior buttock is seen to be distending the perineum, and the vulval and perineal areas swabbed and draped with sterile towels. The bladder is emptied and the perineum is infiltrated with a local anaesthetic in preparation for an episiotomy. This is

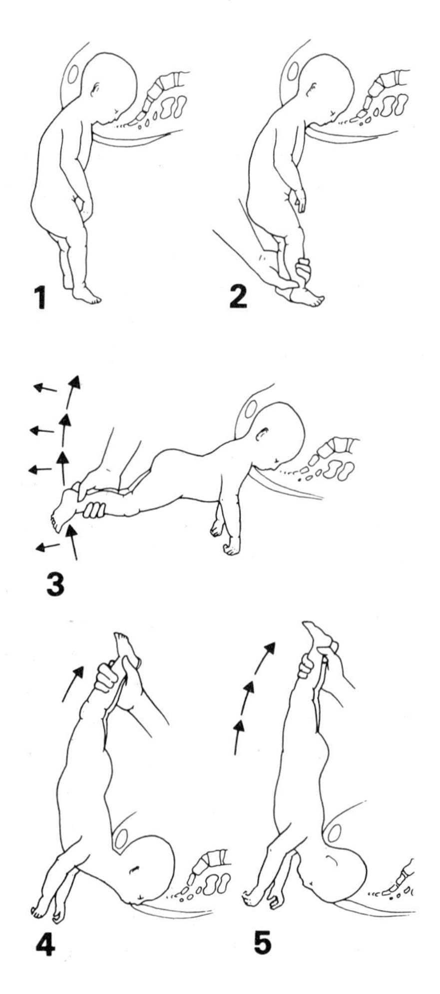

Fig. 8.7 Burns-Marshall technique.

performed when the breech is distending the perineum and immediately the episiotomy is performed the breech will begin to pass through the outlet. As the umbilicus is born, a loop of cord is brought down to prevent traction on the umbilicus. The flexed arms will come down as the shoulders are delivered. The baby is allowed to hang by the weight of its body (Fig. 8.7[1]). In most cases this will cause flexion of the head, and the descent of the body signifies descent of the head. When the hairline is visible the operator grasps the baby's ankle with the right hand (Fig. 8.7[2]) and, exerting a steady traction (Fig. 8.7[3]), draws the body slowly upwards in the arc of a circle towards the mother's abdomen (Fig. 8.7[4,5]). The head is supported by the left hand. When the mouth and nose are delivered the air passages are cleared and the delivery is completed slowly. This method of delivering the flexed head is known as the Burns-Marshall technique.

An oxytocic drug is given as the baby's head is being delivered.

Assisted breech delivery

Complications may present during the course of a breech delivery and assistance is required to facilitate delivery.

Delay in descent of the breech. This may occur due to extension of the legs and, if it occurs, a forefinger is placed on the anterior groin or both groins of the fetus and gentle traction exerted.

Extended arms. If the arms are not across the chest as the trunk is delivered they must be extended and this complication must be dealt with immediately as this will prevent the completion of the delivery. The Lovsett manoeuvre is the method now used for dealing with extended arms and it is based on the knowledge that as the result of the curvature of the birth canal the posterior shoulder must be at a lower level than the anterior shoulder, and that the subpubic arch is the shallowest part of the pelvis. The fetus is grasped by two hands around the pelvic girdle, the thumbs over the back and fingers in the groins. By downward traction, the anterior shoulder is brought to lie behind the symphysis pubis and the posterior shoulder will then lie below the promontory of the sacrum and therefore below the pelvic brim. The fetus is then rotated through 180° so that the back always remains upwards (Fig. 8.8[1]). Moderate traction is used during rotation and by this manoeuvre the posterior shoulder is brought to the anterior and appears beneath the pubic arch (Fig. 8.8[2]). The arm may deliver spontaneously, if not it can be hooked out by digital pressure (Fig. 8.8[3]). The shoulder which was previously anterior now lies posteriorly in the hollow of the sacrum. The fetus is then rotated 180° in the opposite direction, the back again being kept upwards. The remaining arm is thereby delivered (Fig. 8.8[4]).

Delay with delivery of the aftercoming head. When the aftercoming head is delayed at the brim, due to extension the Mauriceau-Smellie-Veit manoeuvre of jaw flexion and shoulder traction may be employed. The baby's trunk is

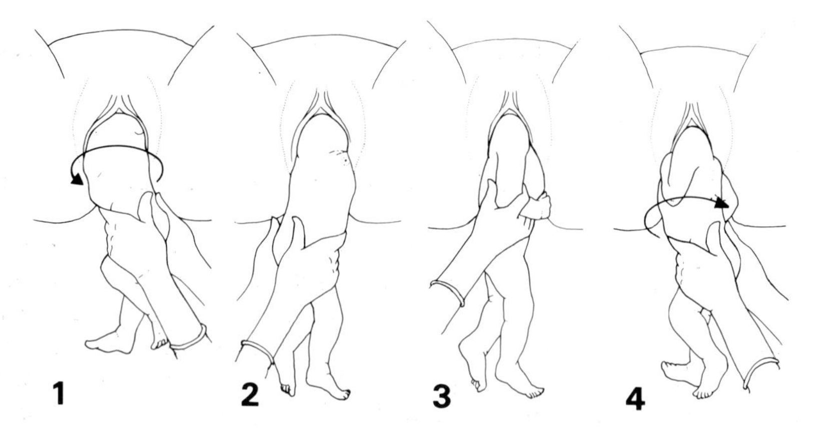

Fig. 8.8 Lovsett manoeuvre.

straddled over the operator's left arm and the hand is passed into the vagina and a finger applies pressure on the jaw to produce flexion (Fig. 8.9[1]). The other hand is passed along the back until the index and middle fingers curve over the shoulders to exert traction. The head will be lying more or less in the transverse diameter of the brim, and it should be drawn through the brim in this diameter by traction on the shoulders (Fig. 8.9[2]). As the head comes down into the pelvic cavity it must be kept flexed then rotated until the neck lies under the pubic arch. Delivery is then completed by lifting the baby's trunk towards the mother's abdomen (Fig. 8.9[3]).

The Burns-Marshall technique and the Mauriceau-Smellie-Veit manoeuvres are rarely used in practice because the majority of breech deliveries are managed by an obstetrician and forceps are used to deliver the aftercoming head.

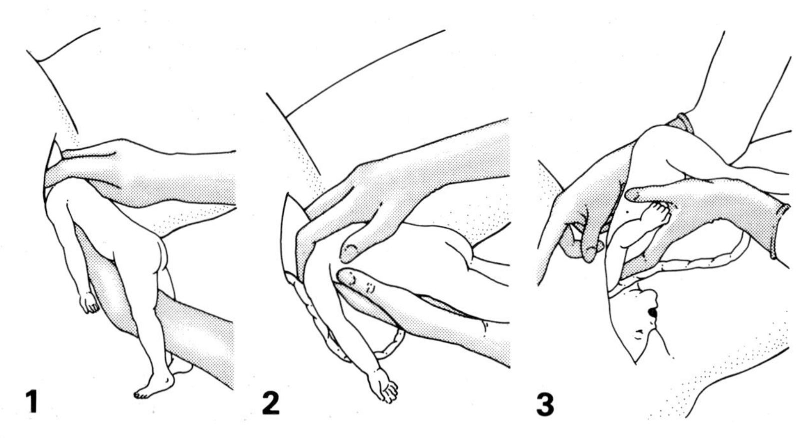

Fig. 8.9 Mauriceau-Smellie-Viet manoeuvre.

Breech extraction
Breech extraction under general anaesthesia is only indicated if immediate delivery is essential because of fetal distress.

DANGERS
The risks to the mother are those related to the operative intervention that may be required.

The perinatal mortality rate varies considerably depending on the expertise of the operator. The fetus is at risk of intracranial haemorrhage which may occur if there is a rapid delivery of the aftercoming head. Anoxia may occur as a result of delay in the delivery and compression of the umbilical cord. Injury can occur to the internal organs if the fetus is grasped around the trunk, and to the limbs if care is not taken with their delivery. Damage to the brachial plexus and sternomastoid muscle may also occur.

Face presentation

Complete extension of the head occurs in approximately 1 in 300 deliveries. Face presentations are either primary or secondary. A primary face presentation is present before and a secondary after the onset of labour.

CAUSE
Increased extensor tone of the fetus may be the cause of this malpresentation. It also occurs in fetal abnormalities such as anencephaly or tumours of the neck. Face presentation may be secondary to a deflexed head accompanying an occipitoposterior position which undergoes extension instead of flexion (see p. 251).

Positions
The mentum is the denominator and the anterior malar bone is the presenting part. The submentobregmatic diameter 9.5 cm presents. Each position relates to a position of the vertex from which they arise thus:
Right mentoposterior is an extended left occipitoanterior position.
Left mentoposterior is an extended right occipitoanterior position.
Left mentoanterior is an extended right occipitoposterior position.
Right mentoanterior is an extended left occipitoposterior position.

The mentoanterior positions are more common because of their origin from occipitoposterior positions.

DIAGNOSIS
Abdominal examination. In a face presentation there is a high prominent occiput felt on the same side as the breech which is prominent in one corner of the fundus. The back is difficult to palpate and the very prominent chest

may be mistaken for it, and the extended head for a well flexed head leading to a mistaken diagnosis of a flexed vertex. The fetal heart is easily heard over the anterior chest wall. X-ray examination may be required to confirm the diagnosis.

Vaginal examination. It may be difficult to reach the presenting part early in labour. Later in labour the orbital ridge may be felt and the nose, mouth and chin identified. Oedema of the face may obscure the landmarks. Care must be taken not to touch the eyes with the examining fingers. The orbital ridge will be felt in either the right or left oblique diameter of the pelvis. The mentum needs to be distinguished to identify the position (Fig. 8.10).

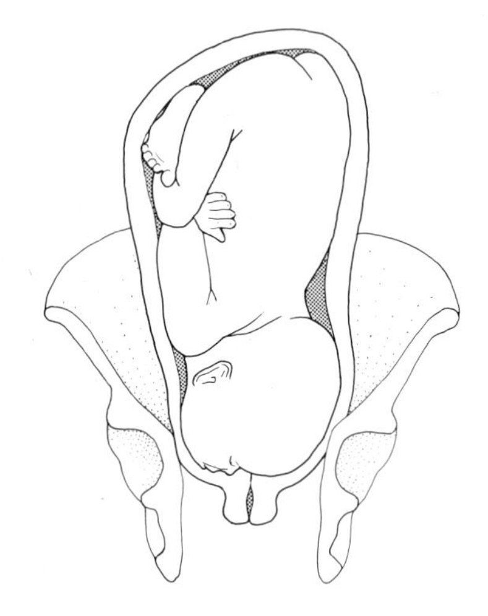

Fig. 8.10 Face presentation.

MECHANISM OF LABOUR

The mechanism is easily understood if the position and the attitude of the head is remembered. At commencement of labour, extension is substituted for flexion and flexion for extension when the head is born (see p. 127).

The movements are:

1 Descent occurs with increased extension.

2 The mentum reaches the resistance of the pelvic floor and undergoes internal rotation through 45° to the anterior and the chin escapes under the pubic arch.

3 The head is born by flexion, the sinciput, vertex and occiput sweep over the perineum. The shoulders enter the pelvis.

4 Restitution and external rotation occurs accompanied by internal rotation of the shoulders.

5 The anterior shoulder escapes under the pubic arch, the posterior shoulder sweeps the pelvic floor and the body is delivered by lateral flexion.

In mentoposterior positions long internal rotation through 135° to the anterior or short posterior rotation through 45° bringing the chin into the hollow of the sacrum occurs. Unless the fetus is small or the pelvis large the direct mentoposterior will be unable to deliver because the relative shortness of the fetal back to the depth of the sacrum necessitates the chest entering the pelvic brim before the chin can reach the pelvic floor. Delay is also likely to occur because the face, due to its irregular features, is a poor stimulus to dilatation, the facial bones are ossified and therefore do not mould, the face is shallow and for the chin to reach the pelvic floor, the shoulders must enter the pelvic cavity. The fetal axis pressure is misdirected to the chin because the head is at a right-angle to the spine.

MANAGEMENT

A vaginal examination must be made as soon as the membranes rupture to exclude prolapse of the umbilical cord.

An episiotomy must be performed to prevent undue delay when the presenting part has reached the pelvic floor and prevent extensive perineal lacerations. If spontaneous delivery occurs, extension is maintained, by pressure on the malar bones, until the chin is born and then the head is flexed to allow the sinciput, vertex and occiput to sweep the pelvic floor. The delivery then proceeds as normal. If the mentum is posterior, time is allowed for spontaneous rotation to occur. If rotation does not occur, manual rotation of the head to the anterior may be attempted under a general anaesthetic, and after rotation, delivery is completed with forceps.

Caesarean section would be necessary if the presenting part fails to descend.

The baby's face is always oedematous and bruised after a face delivery and the parents must be warned what to expect but reassured that it is only temporary.

DANGERS

Because the presenting part is poorly applied to the lower uterine segment prolapse of the umbilical cord is more likely to occur.

Perineal lacerations are more likely to occur because the mentovertical diameter (13.5 cm) and the biparietal diameter (9.5 cm) sweep the perineum.

Brow presentation

This is a cephalic presentation in which the head is neither flexed as in a vertex, nor completely extended as in a face presentation. The attitude is one of partial extension and the longest diameter of the fetal head, the mentovertical diameter (13.5 cm) presents (Fig. 8.11). The incidence is about 1 in 600.

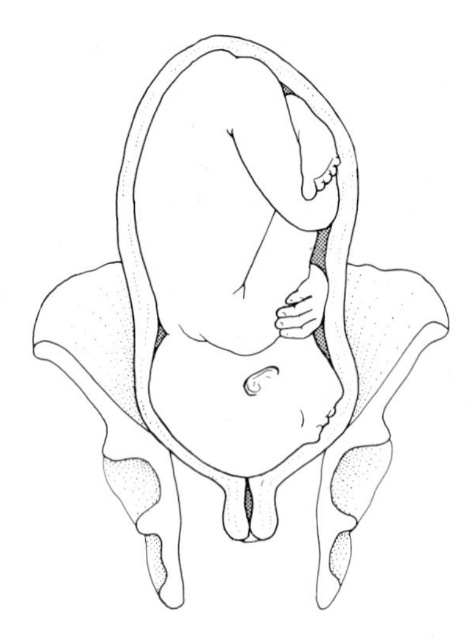

Fig. 8.11 Brow presentation.

CAUSE

The causes of a brow presentation are the same as those of a face presentation. Primary extension of the head may be due to increased fetal extensor tone. Secondary extension may occur in a case in which the descent of the biparietal diameter is prevented by pelvic contraction. More commonly, secondary extension occurs in cases of occipitoposterior position without disproportion. The wide occipital part of the head is arrested in the sacrocotyloid diameter of the pelvis, and the sinciput descends and extension of the head occurs.

DIAGNOSIS

Abdominal examination. The head does not descend into the pelvis and this presentation is suspected if the head fails to engage. The head may be free above the brim or the forepart of the head may become fixed in the brim in labour. The occiput is not so prominent as in a face presentation and the space between the occiput and the back is more marked. This can lead to confusion with a partially flexed head if the fetal back is not carefully identified. The chin may also be felt by dipping the fingers into the pelvis on the opposite side to the occiput.

Vaginal examination. The presenting part is usually very high. If the head can be reached the anterior fontanelle will be felt centrally and the orbital ridge and root of the nose may be identified. If labour has been in progress for some time the landmarks are likely to be obscured by a caput succedaneum.

MANAGEMENT

Because the presenting diameter exceeds all the pelvic dimensions a vaginal delivery is not possible unless the fetus is small and the pelvis is large. Therefore, if labour continues it will become obstructed with considerable risk to the fetus and the mother.

The midwife must inform the doctor as soon as she suspects a brow presentation. In the absence of pelvic contraction a short trial of labour may be undertaken, and this may result in further extension of the head to a face presentation and engagement in the pelvic brim. If the head fails to engage a Caesarean section is performed. If the head enters the pelvic cavity in an occipitoposterior position and undergoes extension within the cavity the chin will be directed anteriorly. The os uteri becomes fully dilated but the head is arrested. In these circumstances, if the occiput is rotated anteriorly, flexion of the head occurs and vaginal delivery with forceps is usually possible. A hand is inserted behind the occiput in the hollow of the sacrum and is flexed and rotated to an occipitoanterior position. Delivery is then completed with the forceps. Alternatively, Kjelland's forceps may be used to effect flexion and rotation.

Abnormal lie and shoulder presentation

Shoulder presentation is the result of a transverse or oblique lie. When the fetus lies with its long axis in the transverse axis of the uterus the lie is transverse, when in the oblique axis of the uterus, the lie is oblique. Oblique lie is more common than transverse in the latter weeks of pregnancy because the transverse lie tends to be converted to an oblique lie as the shoulder occupies the lower pole of the uterus.

Two positions are described, dorsoanterior and dorsoposterior. The fetal head lies in one iliac fossa and the breech on the opposite side of the abdomen in a slightly higher position than the head.

CAUSE

Abnormal lie tends to occur most commonly in multipara with lax uterine and abdominal wall muscles. It may also be found in polyhydramnios and multiple pregnancy or be due to a uterine abnormality such as a bicornuate uterus. By interfering with engagement of the fetal head, placenta praevia and contracted pelvis predispose to an abnormal lie.

DIAGNOSIS

On inspection of the abdomen the uterus appears wider than usual and the fundus not so high as would be expected for the period of gestation. The outline also appears rather asymmetrical. On palpation the fetal head will be felt on one side of the abdomen and the softer more irregular breech on the opposite side in a slightly higher position. The back will be felt across the midline of the abdomen in a dorsoanterior position (Fig. 8.12) and the irregular parts of the limbs felt in a dorsoposterior position.

On vaginal examination the presenting part will be too high to be felt.

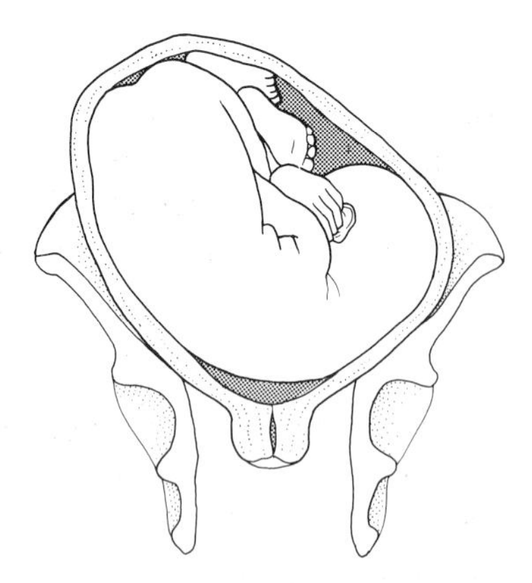

Fig. 8.12 Shoulder presentation—dorsoanterior position.

MANAGEMENT

After the thirty-fourth week of pregnancy the presentation is corrected by external version at each visit to the antenatal clinic. If, however, the abnormal lie persists or the lie is unstable, i.e. varying between longitudinal and oblique or transverse, the woman is admitted to hospital because of the risk of cord or limb prolapse when the membranes rupture or obstructed labour with the risk of uterine rupture if she goes into labour at home.

Following admission, investigations will be made to exclude predisposing causes such as placenta praevia and contracted pelvis which may be interfering with engagement of the fetal head and may influence the management.

LABOUR

After the thirty-eighth week of pregnancy the lie is corrected and a Syntocinon infusion commenced. When the uterus is contracting regularly and the head is over the brim. A forewater rupture of the membranes is performed.

If labour starts spontaneously the lie is corrected by external version if the membranes are intact. If it is not possible to maintain a longitudinal lie, a Caesarean section is performed.

If the woman is admitted to hospital in advanced labour with a shoulder presentation and intact membranes, the membranes may be ruptured under a general anaesthetic and an internal podalic version and breech extraction is performed. Caesarean section is performed if the cervix is not fully dilated.

If labour is neglected the shoulder will become impacted. Labour is now obstructed and uterine rupture and fetal death will occur unless a Caesarean section is performed.

Compound presentation

This term is used to describe prolapse of limbs occurring with a vertex presentation. Commonly it is the hand which comes down, occasionally the foot, and very rarely hand and foot. Conditions in which the head does not fit into the pelvis and lower uterine segment predispose to the presentation as well as intrauterine death.

MANAGEMENT

The arm may go back as the head descends, and active treatment is not required. If the head is small and the pelvis roomy, there may be room for the head to pass, even if the arm remains down. If the progress of the head is delayed the arm may be replaced under a general anaesthetic, the head pushed into the brim and the delivery completed with forceps if the os uteri is fully dilated. When the foot presents with the head, it may be replaced under a general anaesthetic or it may be converted to a footling presentation by pushing up the head. When the head is low in the pelvis, and the os uteri fully dilated, forceps are applied to the head and the foot pushed up out of the way. When the hand and feet come down together, the legs are brought down, and the fetus delivered as a breech.

Cephalopelvic disproportion

Having discussed abnormal pelves and malpositions and malpresentations of the fetus we must now consider the clinical entity cephalopelvic disproportion, that is disproportion between the maternal pelvis and the fetal head that has to pass through it. The disparity between the head of the fetus and the bony pelvis may delay or prevent engagement of head at or before term or in labour.

CAUSE

The cause of cephalopelvic disproportion may be contraction of the pelvis or undue size of the fetus, or of its head.

INDICATIONS

The possibility of disproportion is suspected if there is a history of a previous long labour, difficult delivery or Caesarean section or if the woman is of small stature (less than 1.52 m) especially if she has small hands and feet. The primigravida is an unknown entity and the index of suspicion is increased if she is elderly. The multipara must not be overlooked as the babies' birth weights tend to increase progressively and disproportion can follow several normal deliveries. A history of a previous perinatal death should be investigated carefully as the cause of death may have been a birth injury as a result of cephalopelvic disproportion.

PELVIC ASSESSMENT

A vaginal examination to assess the pelvis is usually performed in the last few weeks of pregnancy when the soft tissues are relaxed (see p. 49).

Assessment of the brim. The diagonal conjugate, which is the distance between the lower margin of the symphysis pubis and the promontory of the sacrum is measured. This is used to indirectly assess the anteroposterior diameter of the brim.

Assessment of the cavity. The concavity of the sacrum, and angle of the sacrosciatic notch and side walls are assessed.

Assessment of the outlet. The prominence of the ischial spines and the interspinous diameter are assessed as well as the angle of the pubic arch and the intertuberous diameter.

ABDOMINAL EXAMINATION

The fetal head is the best pelvimeter at or after the thirty-sixth week of pregnancy. If the head is engaged in the pelvis during the last month of pregnancy inlet disproportion can be excluded. If the head is not engaged an attempt is made to push the head into the brim. This may be achieved by direct pressure backwards on the fetal head when the woman is lying flat or by the woman supporting herself on her elbows at an angle of 45°.

X-RAY EXAMINATION

An erect lateral pelvimetry may be performed and will show not only the anteroposterior diameters of the pelvis but also the general shape and type of pelvis and the relationship of the fetal head to the pelvic brim.

MANAGEMENT

A trial of labour is undertaken for mild to moderate degrees of cephalopelvic disproportion and elective Caesarean section for moderate to severe degrees or if a trial of labour is contraindicated.

Trial of labour

Trial of labour dates from about 1925 and is undertaken in cases where there is a minor degree of cephalopelvic disproportion. It is a necessary procedure requiring great vigilance, for it not only lowers the Caesarean section rate with all its concomitant risks but, if successful, ensures a better obstetric future for the woman.

CONTRAINDICATIONS

Trial of labour is not indicated in the following cases:

1 Elderly primigravida.
2 In the presence of pre-eclampsia or hypertensive disease.

3 Medical complications such as cardiac or pulmonary disease.
4 A true conjugate of less than 9.5 cm.
5 Where there is outlet disproportion.
6 A previous failed trial of labour.
7 Malpresentation of the fetus.

The outcome of the trial of labour depends on the length, strength and frequency of the uterine contractions and the degree of moulding of the fetal head.

MANAGEMENT OF A TRIAL OF LABOUR

A trial of labour should only be undertaken in a major unit where adequate facilities are available for Caesarean section if the outcome is unsuccessful.

Some authorities recommend that labour should be allowed to start spontaneously and that everything should be done to preserve the membranes intact for as long as possible. Other authorities recommend induction of labour at thirty-eight weeks gestation when the fetus is smaller and the head is more malleable. The duration of the trial of labour is variable and depends on the progress being made and the fetal and maternal conditions. Labour is allowed to continue so long as adequate progress is being made, provided there is no fetal or maternal distress. The criteria for progress are the progressive descent of the fetal head and progressive effacement of the cervix and dilatation of os uteri.

A trial of labour may terminate in a spontaneous delivery or a low forceps delivery. If it is unsuccessful a Caesarean section is performed.

The management of a trial of labour is as for that of prolonged labour.

Prolonged labour and active management of labour

We have considered the factors involved with abnormal labour and we will now consider what effects they may have on the length of labour and its outcome, and how these problems can be overcome and their complications prevented.

DEFINITION

Prolonged labour has traditionally been defined as a labour lasting longer than twenty-four hours. This is acceptable as a definition but, with modern management of labour, prolonged labour is unacceptable. The aim is to prevent prolongation of labour by early recognition of signs of delay and active management of labour.

First stage of labour

CAUSES OF DELAY

1 Uterine contractions: hypotonic uterine action; hypertonic incoordinate uterine action.
2 Birth canal: contracted pelvis; cervical dystocia; pelvic tumours.
3 Fetus: malposition of the occiput; malpresentation; congenital malformation—anencephaly or hydrocephaly.

The effects of prolonged labour

Maternal. Exhaustion and maternal distress.

Maternal distress is the result of psychological and physiological changes. Psychologically the woman's morale is low, her threshold for pain is lowered and she may be out of control.

Physiologically the woman is dehydrated and ketotic, there is an increase in the pulse rate, temperature and blood pressure. With good standards of care this condition should not occur however prolonged labour becomes and it must not be confused with the distress shown in response to painful uterine contractions.

Fetal. Intrauterine hypoxia leading to anoxia and death; cerebral trauma due to excessive moulding or hypoxia; caput succedaneum and cephalhaematoma; uterine infection due to prolonged rupture of membranes.

MANAGEMENT

Prevention. Good antenatal care should ensure that the woman approaches labour in a good physical and mental state. Any complications that would lead to prolonged labour should be recognised and, following investigations, the decision regarding the conduct of labour made, i.e. trial of labour or elective Caesarean section.

ACTIVE MANAGEMENT OF LABOUR (ACCELERATED LABOUR)

Active management was introduced in 1969 by Dr Driscoll of Dublin and its aim was to prevent prolonged labour and its dangers. The course of labour is allowed to progress without intervention so long as adequate progress is being made. If progress is slow, active management of labour is substituted. On admission it is determined whether or not the woman is in labour. If it is decided that labour has started, the progress is monitored closely and a vaginal examination performed at approximately four-hourly intervals. If progress is not considered to be adequate the membranes, if intact, are ruptured. If the membranes are already ruptured, a Syntocinon infusion is commenced to stimulate more effective uterine contractions. In this way the majority of women will have completed their labours within twelve hours.

TRIAL OF LABOUR

In an established case of prolonged labour a trial of labour may be undertaken in the absence of maternal or fetal distress or an insurmountable mechanical problem. The management of a trial of labour is as for prolonged labour and involves extreme vigilance and a high standard of physical and psychological care if there is to be a successful outcome.

GENERAL NURSING CARE

This is a very important aspect of the management of prolonged or a trial of labour because the woman's general condition is an essential criterion in the successful outcome. Personal and oral hygiene must receive attention and this includes changes of gown and bed linen as necessary.

Care of the bladder. The woman is offered a bedpan or escorted to the toilet at two-hourly intervals to ensure that the bladder does not become over distended and atonic as this will not only cause discomfort but have an adverse effect on the uterine contractions. The urine is tested for abnormal constituents with particular reference to ketones so that these can be detected and treated to prevent the adverse effects of acidosis on the woman's general condition and on the uterine contractions. The urinary output is recorded.

Diet/hydration. Food is not given in prolonged labour because of the risk of inhalation of stomach contents should a general anaesthetic be required. The woman is allowed sips of water only and this means that an intravenous infusion of 5% Dextrose solution is required to maintain adequate hydration and prevent, or correct ketosis, otherwise the woman feels weak and tired and the contractions become hypotonic. A record is made of the fluid intake. A mixture of magnesium trisilicate, 15 ml is given at two-hourly intervals to counteract gastric acidity and to avoid the risk of acid aspiration if a general anaesthetic becomes necessary.

Prevention of infection. If the membranes are ruptured for longer than eighteen hours there is an increased risk of infection. Frequent changes of pads and the use of the bidet, if the woman is mobile, are recommended. When the membrane rupture–delivery interval exceeds eighteen hours, a high vaginal swab may be taken for culture and sensitivity and a broad spectrum antibiotic prescribed. This will be given intramuscularly as the absorption through the gastric mucosa is reduced during labour.

Bowels. In a prolonged labour it may become necessary to repeat the suppositories or enema that would have been given on admission because the lower bowel will be filling due to food ingested before the onset of labour.

OBSERVATIONS AND RECORDINGS

Extreme vigilance is required in the management of prolonged or trial of labour so that any deviation from normal can be observed and attended to before the mother or fetus is put at risk.

Maternal. The pulse and blood pressure should be recorded at half-hourly intervals as both are good indicators of the maternal condition. Also, hypertension may present for the first time in labour. The temperature is recorded four-hourly unless there is a rise when it would be recorded at more frequent intervals. The woman's physical and mental state is observed.
Fetal. The fetal heart is monitored continuously or, if this is not possible, at fifteen-minute intervals. The rate, rhythm, volume and response to contractions are noted. If the membranes are ruptured the amniotic fluid is observed for signs of neconium.

MONITORING PROGRESS

Careful observations are made of the progress of labour.
Abdominal examination. The descent of the presenting part and the length, strength and frequency of the uterine contractions are noted. Failure of the fetus to descend in the birth canal or the contractions to become progressively longer, stronger and more frequent, indicates lack of progress.
Vaginal examination. The progressive descent of the presenting part and effacement of the cervix are indications of progress in the early or latent phase of labour and continued descent of the presenting part and progressive dilatation of the os uteri in the late or acceleration phase. A graphic method of recording dilatation of the os uteri may be used (see p. 75) and this will demonstrate early any delay in dilatation, and indicate potential prolongation of labour.

SPECIFIC MANAGEMENT

Hypotonic uterine action. Careful examination is made to exclude cephalopelvic disproportion and obstructed labour and this may include an X-ray pelvimetry as well as a vaginal examination. If there is no cephalopelvic disproportion or if there is only a minor degree, an intravenous infusion of Syntocinon is given to improve the uterine contractions (see p. 239).
Hypertonic incoordinate uterine action. This type of uterine action is very painful and distressing to the woman as well as being dangerous to the fetus. The management is aimed at relieving the pain and reducing the tone of the uterus and producing coordination of uterine activity. This may be achieved by the administration of a continuous intravenous infusion of pethidine or an epidural analgesia.
Cephalopelvic disproportion and cervical dystocia. If there is more than a mild degree of cephalopelvic disproportion or if there is cervical dystocia, a Caesarean section will need to be performed.

OPERATIVE INTERVENTION

Maternal or fetal distress, cephalopelvic disproportion, obstructed labour and cervical dystocia are indications for termination of labour by Caesarean section. When there is lack of progress in the absence of the above situations the labour may be terminated by vacuum extraction (see p. 288).

PROGNOSIS

Prolonged labour puts the mother and the fetus at risk.

Maternal

If labour is prolonged due to cephalopelvic disproportion which goes undetected there is a risk of rupture of the uterus due to obstructed labour in the multipara. Uterine rupture is pending if the contractions are very strong and frequent and the interval between contractions is reduced. Eventually there is a continuous contraction and rupture of the uterus is imminent due to the excessive thinning of the lower uterine segment.

Ruptured uterus. The rupture usually occurs obliquely at the junction of the upper and lower uterine segments. At the time of rupture there is severe pain and bleeding may occur into the peritoneal cavity or be lost *per vaginum*. Uterine contractions may expel the fetus into the peritoneal cavity and this will be followed by cessation of contractions which are replaced by a continuous pain due to peritoneal irritation. There are signs of progressive shock due to blood loss and pain.

Treatment must be carried out without delay and involves a laparotomy and removal of the fetus, placenta and amniotic fluid and repair of the uterine rupture.

Maternal mortality. Rupture of the uterus caused fourteen maternal deaths in the three years 1976–78. Seven babies were born alive and five were stillborn. The two remaining cases occurred at the sixteenth week of pregnancy.

Eight of the deaths occurred as the result of spontaneous rupture as described above, three due to scar rupture; two following Caesarean section, one classical and one lower segment, and one following hysterotomy and two following traumatic rupture; one following amniotomy and Syntocinon infusion, and the other after a Kjelland's forceps rotation and delivery.

The mother is also at risk due to operative intervention and general anaesthesia (see p. 291).

Fetus

The dangers to the fetus relate to interference with the placental blood flow leading to hypoxia which if not relieved may progress to anoxia and death.

Excessive moulding may occur and this with the effects of hypoxia predisposes to cerebral injury.

Infection may occur if the membrane rupture-delivery interval is prolonged.

Second stage

If the second stage of labour lasts for longer than half an hour in a multipara or an hour in a primigravida, or if there is lack of progress within these times the following factors may be at fault.

Uterine contractions. Secondary hypotonic uterine action may be the cause of the delay.

Secondary powers. Due to exhaustion, fear, the sedative effects of drugs such as pethidine, or loss of sensation due to epidural analgesia, the woman may be making inadequate use of her accessory muscles, the abdominal wall and diaphragm.

Birth canal. A contracted outlet due to prominent ischial spines or a narrow subpubic arch or a rigid perineum may be delaying progress of the fetus.

The fetus. A large fetus, malpositions of the vertex such as occipitoposterior position and deep transverse arrest, malpresentation or congenital malformation such as anencephaly or hydrocephaly may be at fault. Delay late in the second stage following the birth of the baby's head may occur due to shoulder dystocia.

MANAGEMENT

Observations and recordings

The fetal heart is auscultated between contractions and the maternal pulse and blood pressure are recorded at fifteen-minute intervals.

Assessment of progress

The presenting part should be seen to advance with each contraction. If progress is being made even though it is somewhat slow then, in the absence of signs of fetal distress, the labour is allowed to continue although not longer than half an hour for the multipara or one hour for a primigravida. If, however, no progress is noted after three or four contractions with the mother making good use of her secondary powers, a deep transverse arrest is suspected and the doctor is informed immediately. There is little to be gained by allowing the second stage to continue.

OUTCOME

Episiotomy. If the fetal head is well down on to the perineum a timely episiotomy will prevent further delay (see p. 158).

Forceps delivery. If the head is not low enough for an episiotomy to be performed the doctor is informed and preparations made for a forceps delivery (see. p. 286).

Caesarean section. It is very rare for a Caesarean section to be required but occasionally this is the safest mode of delivery.

Shoulder dystocia. A large bisacromial diameter may lead to failure of the shoulders to deliver and this complication must be dealt with immediately. Delay occurs when the bisacromial diameter of the fetus engages in the anteroposterior diameter of the brim. The posterior shoulder lies just below the promontory sacrum and the anterior shoulder is arrested at the upper border of the symphysis pubis. If an episiotomy has not already been performed this must now be done. If there is already an episiotomy this should be extended to enlarge the outlet and reduce damage to the pelvic floor. The operator then applies suprapubic pressure to the anterior shoulder, pushing it backwards and downwards behind the symphysis pubis. If this is not successful, a gloved hand is passed along the fetal back to the posterior shoulder and rotates it 180° so that the posterior shoulder comes to be under the symphysis pubis. In delivering, avoid putting too much traction on the head as the brachial plexus may be damaged.

DANGERS

There is a danger of overstretching of the pelvic floor and uterine ligaments if the mother is allowed to push too long and this may cause long-term sequelae such as uterine prolapse, cystocele or rectocele.

The risks to the fetus are hypoxia and intracranial injury.

Third stage of labour

Prolongation of the third stage of labour, retained placenta, is discussed in the following section on postpartum haemorrhage.

MATERNAL MORTALITY

There were twenty deaths due to complications of labour in the triennium 1976–78, and although these deaths have been included in the sections dealing with anaesthesia and/or Caesarean section it is worth considering them in this section in relation to the reason for the general anaesthetic or Caesarean section (Table 8.1).

Table 8.1 Deaths due to complications of labour.

Malposition of the fetus in pregnancy	1
Failed induction of labour	1
Delivery complicated by retained placenta	1
Delivery complicated by fetopelvic disproportion	7
Delivery complicated by prolonged labour	6
Fetal distress	4
	20

OBSTETRIC EMERGENCIES

Postpartum haemorrhage

DEFINITION

Postpartum haemorrhage is excessive bleeding from the genital tract after the birth of the baby. Primary postpartum haemorrhage is a loss of 500 ml or more occurring within twenty-four hours of delivery; secondary postpartum haemorrhage is excessive bleeding after twenty-four hours and during the puerperium.

Primary postpartum haemorrhage

Two types of primary postpartum haemorrhage are recognised: haemorrhage from the placental site and haemorrhage from laceration of the genital tract (traumatic haemorrhage).

Haemorrhage from the placental site

To understand the causes of postpartum haemorrhage from the placental site, it is important to have a knowledge of the physiology of the third stage of labour, in particular, separation of the placenta and control of haemorrhage (see p. 77).

In outlining the causes of primary postpartum haemorrhage from the placental site, the women at risk are identified and, therefore, haemorrhage can be prevented by the administration of a quick-acting oxytocic drug such as intravenous ergometrine or intramuscular Syntometrine with the birth of the anterior shoulder.

Causes

Hypotonic uterine action. Weak contractions of the uterus in the third stage of labour may fail to separate the placenta completely, so that it remains in the upper uterine segment and prevents effective retraction of the placental site. In other cases, even though the placenta has completely separated and has been expelled, the weak contractions fail to control the haemorrhage. If the uterus is not completely empty, contraction and retraction will be ineffective. The bleeding may be temporarily controlled by strong contraction following the administration of an oxytocic drug but if a cotyledon is retained or a large blood clot is present in the uterus this will interfere with retraction and bleeding occurs.

Hypotonic uterine action may occur as a result of:

a Prolonged or precipitate labour leading to uterine exhaustion due to prolonged or excessive uterine action.

b Uterine action is less efficient if the bladder is overdistended and atonic.
c Overdistension. If the uterus has been overdistended by a large fetus, polyhydramnios or a multiple pregnancy, there may be loss of retractile power. In a multiple pregnancy the placental site is larger than normal and may also encroach on the lower uterine segment.
d Multiparity. Repeated pregnancies result in fibrous tissue replacing the muscle fibres of the uterus and therefore less efficient uterine action.
e Anaesthesia produces relaxation of muscle and loss of contractile power.
Hypofibrinogenaemia. Associated with concealed placental abruption, amniotic fluid embolism or intrauterine death after an interval of about two weeks. Thromboplastins released into the circulation disrupt the clotting mechanism and intravascular microthrombi occur with excessive utilisation of fibrinogen.
Placental causes. In the case of placenta praevia the placental site is partially or wholly in the lower uterine segment and, because the retractile power in that part of the uterus is poor, control of bleeding is ineffective. If a Couvelaire uterus results, following a concealed placental abruption, the muscle fibres in that part of the uterus may be damaged and fail to contract and retract effectively. In rare cases, failure of the placenta to separate completely may be caused by morbid adherence due to abnormal penetation of the chorionic villi into the basal layer of the decidua or the muscle wall (placenta accreta or percreta).
Mismanagement. If the non-contracted uterus is manipulated, short, irregular contractions of the uterus occur resulting in partial separation of the placenta.

Diagnosis

In the majority of cases the blood loss is escaping from the vagina and the source of bleeding has to be ascertained, i.e. is the bleeding coming from the placental site or from lacerations of the genital tract? Rarely severe bleeding takes place into the cavity of an atonic uterus with little external evidence of blood loss. The situation is recognised if the left hand is kept on the fundus of the uterus.

Management

The management of primary postpartum haemorrhage from the placental site depends on whether the placenta has been delivered or is still *in situ* and whether the woman is in hospital or at home. Postpartum haemorrhage usually occurs suddenly and it is an eventuality that every midwife must be prepared to cope with. Medical help must be summoned at the earliest possible moment and this would involve calling the general practitioner or the Emergency Obstetric Unit if the woman is at home. However, the midwife must continue to cope with the postpartum haemorrhage until medical help arrives.

Bleeding before expulsion of the placenta. The uterus is massaged to stimulate a contraction. This will slow down or stop the bleeding and give the midwife time, if she is on her own, to draw up and give an injection of ergometrine (0.5 mg) intravenously. In an emergency such as this the midwife is permitted to give ergometrine by the intravenous route. As soon as the uterus is contracted, an attempt is made to deliver the placenta by controlled cord traction. If the attempt to deliver the placenta is not successful the first time, a catheter is passed to empty the bladder and, after checking to ensure that the uterus is contracted, a second attempt is made to deliver the placenta by controlled cord traction. If this is not immediately successful an anaesthetic will need to be given and the placenta removed manually (see p. 278).

Bleeding after delivery of the placenta. If bleeding occurs after delivery of the placenta, the uterus is massaged to stimulate a contraction, an injection of ergometrine (0.5 mg) is given intravenously and any blood clot contained in the uterus is expelled. A catheter is passed and the bladder is emptied.

Observations

As soon as the haemorrhage is controlled the mother's condition is assessed and recordings made of the pulse and blood pressure. A fluid balance chart is maintained to record the fluid intake and observe urinary output. The placenta and membranes are examined carefully to ensure that they are complete. The blood loss is measured and the total blood loss is estimated. Blood is taken for cross-matching and if necessary an infusion is commenced.

If bleeding continues bimanual compression of the uterus should be performed.

External bimanual compression of the uterus. A fist is placed on the abdomen above the symphysis pubis, the other hand is placed on the abdomen behind the uterus resting on the posterior surface and the uterus is brought forward and pressed down on to the fist (Fig. 8.13). In this way the posterior wall is pressed against the anterior wall, and the haemorrhage is checked.

Internal bimanual compression of the uterus. One hand is inserted into the vagina, then closed to form a fist with the back of the hand directly posterior and the knuckles in the anterior fornix. The other hand anteverts the uterus in the way previously described (Fig. 8.14).

Occasionally, the uterus does not maintain its tone with the result that

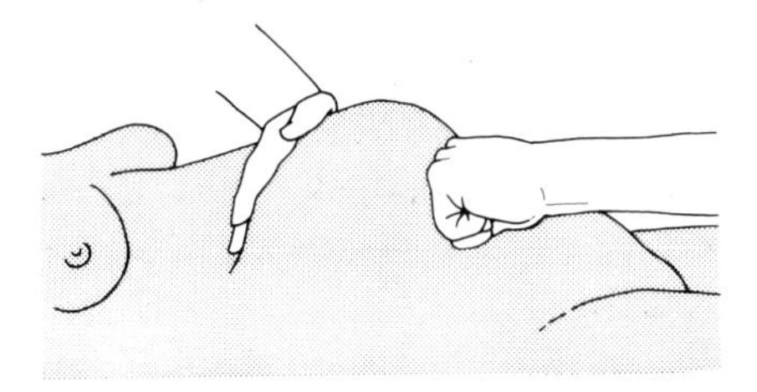

Fig. 8.13 External bimanual compression.

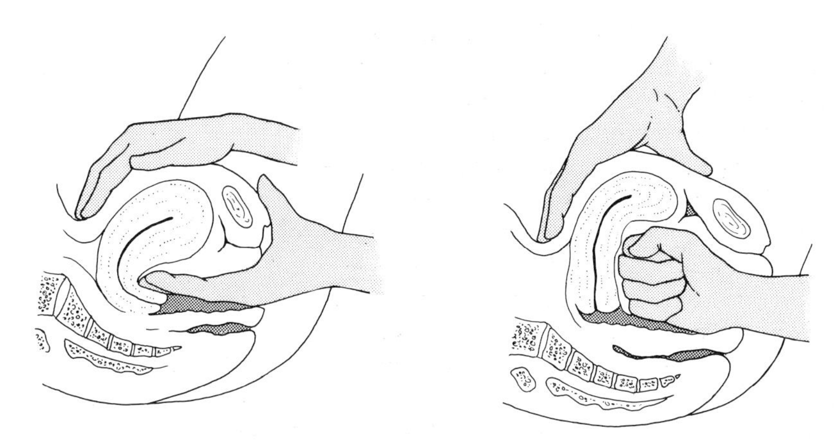

Fig. 8.14 Internal bimanual compression.

haemorrhage recurs. In this event a Syntocinon infusion is commenced. In very severe intractable cases a hysterectomy has to be performed as the only way of stopping the bleeding.

BLEEDING DUE TO A COAGULATION DISORDER

A coagulation disorder is suspected when although the uterus is empty and apparently well contracted there is a steady trickle of blood from the vagina. This blood remains fluid as does blood withdrawn from a vein and allowed to stand.

The cause of the failure of the blood to clot may be due to hypofibrinogenaemia caused by widespread intravascular microthrombi which may cause obstruction of the pulmonary circulation, or fibrinolysis due to excess fibrinolysin in the blood.

Management

Restoration of the fibrinogen level is necessary and fresh blood, or an intravenous infusion of 2–10 g of fibrin or triple strength plasma may be used. The risk of transmission of hepatitis occurs with the latter due to pooling of plasma. An antifibrinolysin, epsilon amino caproic acid (4–6 g) may be given intravenously. This is rapidly excreted in the urine and therefore 1 g requires to be given hourly to replace excretion.

RETAINED PLACENTA

The term retained placenta is used when there is undue delay in delivery of the placenta. The retained placenta may be completely adherent and therefore not accompanied by bleeding or partially or wholly separated when it will be associated with postpartum haemorrhage.

Causes
Uterine atony. Failure of the uterus to contract and retract prevents diminution in the placental site and failure of placental separation.
Constriction ring. The placenta is trapped in the upper uterine segment due to localised tonic contraction.
Morbid adherence. Placenta accreta is a rare cause of retained placenta.

If delay in delivery of the placenta is accompanied by bleeding, the treatment will be that of postpartum haemorrhage before delivery of the placenta. When the delay is not accompanied by bleeding the situation is less urgent.

MANUAL REMOVAL OF PLACENTA

This procedure is performed under a general anaesthetic and therefore the midwife is required to prepare the equipment for a manual removal of placenta and the woman for a general anaesthesia. Prior to the procedure, blood will be taken and an intravenous infusion commenced because of the risk of severe bleeding during the procedure.

Technique
One hand is placed on the fundus of the uterus through the abdominal wall to apply counter-pressure, and the other hand is inserted into the vagina and follows the umbilical cord to its insertion. The edge of the placenta is identified, and then the placenta is gradually separated with the fingers.

Following the procedure an intravenous injection of ergometrine (0.5 mg) is given.

Haemorrhage from laceration

Traumatic haemorrhage may occur as the result of laceration of the vagina and perineum, episiotomy, cervical laceration or rupture of the uterus.

Lacerations would be suspected as the source of haemorrhage if the loss commences immediately the baby is born and continues, although the uterus is contracted.

Management
The midwife must control the bleeding point by use of an artery forceps or pressure. The doctor is summoned and the bleeding point is ligated and the tear sutured. If the cause of the bleeding is a cervical laceration or suspected uterine rupture, the exploration and repair is performed under a general anaesthesia.

SECONDARY POSTPARTUM HAEMORRHAGE (see p. 299)

Table 8.2 A summary of the factors involved in the three stages of labour as they relate to normal and abnormal labour.

Factors involved	*Normal*	*Abnormal*
Powers		
Primary: uterine contractions (first, second and third stage)	Progressive increase in strength, length and frequency	Hypotonic uterine action Hypertonic uterine action Bandl's ring Tonic contraction Constriction ring
	Coordinate uterine action	Incoordinate uterine action
Secondary: diaphragm; abdominal muscles (second stage)	Well utilised	Poorly utilised: maternal exhaustion; non-cooperation—fear; loss of sensation—epidural
Passages		
Cervix (first stage)	Progressive: effacement dilatation	Cervical dystocia
Vagina (second stage	Elastic—distensible	Lack of elasticity
Pelvic floor (second stage)	Stretches, perineal body flattens and elongates	Failure to stretch Rigid
Pelvis (first and second stage)	Gynaecoid	Justominor Android Anthropoid Platypelloid
Passengers		
Fetus (first and second stage)	Normal { lie, presentation, position	Abnormal lie Malpresentation Malposition
	Singleton	Multiple pregnancy
	No abnormality	Abnormality: anencephaly; hydrocephaly
Placenta and membranes (third stage)	Complete separation and expulsion	Retained placenta/ products of conception
	Control of bleeding	Postpartum haemorrhage

Pituitary necrosis

Severe postpartum collapse due to haemorrhage may be followed by ischaemic necrosis of the anterior lobe of the pituitary gland. Death may occur soon after delivery, but if the woman survives she will show clinical signs of Sheehan's disease. The endocrine functions of the anterior lobe of the pituitary gland are disturbed. There is failure of lactation due to lack of prolactin, lack of gonadotrophic hormones will lead to amenorrhoea, atrophy of the breasts and genital atrophy. Lack of the thyrotrophic hormone causes lethargy, weight gain and abnormal sensitivity to cold and lack of corticotrophic hormone results in hypotension and a poor response to infection. Prompt and adequate treatment of blood loss should prevent this complication. Once necrosis has occurred replacement therapy is necessary.

MORTALITY

There were eighteen deaths directly due to postpartum haemorrhage in the triennium 1976–78. In addition there were nine deaths from other causes in which postpartum haemorrhage contributed to the fatal outcome. In these nine deaths there were three cases due to amniotic fluid embolism, three due to severe pre-eclampsia, two to complications of anaesthesia and one to a drug overdose.

Amongst the twenty-seven deaths in which postpartum haemorrhage caused or contributed to the cause of the death, a blood coagulation disorder was demonstrated in twelve.

Obstetric shock

Shock is a term used for a syndrome associated with peripheral circulatory failure and depression of vital functions. Many conditions are associated with obstetric shock, it is not an entity on its own. However, certain conditions are peculiar to obstetrics although some may also occur in other situations. Shock in obstetric practice may be haemorrhagic or non-haemorrhagic in origin or a combination. Most cases of shock in obstetrics are associated with haemorrhage (Tables 8.3 and 8.4).

MANAGEMENT

The management of shock is primarily the treatment of the cause and will therefore be discussed in relation to that cause.

Table 8.3 Shock in obstetrics 1.

Haemorrhagic (hypovolaemic shock)	*Non-haemorrhagic (normovolaemic shock)*
Abortion	Eclampsia
Ectopic pregnancy	Embolism { blood; amniotic fluid; air }
Placenta praevia	Inverted uterus without bleeding
Placental abruption	Postoperative shock
Postpartum haemorrhage	Anaesthetic accidents
Ruptured uterus	Cardiac failure
Inverted uterus	Adrenal insufficiency
	Anaphylactic shock
	Septic shock

Table 8.4 Shock in obstetrics 2.

Hypovolaemic shock: blood loss—abortion; antepartum haemorrhage; postpartum haemorrhage

Trauma: release of histamine due to tissue damage—Couvelaire uterus; ruptured uterus; inverted uterus

Oxygen deprivation:
Obstruction of pulmonary artery: embolism—blood; amniotic fluid; air
Anaesthesia: inhalation of gastric contents—obstruction; Mendelson's syndrome

Endotoxic shock: invasion by virulent toxins, e.g. *Clostridium welchii*—septic abortion; intrauterine death

Presentation and prolapse of the umbilical cord

Abnormalities involving the umbilical cord constitute a grave risk to the fetus because of the danger of impairment of the cord circulation.

There are three conditions involving the umbilical cord.

Cord presentation. A loop of umbilical cord lies below the level of the presenting part within the intact membranes.

Cord prolapse. The umbilical cord descends out of the uterus into or outside the vagina when the membranes rupture.

Occult cord prolapse. The umbilical cord is at the side of the presentation but not usually within reach of the fingers during vaginal examination. This may also cause fetal distress.

In clinical practice it is simpler to consider these conditions as three degrees of cord prolapse.

The incidence of prolapse of the umbilical cord is about 1 in 400 pregnancies.

CAUSES

Any factor which interferes with the close application of the presenting part to the lower uterine segment predisposes to presentation and prolapse of the umbilical cord. Therefore, a well flexed vertex presentation which engages before the onset of labour or soon after tends to prevent prolapse of the cord. The causes include:

Malpresentation. Cord prolapse is particularly associated with a flexed breech or shoulder presentation although it may also occur with a face or brow presentation.

Polyhydramnios. When the membranes rupture a sudden gush of amniotic fluid may bring down the cord.

CORD PROLAPSE

This is more likely to occur if the fetus is small, and may therefore complicate a multiple pregnancy if labour is premature.

Other factors associated with cord prolapse are first and second degrees of placenta praevia and velamentous and battledore insertions of the cord. In these conditions the cord is more likely to be lying low in the uterus. A long cord may also predispose to prolapse. Cephalopelvic disproportion causing non-engagement of the fetal head will also predispose to prolapse of the cord as may multiparity which is often associated with a high head.

DIAGNOSIS

A presenting cord may be felt pulsating through the intact membranes although this condition may be missed. Pulsation may also be felt in vasa praevia in which there is a velamentous insertion of the cord and the velamentous portion crosses the membranes covering the internal os. In prolapse of the cord, the diagnosis presents no difficulty as a loop of cord is felt in the vagina, and may even present at the vulva. A vaginal examination should be performed as soon as possible after rupture of the membranes to exclude or diagnose prolapse of the cord, unless, on previous examination the fetal head was well applied to the cervix.

Slowing of the fetal heart during a contraction or when the woman lies on her side may indicate compression of the cord that is lying beside the presentation. In the case of occult prolapse the fetal heart returns to normal when the woman is turned on to her back or the other side.

PROGNOSIS

The maternal risk is related to the need for emergency operative intervention such as forceps delivery, breech extraction or Caesarean section in order to save the baby. The prognosis for the fetus depends on early diagnosis and intervention and has been improved by more frequent use of Caesarean section. The perinatal mortality rate associated with cord prolapse and presentation is about 20%.

MANAGEMENT

The treatment depends on whether the fetus is alive or dead, and on the degree of dilatation of the os uteri.

Os uteri incompletely dilated and a live fetus

If a cord presentation or prolapse is diagnosed when the os uteri is not fully dilated and the fetus is alive, an emergency Caesarean section is performed. In a case of presentation of the cord the membranes must not be ruptured as intact membranes prevent cord prolapse and also make it unlikely that compression of the cord will occur.

If pulsation is not felt in a prolapsed cord it must not be assumed that the fetus is dead since the fetal heart may still be audible on auscultation.

Immediate action is required to relieve the compression of the cord. This may be achieved by placing the woman in an exaggerated Sim's position and elevating the foot of the bed or the buttocks by use of pillows. A firm pad is placed over the vulva to prevent the cord from emerging, but if the cord is outside, replacement into the vagina may prevent spasm due to exposure. Another method to relieve cord compression is to push the presentation up by digital pressure from the vagina and to elevate the buttocks or foot of the bed. Auscultation of the fetal heart will confirm that compression has been relieved. One of these methods is used whilst preparations for Caesarean section are being made. Replacement of the cord is of no practical value and the knee-chest position causes the woman considerable discomfort and is therefore not recommended.

Os uteri incompletely dilated and a dead fetus

If the os uteri is not fully dilated and the fetal heart cannot be heard it must be assumed that the fetus is dead. Caesarean section is not justified and there is no indication for interference unless a shoulder presentation or a contracted pelvis makes it necessary.

Os uteri fully dilated

If prolapse of the umbilical cord occurs when the os uteri is fully dilated immediate vaginal delivery is indicated. Delivery should be expedited by forceps delivery if the head presents, or a breech extraction if a breech presentation. If a prolapsed cord occurs with a shoulder presentation, internal version and breech extraction or Caesarean section may be performed. A Caesarean section may also be performed in the rare circumstances of pelvic contraction.

Because of the grave risk to the fetus a paediatrician should be present at delivery so that resuscitative measures can be commenced without delay if the baby is asphyxiated.

Inversion of the uterus

Inversion of the uterus is a rare complication occurring in about 1 in 200000 deliveries.

There are three degrees of inversion (Fig. 8.15).

First degree. The fundus is turned inside out but does not protrude through the cervix.

Second degree. The fundus protrudes through the cervix and lies within the vagina.

Third degree. The entire uterus is turned inside out and protrudes outside the vagina.

Inversion may take place either before or after separation of the placenta.

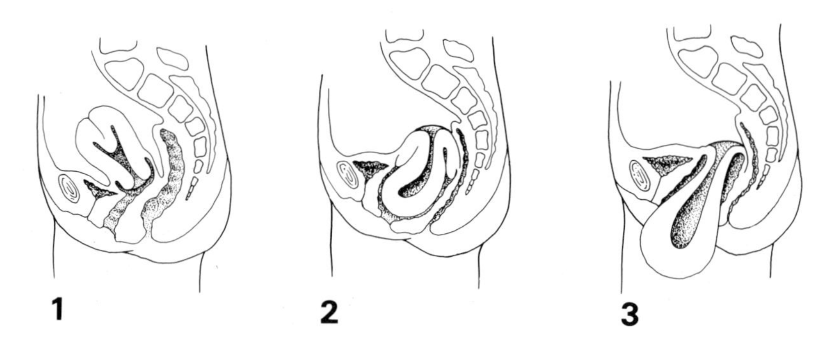

Fig. 8.15 Inversion of the uterus; 1, first degree; 2, second degree; 3, third degree.

CAUSES

The commonest cause of inversion of the uterus is mismanagement of the third stage of labour by applying traction on the cord or fundal pressure when the uterus is not contracting. The risk of inversion is increased if the placenta is attached to the fundus. On rare occasions the inversion may occur spontaneously.

SIGNS AND SYMPTOMS

The main signs are shock and haemorrhage. The shock is usually severe and greater than the blood loss indicates. Unexplained shock during the third stage of labour should always suggest that inversion of the uterus may have occurred. The amount of bleeding will vary according to whether the placenta is separated or not.

DIAGNOSIS

The diagnosis is made by the body of the uterus not being palpable on abdominal examination and a rounded mass being felt through the cervix. Rarely the signs and symptoms are so slight that the inversion is not diagnosed until the condition of chronic inversion is present.

PROGNOSIS

Acute inversion may cause extreme shock and death may occur rapidly due to shock or blood loss when the placenta has separated. The mortality rate is over 40%.

MANAGEMENT

The woman's life is in danger due to the shock and bleeding, and both of these will continue until the uterus is replaced, therefore, this should be undertaken at once. The mortality is higher if replacement is delayed while treatment for shock is being carried out. Following diagnosis an injection of morphine (15 mg) is given and the woman is anaesthetised. The vulva, vagina and inverted uterus are cleansed and the placenta, if attached, is removed. The uterus is then replaced, the part which became inverted last being replaced first, and the fundus last of all. Counterpressure is maintained on the abdomen with the other hand throughout the manipulation.

Intravaginal fluid pressure is an alternative method. Sterile water is run into the vagina from a douche can suspended above the woman. By closing the entrance of the vagina with the hand the intravaginal pressure is raised sufficiently to replace the uterus.

Following replacement, an intravenous injection of ergometrine (0.5 mg) is given to control bleeding, improve uterine muscle tone and therefore, prevent recurrence of the inversion.

Treatment for shock is given concurrently because shock and bleeding will continue until the uterus is replaced, therefore it is not appropriate in this situation to resuscitate the woman before replacing the uterus.

Amniotic fluid embolism

Blockage of the small pulmonary arterioles and alveolar capillaries by amniotic fluid. The amniotic fluid enters the maternal circulation through a hole in the membranes usually when uterine contractions are very strong.

CLINICAL FEATURES

Severe shock with dyspnoea, cyanosis and tachycardia occurs and, if not immediately fatal, hyperpyrexia. Hypotension, vomiting and convulsions may also occur. An X-ray of the chest shows widespread opacities, the central venous pressure is raised, and an electrocardiograph gives evidence of right-sided heart failure. Death frequently occurs and may occur immediately or within a few hours. Haemorrhage manifestations associated with hypofibrinogenaemia due to intravascular microcoagulation occur.

DIAGNOSIS

The diagnosis can only definitely be established at autopsy when the embolus is found to contain epithelial squames, fat, lanugo and meconium, all being constituents of amniotic fluid.

DIFFERENTIAL DIAGNOSIS

Acute pulmonary oedema, pulmonary embolism and inhalation of vomit may present in a similar way to amniotic fluid embolism.

MANAGEMENT

Oxygen is given to relieve the cyanosis and intravenous infusion of heparin to correct the intravascular microthrombi. The shock must be treated immediately.

MATERNAL MORTALITY

There were eleven confirmed and eight suspected deaths from amniotic fluid embolism in the triennium 1976–78 including five with a coagulation defect.

Air embolism

The air embolus may enter the circulation via the placental sinuses or during an infusion. A massive air embolus may be instantly fatal or manifest as severe shock which must be treated at once.

Pulmonary embolism

Obstruction of the pulmonary artery or one of its branches by a blood clot (see p. 301).

OPERATIVE PROCEDURES

Episiotomy

An incision in the perineum to enlarge the introitus. It is a minor operative procedure which is used to increase the safety of many obstetric procedures (see p. 158).

Forceps delivery

The obstetric forceps is an instrument designed for applying traction to the head of the fetus to assist delivery.

This procedure does not fall within the midwife's practice in Great Britain, but all midwives should understand the constuction of and indications for using forceps as they will be assisting the obstetrician at forceps delivery.

Types of obstetric forceps

The obstetric forceps in use today are very varied, but they none the less fall into four main categories (Fig. 8.16): short curved (low cavity) forceps; long curved (midcavity) forceps; Kjelland's (rotation) forceps; axis traction forceps.

Every type of forceps consists of two halves. The parts common to all types of forceps are the handle, shank, lock and blade. The blades have two curves; the cephalic curve in which the blade is curved to correspond with that of the fetal head; and a pelvic curve to correspond with that of the pelvis.

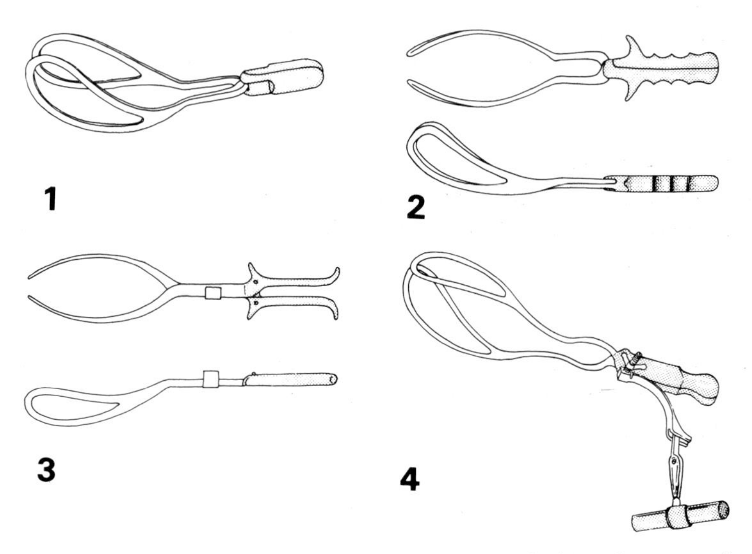

Fig. 8.16 Obstetric forceps; 1, short curved (Wrigley's); 2, long curved; 3, Kjellands; 4, traction.

SHORT CURVED FORCEPS (WRIGLEY'S FORCEPS)

This instrument is for use in low or outlet forceps deliveries and for disengaging the head from the pelvis at Caesarean section. This is a light instrument with short handles and shanks, a fixed lock and blades with well defined cephalic and pelvic curves.

LONG CURVED FORCEPS

This instrument is used for application when the head is in the midcavity and the occiput anterior. The handles and shanks are long, the lock fixed and the blades also have well defined cephalic and pelvic curves.

KJELLAND'S FORCEPS

This instrument can be used when the occiput is posterior or lateral to rotate the head bringing the occiput anteriorly. This is made possible because it has a sliding lock which allows one blade to slide on the other in the long axis of the pelvis and in this way permits the blades to lie at different levels when applied to a head which is lying transversely. The forceps also has only a slight pelvic curve and it is this feature which makes rotation by forceps possible.

AXIS TRACTION FORCEPS

This instrument is fitted with a device which enables the operator to exert traction in the direction of the axis of the pelvis. This type of forceps is now rarely used.

Indications for forceps delivery

1 Delay in the second stage of labour due to:
   - **a** Secondary hypotonic uterine action and poor utilisation of secondary powers.
   - **b** Malposition of the occiput, occipitoposterior and deep transverse arrest.
   - **c** Large fetus.
   - **d** Rigid pelvic floor and perineum.
   - **e** Mild contraction of the pelvic outlet.
2 Fetal distress.
3 Maternal conditions such as hypertension or cardiac disease.

Preparation for forceps delivery

To apply forceps safely and successfully certain basic conditions must be fulfilled.

1 The os uteri must be fully dilated.
2 The membranes must be ruptured.
3 The head must be in the mid or low cavity.

4 The pelvic outlet must be adequate.
5 The uterus must be contracting.
6 The presentation must be deliverable.
7 The bladder and rectum must be empty.
8 An episiotomy is performed.
9 An anaesthetic, usually a pudendal block, is required.
The woman is placed in the lithotomy position for the procedure.

Vacuum extractor (Ventouse)

This procedure involves the application of a suction cup to the fetal scalp to expedite delivery.

The apparatus consists of a metal cup containing a plate attached to a metal chain inside the lumen of the tubing, which attaches the cup to a glass container with a pressure gauge and a pump (Fig. 8.17). A traction bar is attached to the chain in the tubing by means of a pin. The metal suction cups are made in three sizes 40, 50 and 60 mm in diameter. The largest possible cup is used depending on the degree of dilatation of the os uteri.

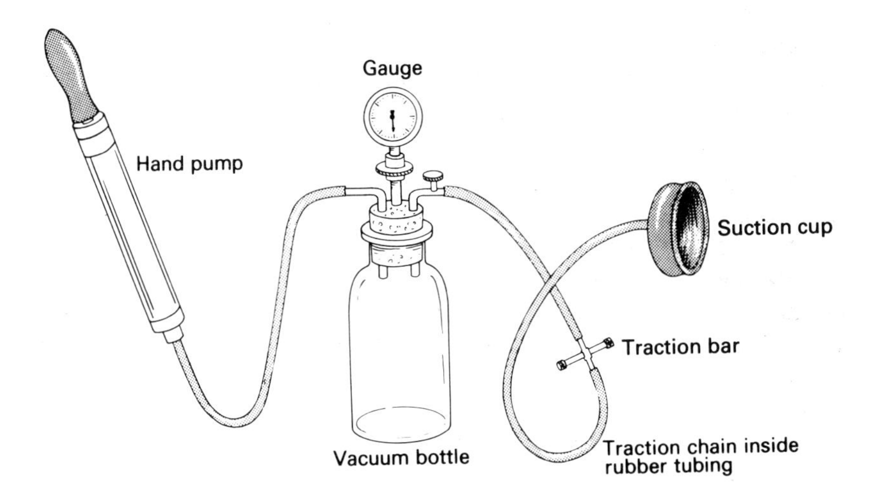

Fig. 8.17 The vacuum extractor.

Indications for vacuum extraction
The indications for using the vacuum extractor are similar to those for which the obstetric forceps are used. However, unlike the forceps, it may also be used to accelerate dilatation of the cervix in cases of prolongation of the first stage of labour or fetal distress when the alternative would be a Caesarean section. The os uteri must be sufficiently dilated to allow application of the suction

cup. The vacuum extractor has the advantage of not effectively increasing the presenting diameter because the cup is applied to the upper part of the fetal scalp.

An artificial caput succedaneum or 'chignon' is formed within the cup. The swelling usually disappears within a few hours and leaves a discoloured area which fades within about a week (see p. 347).

Caesarean section

Caesarean section is the delivery of the fetus through an incision in the uterine wall after the twenty-eighth week of pregnancy. The term hysterotomy is used for a similar procedure before that time.

Two types of Caesarean section are performed:

1 LOWER SEGMENT

A transverse incision is made in the lower uterine segment. This is the method most commonly used because the risk of rupture of the scar in a subsequent labour is low.

2 CLASSICAL

A longitudinal incision is made into the upper uterine segment. This method is rarely used now because of the risk of subsequent rupture of the scar.

The procedure of Caesarean section may be elective or emergency. An elective Caesarean section is performed prior to the onset of labour as a planned procedure with good preoperative preparation. As the name suggests, an emergency Caesarean section is performed as the result of a sudden complication occurring before or after the onset of labour and, because there is inadequate time to fully prepare the woman for anaesthesia the risk of complications are increased.

The national incidence of Caesarean section is between 11–12%.

Indications for Caesarean section

1 Cephalopelvic disproportion.
2 Major degrees of placenta praevia.
3 Fetal distress before the onset of labour or in the first stage.
4 Malpresentation such as brow or shoulder presentation.
5 Prolapse of the umbilical cord before full dilatation of the os uteri.

The indications for Caesarean section have tended to change in recent years. The more effective methods for inducing and actively managing labour has reduced the incidence of Caesarean section for failure of induction and prolonged labour, whereas the more efficient methods of monitoring the fetus have increased the number of Caesarean sections performed for fetal distress. There has been a trend in recent years to perform an elective Caesarean section, more or less as a routine, for a breech presentation, and this has not only increased the incidence of Caesarean section but, because breech presentation is more common in primigravidae, it will also affect the rate in the future as repeat Caesarean sections are common.

The procedure of Caesarean section is usually performed under general anaesthesia although epidural anaesthesia may be used.

MATERNAL MORTALITY

There were ninety deaths recorded as being associated with, but not necessarily due to, Caesarean section during the three years 1976–78. Sixty-five of these deaths were classified as true maternal deaths. In the remaining twenty-five, the women died from an associated illness (Table 8.5).

Table 8.5 Immediate causes of death and percentage of total deaths.

Immediate cause	*Number*	*Percentage of total deaths*
Haemorrhage	10	11%
Pulmonary embolism	9	10%
Sepsis	8	9%
Hypertensive diseases of pregnancy	12	13%
Anaesthesia	20	22%
Other true causes	1	7%
Associated diseases	2	28%
Total	90	100%

RISK TO THE FETUS

The average baby born by Caesarean section does not breathe as spontaneously or as quickly as a baby born vaginally. The anaesthesia causes depression of the fetal respiratory centre which predisposes to asphyxia neonatorum. The indication for performing the Caesarean section is also an important factor. If fetal distress is the cause then a degree of intrauterine hypoxia is likely to have existed prior to the anaesthetic.

A paediatrician should be present at the delivery with resuscitation apparatus available.

In addition to the risks associated with Caesarean section (see Table 8.5), other factors need to be taken into account. Following Caesarean section, the mother usually has a longer stay in hospital and this may involve prolonged separation from her other children. It may also cause feelings of guilt and failure that may adversely affect the mother's response to her baby and, if performed under a general anaesthesia she and her husband miss the actual birth and the important initial contact with their baby is delayed.

The mother who has an abdominal wound will have difficulty in coping with her baby during the initial period of discomfort, and this may not only lead to a problem in establishing a satisfactory mother–baby relationship, but may also create difficulties with breast feeding which may lead to lack of success and further feelings of guilt and failure.

ANAESTHETIC HAZARDS

There were forty maternal deaths associated with complications of anaesthesia in the triennium 1976–78 compared with a total of thirty-one in 1973–75. Twelve of the deaths occurred in 1976, nineteen in 1977 and nine in 1978.

Table 8.6 Deaths associated with anaesthesia.

Complications		*Number of deaths*
Pulmonary complications of anaesthesia		16
Inhalation of stomach contents	5	
Inhalation of stomach contents and endotracheal wrongly placed	9	
Pulmonary oedema and endotracheal tube wrongly placed	1	
Respiratory arrest	1	
Cardiac complications of anaesthesia		6
Cardiac arrest	4	
Cardiac arrest and failure of apparatus	1	
Cardiac failure and endotracheal tube wrongly placed	1	
Central nervous system complications of anaesthesia		7
Cerebral anoxia	2	
Cerebral anoxia and endotracheal tube wrongly placed	5	
Other complications of anaesthesia		1
Gas embolism and failure of apparatus	1	
Total		30

Causes of death

INHALATION OF STOMACH CONTENTS

Fourteen deaths were associated with inhalation of stomach contents, five leading to obstructive asphyxia and the others to Mendelson's syndrome.

MENDELSON'S SYNDROME

Mendelson (1946) differentiated two types of aspiration of vomit; the obstructive type due to solid particles of food and the 'asthmatic' type which is more common in obstetrics and is due to inhalation of highly irritant acid gastric contents. Inhalation occurs at the time of induction or recovery from anaesthesia. The woman's condition may at first appear to be satisfactory but

Table 8.7 Operative procedures for which anaesthesia was given.

Operation	*Indication*	*Number of Deaths*
Vacuum aspiration	Legal termination	2
Evacuation of uterus,	Incomplete abortion	1
dilatation and curettage	Legal termination	1
Hysterectomy	Legal termination	1
Pain relief in labour		1
Forceps delivery	Persistent occipitoposterior position	1
Proposed emergency Caesarean section (died during induction of anaesthesia)	Prolonged labour	1
Elective Caesarean section	Pre-eclampsia	1
	Placenta praevia	1
	Pre-eclampsia and disproportion	1
Emergency Caesarean section	Failed induction of labour	1
	Disproportion	6
	Fetal distress	4
	Prolonged labour	5
	Antepartum haemorrhage	1
Manual removal of placenta	Retained placenta	1
Laparotomy	Ectopic pregnancy	1

soon cyanosis, dyspnoea and marked tachycardia and hypotension occur. A type of pulmonary oedema with bronchospasm sometimes presents and death may occur within twelve hours in the more severe cases and sometimes four or five days later if an aspiration bronchopneumonia supervenes.

Prevention

In order to minimise the hazard of acid aspiration a mixture of magnesium trisilicate (15 ml) is given at two-hourly intervals throughout labour and prior to general anaesthesia. Some anaesthetists prefer the stomach contents to be emptied by means of a stomach tube in the event of an emergency when inadequate preoperative preparation occurs.

Anaesthesia for obstetric procedures should be administered by an experienced anaesthetist in view of the risk involved and the routine use of a cuffed endotracheal tube is recommended.

Management

Should vomiting occur the head must be lowered immediately so that the vomit can flow out of the mouth rather than down the trachea. Suction apparatus must be available to clear the nasopharynx. If inhalation has occurred a bronchial wash-out is undertaken. The woman is closely observed if there has been any vomiting during anaesthesia. If Mendelson's syndrome develops an intravenous injection of hydrocortisone 500 mg is given and oxygen is used as required. Further injections of hydrocortisone 250 mg six-hourly, may be required, and prophylactic antibiotics are prescribed. Digoxin may be given in an attempt to control the trachycardia and intravenous aminophylline (250 mg) may be used if bronchospasm occurs. If hypotension is severe noradrenaline (Levophed) 2–4 mg in 500 ml of 5% Dextrose solution may be used.

HYPOXIC CARDIAC ARREST

Eighteen women died of hypoxic cardiac arrest and the cause was often obscure. Cardiac arrest and difficulty in tracheal intubation and ventilation were problems encountered by the anaesthetist. Hypoxic cardiac arrest is almost invariably preceded by irreversible brain damage.

MISUSE OF APPARATUS

Misuse of the anaesthetic apparatus resulting in asphyxia caused the death of three women. This included misdirection of gases and misconnection of a valve in the breathing circuit.

INTUBATION DIFFICULTY

This was encountered in five cases, twice in association with inhalation of stomach contents and three times in association with cardiac arrest.

Women requiring an anaesthetic for an obstetric emergency are gravely at risk and require the skill and knowledge of an experienced anaesthetist.

An avoidable factor was present in twenty-eight (75.5%) of the thirty-seven deaths.

Chapter 9
Abnormal Puerperium

The abnormalities of the puerperium will be considered under the following headings: puerperal infection; secondary postpartum haemorrhage; thrombo-embolic disease; puerperal psychosis.

Puerperal infection

The causes of puerperal pyrexia are genital tract infection (puerperal sepsis); urinary tract infection; breast infection; thrombophlebitis; respiratory tract infection.

GENERAL PREDISPOSING CAUSES

Anaemia, haemorrhage, prolonged labour, and bruising and trauma.

GENERAL SIGNS AND SYMPTOMS

Pyrexia and tachycardia; general malaise, headaches, shivering and rigors.

GENERAL MANAGEMENT

When the mother presents with signs and symptoms of an infection she and her baby are isolated and the doctor is informed. A general examination is performed by the doctor in an attempt to find the cause, and swabs are taken from the nose, throat and vagina and a midstream specimen of urine is obtained for culture and sensitivity.

General nursing care includes four-hourly recordings of temperature, pulse and respirations. Fluids are encouraged and a fluid balance chart is maintained. Sleep and rest is encouraged and analgesics to relieve pain and sedatives to ensure rest may be required. An aperient may be required as constipation often results.

Genital tract infection (puerperal sepsis)

Following placental separation an extensive raw area remains on the uterine wall. Wounds of the vagina, vulva and perineum may be present as the result of laceration or episiotomy. These wounds may become infected like wounds anywhere else and the symptoms and physical signs constitute the condition which is termed puerperal sepsis.

Causative organisms found in genital tract infections are anaerobic streptococcus, *Staphylococcus aureus*, *Streptococcus faecalis*, haemolytic streptococcus (group A), *Clostridium welchii*, coliform organisms.

Puerperal sepsis is more common after interference in labour by manipulation or instrumental delivery, particularly if there is soft tissue damage. Trauma partially devitalises the tissues and lessens their resistance, thus making invasion by organisms easier. Retained products of conception also predispose to uterine infections.

The source from which the organisms are derived may be either endogenous, caused by organisms already in the woman's body prior to the onset of labour, or exogenous, caused by organisms introduced from some outside source.

SPECIFIC SIGNS AND SYMPTOMS

The uterus may be subinvoluted and tender and the lochia profuse and offensive or in very severe cases of uterine infection, scanty. The time of onset is usually between the third and seventh postpartum days.

SPECIFIC MANAGEMENT

A broad spectrum antibiotic such as ampicillin may be given whilst the bacteriological report is awaited in more severe cases.

Vulval toilet and frequent changes of pads are important aspects of care in puerperal sepsis.

Complications

Infection from the uterus may spread to involve the Fallopian tubes causing salpingitis or to the peritoneum giving rise to peritonitis, or to the pelvic cellular tissue with resultant parametritis. Generalised spread involves entry of the organisms into the bloodstream, producing septicaemia.

MATERNAL MORTALITY

There were twenty-four deaths attributed to infection of the genital tract in the three years 1976–78. Seven deaths were due to sepsis following abortion, eight due to puerperal sepsis and nine due to sepsis after surgical procedures. Of the eight women who died from puerperal sepsis the membranes ruptured spontaneously in six cases; all were delivered in less than twenty-four hours from the time of rupture of the membranes. One of the eight women had labour induced by artificial rupture of the membranes, the other had the membranes ruptured in labour.

Urinary tract infection

Infection of the urinary tract may recur in the puerperium the previous infection having occurred during pregnancy. Predisposing causes include retention of urine which may be due to loss of bladder tone or bruising and oedema of the bladder or urethra. The infection may have been introduced by catheterisation which is sometimes necessary in labour. The causative organism is generally the *Escherichia coli* and the infection can present at any time.

SPECIFIC SIGNS AND SYMPTOMS

Frequency of micturition, dysuria and pain in the loins radiating to the groin and a fluctuating temperature may present.

The diagnosis is confirmed by examination of a midstream specimen of urine or on a specimen obtained by suprapubic bladder puncture.

Treatment includes an increased fluid intake and chemotherapy such as Sulphadimidine or ampicillin.

Anaemia is a common complication associated with infections of the urinary tract and therefore the haemoglobin concentration is estimated and iron therapy given. Tepid sponging may be necessary if the temperature is very high.

Other problems of the urinary tract that may be encountered during the puerperium are:

Retention of urine. If the bladder becomes overdistended and atonic during labour or the early puerperium the woman is unable to pass urine. Difficulty in passing urine may also be associated with bruising and oedema of the bladder or urethra due to pressure from the fetal head. The woman may also be reluctant to pass urine because of a painful perineum.

Incontinence. Paradoxical incontinence may occur as the result of retention with overflow. Stress incontinence is due to laxity of the pelvic floor and urethral sphincter and is seen most commonly in the multiparous woman. Incontinence may very rarely be due to a fistula between the urinary and genital tracts usually the bladder and the vagina. A vesicovaginal fistula occurs as the result of a vascular necrosis due to prolonged pressure which may still be seen in countries where prolonged and obstructed labour still occur.

Breast infections

Mastitis is the term used for inflammation of the breast tissue.

Predisposing causes

Engorgement. Imperfect emptying of the breasts may lead to stasis of milk and engorgement. This is prevented by ensuring that the breasts are emptied following each feed.

Cracked nipple. The infection enters the breast tissue through a crack in the nipple. This can be prevented by ensuring that the baby is fixed correctly on

to the breast and is not allowed to suckle too long. The nipples should be inspected before and after each feed and, if sore, the nipples are rested and the milk expressed and given to the baby by bottle.
Bruising. If the breasts are roughly handled as can occur if great care is not taken during hand expression of milk, the traumatised tissue will be less resistant to invasion of organisms.

The most usual time of onset of mastitis is in the second week following delivery and the causative organism in the majority of cases is the *Staphylococcus aureus.*

SIGNS AND SYMPTOMS

There is often a sharp rise in temperature to between 38.3 °C and 40 °C and a rapid pulse rate. The breast will be tender and throbbing and a wedge-shaped reddened area can be seen over the infected lobe.

Investigations include sending a specimen of expressed breast milk to the laboratory for culture and sensitivity. Breast feeding is discontinued on the infected breast and the milk is expressed and discarded or lactation may be suppressed. The breasts are well supported by a brassiere or binder and analgesics given to relieve the pain. A broad spectrum antibiotic is given until the sensitivity is known when the appropriate drug is prescribed.

If breast feeding is continued after the infection is clear there must be a gradual return to the full feeding time to avoid sore nipples.

DANGER

Breast abscess is a serious complication of a neglected mastitis. The area is red, shiny and swollen and there is pain over the abscess formation. In this situation, in addition to the treatment mentioned above, lactation is suppressed and the abscess incised and drained under a general anaesthetic.

Thrombophlebitis

This condition will be discussed under the heading thromboembolic disease (see p. 299).

Respiratory infections

If a general anaesthetic has been given during labour, postanaesthetic chest complications, such as bronchopneumonia may occur. Acute specific infections, such as tonsillitis or influenza may also occur in the puerperium.

Secondary postpartum haemorrhage

The causes of excessive bleeding occurring more than twenty-four hours after delivery and during the puerperium are:

a Retained products of conception: placental tissue or membranes.

b Uterine infection.

Most secondary postpartum haemorrhages occur within a week to ten days of delivery but sometimes much later.

Indications that the woman is at risk of a secondary haemorrhage are: heavy red lochial loss sometimes containing clots; offensive lochia indicating a genital tract infection; soft, bulky uterus that is slow to involute; a low grade pyrexia and tachycardia.

MANAGEMENT

The condition is potentially dangerous as a large fatal haemorrhage may occur. The midwife must inform the doctor if the bleeding is slight, and, if the mother is at home, she is transferred to hospital accompanied by her baby. If bleeding is severe an intravenous injection of ergometrine (0.5 mg) is given and the Emergency Obstetric Unit is summoned so that the mother's condition can be restored prior to transfer to hospital. On admission blood is taken for cross-matching and a high vaginal swab to exclude or confirm infection. The uterine cavity is explored under a general anaesthesia. Within seven days of delivery, instrumental dilatation of the cervix is not usually required and a curette must be used with caution because there is a risk of perforation. The appropriate antibiotic therapy is given in infected cases.

Thromboembolic disease

Although this condition has been included in this chapter relating to the abnormal puerperium, there has been an increase in the number of cases presenting during pregnancy. The physiological changes which occur during pregnancy include an increase in the plasma fibrinogen levels and a decrease in the plasma fibrinolytic activity. These changes together with the increased blood volume reduce the risk of haemorrhage during and after placental separation but also increase the risk of thromboembolic disorders.

Thrombophlebitis

This is the term used to describe clot formation that occurs in association with inflammation of the vein wall. If the wall of a vein is damaged, repair takes place by formation of small thrombi which may enlarge to form a clot. The clot is adherent to the vein wall and rarely becomes detached, therefore, the risk of pulmonary embolism is minimal. The clot causes partial or complete occlusion of the vein.

Thrombophlebitis may occur in the superficial or deep veins although a superficial thrombophlebitis is more common than a deep thrombophlebitis.

CAUSES

Infection and trauma of the vein wall will cause thrombophlebitis and varicose veins and anaemia will predispose to its cause.

SIGNS AND SYMPTOMS

There is pain and oedema of the leg and tenderness and redness over the affected area. There is usually a slight increase in the temperature and pulse rate.

MANAGEMENT

The affected leg is supported by a firm bandage or elastic stocking. The leg is elevated and active exercises performed. Analgesics may be required to relieve the pain and a local anti-inflammatory agent such as glycerine and icthymal, used.

Phlebothrombosis

Clot formation in the deep veins not associated with inflammation of the vein wall. It is also referred to as deep vein thrombosis. The cause of this condition is venous stasis and the incidence increases with age (over thirty years of age), parity, operative intervention and suppression of lactation with oestrogens.

SIGNS AND SYMPTOMS

In about 50% of cases there are no signs and symptoms. Homan's sign, i.e. pain in the calf and popliteal region on passive dorsiflexion of the foot with the knee flexed, may be positive but is not a reliable sign. The affected leg may be oedematous, cold and white, a condition known as phlegmasia alba dolens.

MANAGEMENT

Thrombosis after delivery is a preventable condition in the majority of cases. Prevention of anaemia and treatment of varicose veins in the antenatal period, early ambulation following delivery and exercises if the woman is confined to bed are recommended to reduce the risk.

When thrombosis occurs, the affected leg is elevated and exercises performed to encourage venous return.

Intravenous anticoagulants. Heparin may be given to inactivate thrombin and increase the clotting time from the normal of five to eight minutes to twelve to twenty minutes. A heparin infusion of 20000 units to 500 ml of dextrose saline solution is given in twelve hours. The anticoagulant effect of heparin can be rapidly reversed by protamine sulphate. Long-term heparin treatment, self-administered by the subcutaneous route, is being recommended when thrombosis presents for the first time in pregnancy and this is continued until six weeks following delivery. The dosage is carefully monitored by laboratory tests because levels of plasma heparin do not remain constant but vary at different stages of pregnancy.

Oral anticoagulants. Warfarin sodium (Marevan) is the most commonly used and prevents the synthesis of prothrombin. Oral anticoagulants are not effective until approximately forty-eight hours after administration of the initial dose. An initial dose may be given simultaneously with the commencement of heparin therapy and a maintenance dose of between 2 and 20 mg a day is controlled by estimation of the prothrombin time.

Warfarin crosses the placenta and is secreted in the breast milk and may cause haemorrhage in the fetus during labour and in breast fed babies. Heparin has a larger molecule and does not cross the placenta and is not secreted in the breast milk.

DANGER

Phlebothrombosis and occasionally thrombophlebitis may result in the very serious complication of pulmonary embolism.

Pulmonary embolism

There is obstruction to the pulmonary artery or one of its branches by a clot of blood which may have originated from veins in the legs or pelvis. Less than 25% of cases of massive pulmonary embolism are preceded by any warning signs.

SIGNS AND SYMPTOMS

The signs and symptoms vary according to the size of the clot. There may be a massive fatal embolism with no warning signs. Chest pain occurs due to ischaemia of the lungs, there is breathlessness and cyanosis due to the obstruction of lung tissue and frothy bloodstained sputum may present.

MANAGEMENT

The woman is sat up and inclined towards the affected side. Oxygen is given and the doctor informed immediately. Anticoagulant therapy is commenced as already outlined and a chest X-ray is performed.

MATERNAL MORTALITY

There were forty-five deaths due to pulmonary embolism during the three-year period 1976–78. This is the most common cause of maternal death. Fourteen deaths occurred during pregnancy and thirty-one occurred after delivery, nine of these after Caesarean section and twenty-two after vaginal delivery. In addition there were two deaths coded as due to abortion.

Puerperal psychosis

Childbirth is the most important event in the life of the woman and her family. No other event has such obvious physical, emotional and social repercussion on the woman or her immediate associates. It is not surprising that such an event should be surrounded with a multitude of myths, old wives' tales and prejudices.

There is no such specific entity as puerperal psychosis the usual psychiatric illnesses are precipitated and modified by the particular stresses associated with childbirth. Not all women are well balanced or emotionally mature and reactions to pregnancy will vary.

Influencing factors: distress about an unplanned pregnancy; fear of an abnormal baby; financial or accommodation problems; fear of rejection by husband; insufficient explanation given by medical and midwifery personnel; effect of the media; depression for no apparent reason.

Indication of pending mental illness

1 Prolonged postnatal depression.
2 Restlessness and agitation.
3 Non-response to reassurance.
4 Withdrawn, quiet and non-communicative.
5 Unnatural sleeplessness.
6 Sudden refusal of food.
7 Strange, irrelevant remarks.
8 Inability to cope with or rejection of baby.
9 Paranoia.
10 Accusations against husband, other mothers or the staff.

The midwife should be suspicious if the mother presents with any of these signs and should inform the doctor without delay so that a psychiatrist can be asked to see her.

CONDITIONS

Neuroses are more common than psychotic illness and a family history is common, particularly in the obsessional states. There is often a family history of personality traits predisposing to neurosis but it is often difficult to know if these personality traits are inherited or acquired.

TYPES OF NEUROTIC STATES

Anxiety states. The most common of the neurotic states presenting with a wide variety of symptoms which last for a few weeks with a tendency to spontaneous recovery. Symptoms include anxiety, a tendency to overrespond to small stimuli, irritability and general emotional lability, sleeplessness, tension, muscular pains and palpitations.

Reactive depression. A mild type of endogenous depression an example of which is postnatal depression.

Hysteria. This must not be confused with histrionics.

Obsessional states. There are two kinds but they may be mixed.

a Obsessional ruminations which are the recurring presence of unwelcomed thoughts.

b Obsessional compulsions which may be based on an attempt to control ruminations.

Duration of obsessional illness is usually months but may be a year or two. If obsessional symptoms appear in a woman who has not shown previous obsessional personality traits or symptoms, an underlying endogenous depressive illness is suspected.

TREATMENT

The treatment of this type of mental illness is behavioural therapy.

Psychoses

These are the more major forms of mental illness in which there is an effect on the woman's personality and all aspects of her behaviour are involved.

The main diagnoses within the category of psychosis are schizophrenia, manic-depressive psychosis and depressive psychosis.

SCHIZOPHRENIA

This is the commonest mental illness. There are no signs only symptoms and these have to be elicited from the woman. Symptoms include:

a Auditory hallucinations. The woman hears voices commenting on her thoughts or behaviour.

b The experience of alien thoughts being put into her mind by some external agency.

c The experience that her thinking is no longer confined within her own mind, but is accessible to others.

d The experience of feelings, impulses or acts being experienced or carried out under external control.

e The experience of being a passive recipient of bodily sensations imposed by some external agency.

f Certain types of delusion.

Definitions
An hallucination is a perception without an external stimulus, i.e. a person hears a voice speaking to her when in fact there is no voice.

A delusion is a false belief which is held with great conviction despite evidence to the contrary and is generally out of keeping with the person's social, cultural and educational background.

MANIC-DEPRESSIVE PSYCHOSIS

A disorder of mood characterised by alternating attacks of mania and depression.

Mania is an elation of mood where the woman feels euphoric and disinhibited. 'Flights of ideas' is characteristic of this condition and in this state the woman's ideas rush along with little apparent logical connection. She uses a great deal of energy rushing around, usually to little purpose as her energies are poorly organised.

DEPRESSIVE PSYCHOSIS

An illness characterised by extreme lowering of mood to the extent that suicide may follow. The woman often feels life is not worth living and generally shows signs of physical depression in addition. The appetite is very poor often leading to serious malnutrition in chronic cases. A characteristic sleep disturbance occurs in which the woman wakes early in the morning and feels depressed on waking.

The cause of psychosis, both schizophrenia and manic-depressive psychosis, is thought to be biochemical and may involve disturbances of cerebral amine metabolism, and therefore the treatment of psychosis is largely by physical and chemical means.

TREATMENT

The treatment of schizophrenia is by use of drugs such as chlorpromazine (Largactil) and trifluoperazine (Stelazine).

Lithium medication, which alters cerebral metabolism has been introduced into the management of manic-depressive psychosis. Acute attacks of mania are managed by the administration of major tranquillisers such as chlorpromazine and haloperidol.

Antidepressant drugs such as imipramine and amitryptiline are used for depressive states, but if severe, electrotherapy may be used.

MATERNAL MORTALITY

There were eighteen cases of suicide in the three years 1976–78, one during pregnancy and seventeen postpartum. Eleven of the deaths were classified as indirect maternal deaths although five occurred more than six weeks after delivery. All five had shown evidence of depression during pregnancy or the puerperium for which they had received treatment. In two of the remaining cases the women had appeared to be only mildly anxious about feeding difficulties and their suicides were quite unexpected. Two cases of suicide were in unmarried mothers.

Seven deaths were considered to be fortuitous as they did not appear to have been related to pregnancy or childbirth. Six of the deaths occurred between two and eleven months after delivery. Five of the women had long histories of psychiatric illness, two of the women were Asian.

THE BABY

In the majority of cases the baby is admitted to hospital with its mother and she continues to undertake its care. If she is breast feeding the baby, the advisability of continuing this is determined by the mother's condition and the medication she is receiving. If the baby cannot be admitted to hospital with its mother or if she is unable to undertake its care, fostering may need to be arranged if the baby cannot be cared for by relatives.

Further reading

BAKER A.A. (1967) *Psychiatric Disorders in Obstetrics.* Blackwell Scientific Publications, Oxford.

DE SWIET M. (ed.) (1984) *Medical Disorders in Obstetric Practice.* Blackwell Scientific Publications, Oxford.

DONALD I. (1979) *Practical Obstetric Problems.* Lloyd-Luke, London.

MCCLURE BROWNE J.C. & DIXON G. (1970) *Browne's Antenatal Care.* Churchill, London.

SECTION III

THE FETUS AND NEONATE

Chapter 10
The Fetus

The fertilisation, development and implantation of the ovum to the blastocyst stage has been described elsewhere (see p. 85). As the trophoblast is developing into the placenta and chorion (see p. 90), the inner cell mass is developing into the fetus and amnion. The intrauterine development of the human individual takes place, on an average, over a period of 280 days. The growth is divided into three stages. The first stage is the pre-embryonic stage lasting fourteen days, in which the fertilised ovum consists of a mass of dividing cells. The embryonic stage, from the fourteenth day to the end of the second month, is the stage in which the embryo has not yet assumed a human form. The fetal stage, from the end of the second month until birth is the stage when the embryo has assumed a human shape and is known as the fetus. During this stage, the various parts of the embryo which were formed and differentiated during the embryonic stage, develop and grow. It is when tissues and organs are actively differentiating, that they are particularly vulnerable to harmful substances such as infective organisms and drugs. It is during the first three months, and particularly the first two months of pregnancy that malformations are liable to occur. This is why it is so important not to expose expectant mothers to these risks in early pregnancy.

Development of the fetus

The inner cell mass projects into the cavity of the blastocyst. The cells in the inner aspects of the mass become flattened and are known as endodermal cells. These cells spread out round the inner aspect of the trophoblastic capsule and the blastocyst becomes a two-layered structure; trophoblast on the outside, endoderm on the inside. The enclosed capsule is now known as the yolk sac. A division occurs within the inner cell mass and the resulting cavity is known as the amniotic cavity, and separates the trophoblast from the embryonic disc.

The central cells of the inner cell mass form the embryonic disc from which the embryo develops. It consists of three germinal layers; an upper layer of ectoderm continuous with the cells lining the amniotic cavity, an inner layer of endodermal cells and mesoderm which develops between the trophoblast and the endoderm of the yolk sac, extending also round the amnion. The mesoderm proliferates to form a thick layer of loosely arranged primitive connective tissue called mesenchyme. A division appears in the mesenchyme and extends almost the whole way round the yolk sac and amniotic cavity.

The division does not extend round completely and the region where the mesoderm is not divided is known as the connecting (body) stalk. The trophoblast and the layer of mesenchymatous mesoderm related to it constitute the chorion. Soon after the establishment of the body stalk, an outgrowth from the yolk sac endoderm grows into it, this is the allantois.

Marked and uneven proliferation of the cells takes place in the embryonic disc. The anterior (cephalic) end of the disc, is soon broader than the posterior (caudal) end and the growth in length is greater initially than the growth in breadth, this causes the anterior and posterior ends to bulge into the enlarging amniotic cavity. At the same time the lateral surfaces of the embryonic disc fold inwards on the ventral surface. By twenty-five days the embryo has reached a stage of development which enables the future fetal structures to be recognised. The embryo is growing rapidly during this stage and is dependent on oxygen and nutrients from the mother's blood conveyed via the developing placenta. It is therefore necessary for the structures required for this function to rapidly develop.

The cardiovascular system is derived from mesoderm and within four weeks of conception, the embryo has a rudimentary vascular system and a heart which is already beating.

The second month of embryonic life is involved with converting the embryo into a fetus, which will measure about 15 mm from crown to rump and has a form which is clearly recognisable as a human fetus. By this stage the head and face are well formed and the limbs are well differentiated into arms and legs with hands and feet with fingers and toes. The embryo begins its earliest movements at this stage. The heart is now well developed and beating strongly and the brain, which is already well developed is thought to be sending out impulses to different parts of the body. The kidneys are thought to begin their excretory function at this time and also the internal reproductive organs begin to differentiate according to the sex of embryo. The liver produces blood cells.

The developing parts of the fetus are very soft at this stage and the skeleton is laid down early to reinforce and support the developing structures. At first the skeleton consists of cartilage but from the eighth week of intrauterine life there is a progressive conversion to bone.

During the third month of pregnancy, the process of differentiation nears completion in most organs and systems. It is now that the external differences between the developing male and female fetuses become apparent. There is the appearance of eyelids, which close the eyes, nails also appear during this time and the ears come to lie in at their proper level on the sides of the head. The fetus measures approximately 50 mm from crown to rump by the end of the third month after conception and most of the organs are developed and more or less in position.

The remaining two-thirds of pregnancy are concerned with the growth of the fetus and maturing of the various organs so that the fetus becomes progressively better able to live an extrauterine life.

Physiology of the fetus

To understand the adjustments the baby has to make at birth it is necessary to have an insight into the fetal environment and the behaviour of the fetus *in utero*. The fetus is suspended in a fluid environment with a temperature that is 0.5 °C higher than the maternal temperature. The fetus usually adopts an attitude of flexion due to limitation in the space available, and this attitude is usually maintained by the baby after birth.

The fetus moves freely within the amniotic fluid during early pregnancy but as pregnancy advances and there is less space available these movements are limited. Although the limbs are skeletal, muscles are developed by about the eighth week of pregnancy, and therefore movements are being made. They are not sufficiently vigorous to be felt by the mother until between sixteen and twenty-two weeks.

The fetus swallows the amniotic fluid and this is an important factor in relation to the circulation of the amniotic fluid. This fact is further proved by the presence of some of the constituents of the amniotic fluid in the meconium.

Meconium is present in the fetal bowel, but under normal circumstances the anal sphincter remains closed and meconium is not passed into the amniotic fluid. The fetal kidneys secrete urine in increasing amounts as pregnancy progresses and the constituents of the amniotic fluid reflect this activity. Constituents of the fetal urine, e.g. creatinine, found in the amniotic fluid can be measured to assess fetal maturity. The concentrations of creatinine increase steadily after thirty weeks gestation and are about 1.8 mg% after thirty-six weeks gestation.

Although the fetal lungs are not required for gaseous exchange respiratory movements take place *in utero* and measurements of fetal breathing are used to assess the wellbeing of the fetus at risk. Maturity of the lung tissue is important in relation to survival in an extrauterine environment and the presence of surfactant is indicated by increasing amounts of the phospholipids, lecithin and sphingomyelin in the amniotic fluid.

Lanugo, which is the name given to the fine hair on the fetal skin, appears at about twenty weeks gestation and until the twenty-eighth weeks covers the entire body. After this time it begins to disappear and is not present after thirty-eight weeks gestation.

Vernix caseosa, the greasy substance covering the fetal skin, appears at about twenty-four weeks gestation and covers the entire body until about thirty-nine weeks gestation when it begins to decrease. Vernix caseosa is secreted by the sebaceous glands of the skin.

Subcutaneous fat is present from about twenty-eight weeks gestation and gradually increases in thickness as pregnancy advances. The fetal fat line can be identified on radiological examination.

Fetal circulation

Cardiovascular development results in a system which is adequate for intrauterine needs and yet is capable of undergoing changes at birth which make it suitable for an extrauterine existence (Fig. 10.1).

Fetal blood is oxygenated and receives nutrients in the extensive capillary network in the placenta. The deoxygenated fetal blood reaches the placenta

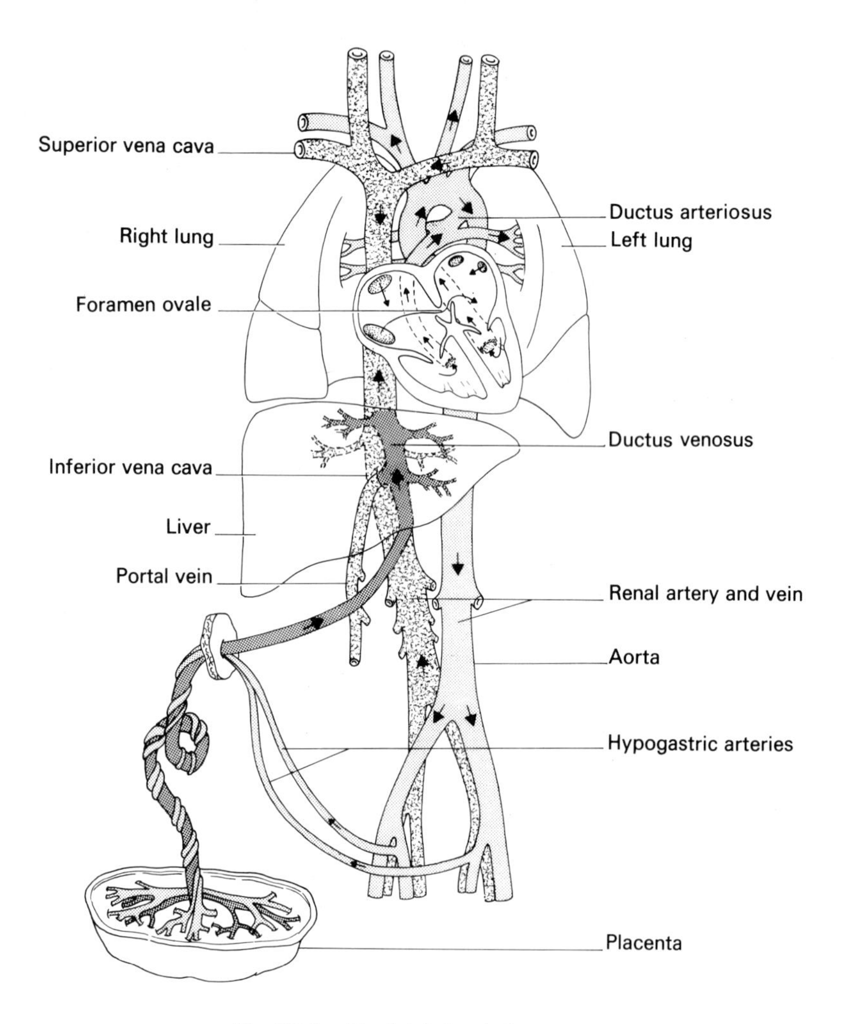

Fig. 10.1 The fetal circulation.

through the two umbilical arteries in the umbilical cord, circulates through the capillary network in the placenta and the oxygenated blood returns to the fetus in the umbilical vein. The umbilical vein passes through the umbilicus and, as the abdominal portion of the umbilical vein, passes in the edge of the falciform ligament to the portal vein. A small amount of blood passes in the portal vein for the nutrition of the liver but the greater part is diverted through the ductus venosus, which passes upwards behind the liver to the inferior vena cava (Fig. 10.2).

The oxygenated blood from the umbilical vein is mixed with the de-oxygenated blood in the inferior vena cava from the abdomen, lower limbs and hepatic veins. The volume of blood is relatively small, however, so the blood remains well oxygenated. The blood in the inferior vena cava enters the right atrium of the heart and the majority is directed through the foramen ovale in the interatrial septum into the left atrium. A large volume of deoxygenated blood from the head, neck and upper limbs also enters the right atrium via the superior vena cava and, although there is some mixing of this deoxygenated blood with the oxygenated blood passing from the inferior vena cava, the orifices are so placed that the two streams remain substantially separate. The oxygenated blood in the left atrium is mixed again, this time with blood from the pulmonary veins before passing downwards through the mitral valve into the left ventricle and thence into the ascending aorta. The branches of the aorta thus have a good supply of oxygenated blood for the developing heart and brain. Some oxygenated blood will spill over into the descending aorta (Fig. 10.3).

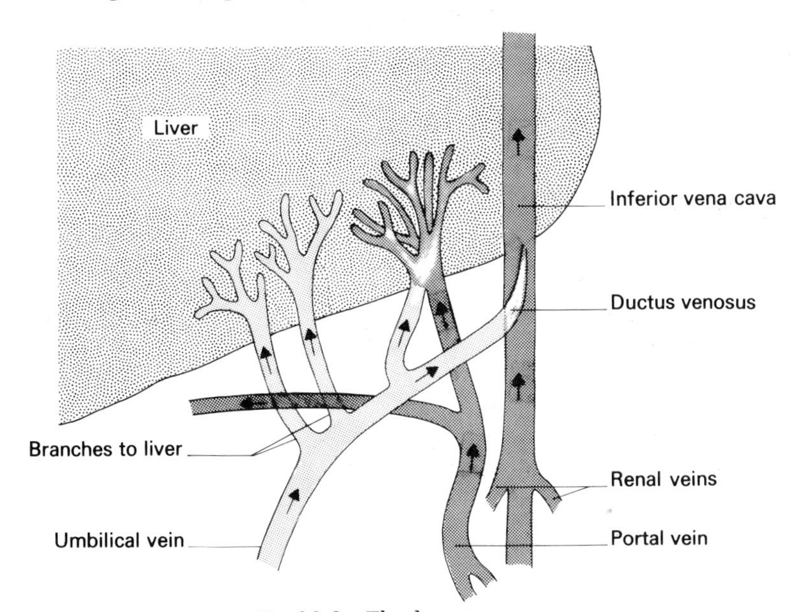

Fig. 10.2 The ductus venosus.

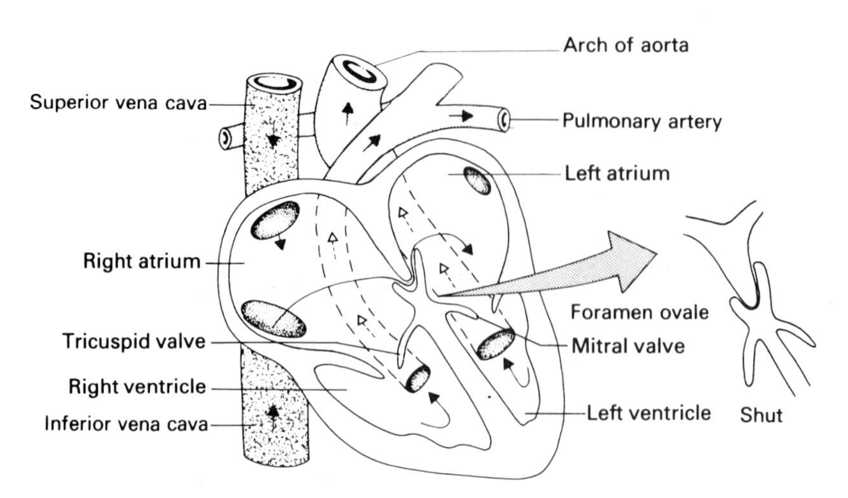

Fig. 10.3 The heart, the inset shows the foramen ovale in shut position.

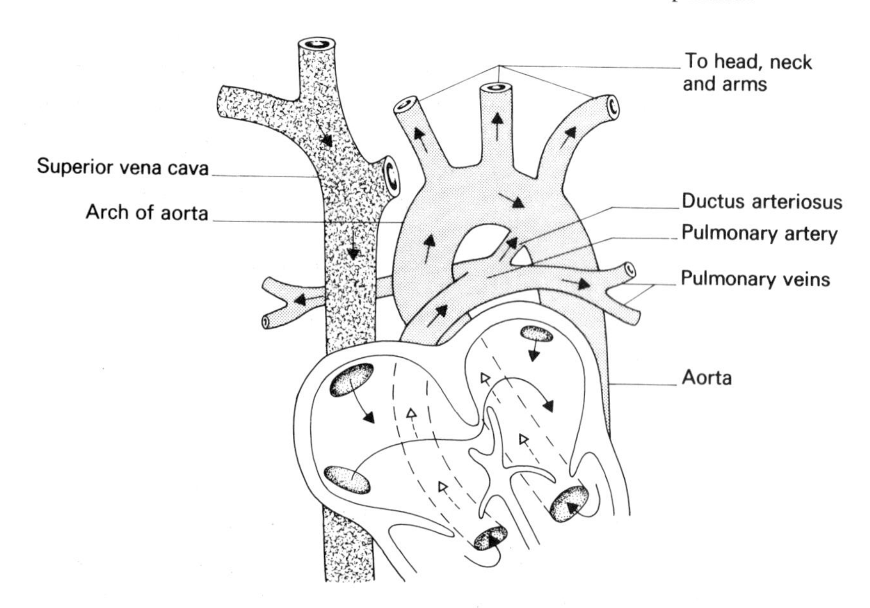

Fig. 10.4 The ductus arteriosus.

Deoxygenated blood from the head, neck and upper extremities returns via the superior vena cava to the right atrium, passes through the tricuspid valve into the right ventricle and thence into the pulmonary artery. The lungs before birth require only a small quantity of blood and, therefore, most of the blood from the pulmonary artery is diverted into the descending aorta via the ductus arteriosus (Fig. 10.4).

Here it mixes with some of the blood that entered the aorta from the left

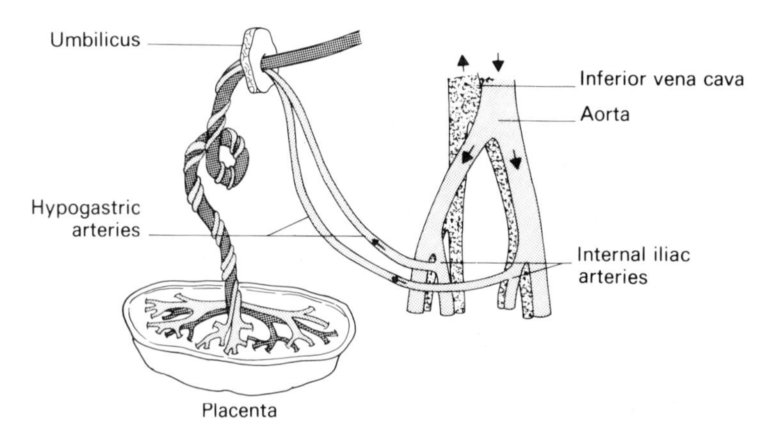

Fig. 10.5 The hypogastric arteries.

ventricle and passes downwards to supply the abdomen, pelvic viscera and lower limbs. Most of the blood passes back to the placenta, to be reoxygenated and recharged with nutrients by the two hypogastric arteries, which are terminal branches of the common iliac arteries. These vessels are situated along the lower anterior abdominal wall and leave the fetus at the umbilicus. They enter the umbilical cord as the umbilical arteries (Fig. 10.5).

TEMPORARY STRUCTURES OF THE FETAL CIRCULATION

1 Abdominal portion of the umbilical vein.
2 Ductus venosus.
3 Foramen ovale.
4 Ductus arteriosus.
5 Hypogastric arteries.

Growth and maturity of the fetus

The growth and maturity of the fetus is taking place from the end of the second month of pregnancy, during the fetal stage of intrauterine development.

At twelve weeks gestation the fetus is about 8.2 cm in length and weighs approximately 14.2 g. The fetus is viable, i.e. capable of leading an extrauterine existence, by the end of the twenty-eighth week of pregnancy and is approximately 35.6 cm long and weighs 1.4 kg. By the thirty-sixth week of pregnancy the fetus is 45.7 cm long, weighs 3 kg and has a head circumference of 33 cm. At forty weeks gestation the fetus is fully matured, weighs 3.54 kg, is 50 cm long and has a head circumference of 35.0 cm (Table 10.1).

Table 10.1 The fetus—growth.

Weeks (completed)	*Weight (kg)*	*Length (cm) (crown to heel)*	*Head circumference (cm)*
32	2.0	40.5	30.0
33	2.25		30.8
34	2.5		31.6
35	2.75		32.4
36	3.0	45.7	33.0
37	3.15		33.4
38	3.3		34.0
39	3.4		34.6
40	3.54	50.0	35.0
41	3.51		35.6
42	3.54		36.2

Assessment of fetal growth and maturity

In modern obstetric practice the fetus receives as much care and attention as does the expectant mother. The term 'fetal medicine', which refers to all aspects of care of the fetus, is now used and highlights the greater understanding of the hazards of the intrauterine environment and the accessibility of the fetus which was previously very limited.

The continuing use of radiology, the introduction of ultrasound and amniotic fluid studies have added to the accuracy of clinical assessment.

CLINICAL ASSESSMENT

The most accurate estimation of the period of gestation is made in the first trimester of pregnancy. A bimanual pelvic examination is performed to assess the size of the uterus and to compare this with the last normal menstrual period with an allowance being made for the length of the menstrual cycle. Thereafter, the growth of the uterus is estimated at each antenatal examination and compared with the period of gestation. Fetal growth is implied by uterine growth although as pregnancy advances the size of the fetus can be estimated. This method is satisfactory in normal pregnancy but if failure of fetal growth is suspected then clinical assessment is rather an imprecise index of fetal growth. The margin of error is reduced if the same person performs the examinations.

RADIOLOGY

The use of X-rays is not without risk as the fetus is sensitive to irradiation by X-rays. Therefore, the hazards of radiology must be balanced against the value of the information obtained and the risks involved if the information is not known, e.g. premature induction of labour.

Table 10.2 The fetus—growth and maturity.

Weeks	*Length (mm) (crown-rump)*	*Biparietal diameter (mm)*	*Epiphysis*
8	15		
10	30		
12	50		
14	90	25	
26		70	Talus
28		75	Calcaneum
32		85	
36		90	
37			Lower femoral
38			Upper tibial
40		95	Tarsal cuboid

A straight X-ray of the woman's abdomen provides a good view of the fetus.

Assessment of fetal maturity/gestational age is based on the osseous development of the fetus as shown by the appearance of the centres of ossification as seen in Table 10.2.

ULTRASOUND

The use of ultrasound has extended the scope of fetal monitoring by making it possible to safely monitor the fetus from an earlier stage of pregnancy than has been previously possible by any method other than clinical assessment. The gestational age can be estimated in the first trimester of pregnancy by measuring the crown-rump length, and from the second trimester by serial estimation of the biparietal diameter (Table 10.2).

AMNIOTIC FLUID STUDIES

Biochemical and cytological studies of the amniotic fluid obtained by amniocentesis are used in the third trimester of pregnancy to estimate fetal maturity (see p. 474).

Biochemical

The maturing fetal kidneys make an increasing contribution to the contents of amniotic fluid and concentrations of creatinine and urea increase. Creatinine levels of 1.8 mg% are an indication that the fetus is more than thirty-six weeks gestation.

Cytology

The mature fetal skin sheds increasing numbers of cornified cells and anucleated squames into the amniotic fluid. Some of the anucleated squames are derived from sebaceous glands and contain lipid which stains orange with Nile blue sulphate. If 10% of the amniotic fluid cells stain orange the pregnancy has reached thirty-eight weeks and if in excess of 40% the fetus is thirty-eight weeks gestation or more. In some cases there are few or no orange-staining cells at or even after term.

PULMONARY SURFACTANT

Maturity of the fetal lungs is determined by the presence of surfactant. Lecithin is a phospholipid component of surfactant and it is formed in increasing amounts in the amniotic fluid as the lungs mature. Lecithin concentrations or lecithin:sphingomyelin ratio can be measured. A lecithin concentration of more than 3.5 mg/100 ml and a lecithin:sphingomyelin ratio of 2:1 are an indication of fetal lung maturity.

The 'at risk' fetus

Identifying the fetus at risk is an important factor of antenatal care and in reducing perinatal morbidity and mortality (see p. 448). The 'at risk' fetus is one that is subject to stress due to complications occurring during the pregnancy. In 1982, the number of stillbirths and deaths in the first week of life was 11.3 per 1000 registered live and stillbirths. The majority of these deaths, 6.3 per 1000, as in all previous years, occur before birth. Some risk factors are present before pregnancy or are recognised early in pregnancy but others will become apparent as pregnancy progresses.

Maternal factors

Primigravida. The first pregnancy is associated with higher risks than the second or third. The primigravida is also more likely to develop pre-eclampsia and to have a difficult labour.

Parity. After the third pregnancy the hazards rise steadily. Increasing parity usually implies increasing age.

Age. This has an independent influence upon reproductive efficiency although increasing age may also be associated with high parity and the very young tend to come from the lower social classes.

Socioeconomic status. Low socioeconomic status is associated with high fetal risk.

Stature. In women who measure less than 1.52 m there is a risk of difficult labour and birth trauma.

Smoking. Cigarette smoking during pregnancy increases the chances of the fetus being underweight or dying (see p. 9).
Drugs. Some drugs taken by a woman during pregnancy have a harmful effect on the growth and development of the fetus (see p. 9).
Alcohol. Maternal alcohol consumption is now recognized as potentially harmful to the fetus. Alcohol readily crosses the placenta and circulates in the fetal blood in the same concentrations as in the expectant mother's blood (see p. 41).
Illegitimacy. There is an increased risk associated with illegitimacy, the reason for which is not clearly understood. The majority of illegitimate births, however, occur among young unmarried girls having a first pregnancy who are not able to provide a satisfactory environment for themselves and who do not take advantage of the medical services available.

MATERNAL DISEASES

Diabetes mellitus. This is associated with a considerably increased risk to the fetus although this can be minimised by good care of the woman with diabetes mellitus during pregnancy.
Hypertension. A rise in the blood pressure to 140/90 mmHg or more is associated with diminution in blood flow to the placenta.
Chronic renal disease. Indicates an increased hazard to the fetus.

PREVIOUS OBSTETRIC HISTORY

Where there is a history of abortion or ectopic pregnancy, premature live births, stillbirths, pre-eclampsia, antepartum haemorrhage or Caesarean section there is an increased risk in a subsequent pregnancy.

COMPLICATIONS OF PREGNANCY

1 Threatened abortion and antepartum haemorrhage lead to an impairment of placental function to a greater or lesser degree and are a potential hazard to the fetus.
2 Hypertension predisposes to placental insufficiency and therefore puts the fetus at risk.
3 Blood group incompatibilities, especially resulting in Rhesus haemolytic disease, put the fetus at risk.

Fetal factors

Intrauterine growth retardation. This may be associated with maternal disease or a complication of pregnancy, or may occur for no apparent reason.
Multiple pregnancy. This is associated with an increased fetal risk.
The pre-term fetus. There is a greater risk of trauma during labour.

Postmaturity. Prolonged pregnancy resulting in postmaturity of the fetus and placenta increases the risk to the fetus especially if another complication exists.
Malpresentation and malposition. These have implications for difficult labour and an increased risk of complications such as prolapse of the umbilical cord.
Fetal abnormality. This is associated with an increase in mortality.
Intrauterine infection. This may occur as a result of maternal infections such as rubella, cytomegalic inclusion disease, toxoplasmosis or syphilis, or as a result of premature rupture of the membranes, and increase the hazards of the fetus.

OTHER FACTORS
Drugs. Medication given to the mother immediately prior to or during pregnancy may adversely affect the fetus.
Rhesus incompatibility. There is a risk to the fetus where there is incompatibility between the maternal and fetal blood.

Assessment of placental function and fetal wellbeing

Assessment of placental function and fetal wellbeing forms an important part of antenatal supervision, and in addition to clinical assessment there are now many tests and investigations that can be performed.

Clinical assessment

A reliable estimate of the period of gestation must be known before the placental function can be estimated with any degree of accuracy.
1 Last menstrual period and length and regularity of the menstrual cycle. These may be misleading if the woman has not established a normal cycle following either pregnancy or cessation of oral contraception.
2 Bimanual pelvic examination in early pregnancy gives an accurate estimation of uterine size in relation to the period of amenorrhoea. Uterine growth is less reliable as a means of determining the period of gestation as pregnancy progresses.
3 Fetal movements can be helpful in conjunction with other factors (see p. 321).

If there is a disparity between the period of gestation and the clinical findings an ultrasound examination can be performed (see p. 317).

When the period of gestation is known, clinical observations can be of considerable value in assessing placental function and fetal wellbeing.
Maternal weight gain. The fetus, placenta and amniotic fluid contribute to the maternal weight gain. Therefore, if the woman fails to gain weight or loses

weight it may indicate failure of intrauterine growth. Other factors such as vomiting or dieting must of course be excluded.

Uterine size. Estimation of uterine growth assumes intrauterine growth, and in most cases is reliable, especially when the examination is made by the same observer. The degree of accuracy can be increased by serial measurement of the girth from the thirty-fourth week of pregnancy.

Amount of amniotic fluid. Placental insufficiency is often accompanied by diminution in the amount of amniotic fluid. This would usually be associated with static or falling maternal weight and girth.

The wellbeing of the fetus may also be assessed in the following ways.

Fetal movements. The woman is asked to note the number of times the fetus moves during the day. Reduced fetal activity is thought to be associated with a deterioration in the fetal condition and poor prognosis.

Fetal heart monitoring. Continuous monitoring of the fetal heart may be undertaken in high risk women at intervals during the antenatal period. The recordings are made using an ultrasound transducer strapped to the maternal abdomen. Fetal response to Braxton Hicks contractions are also observed.

Fetal breathing movements. These are being detected using an ultrasound transducer strapped to the maternal abdomen. A quantitative measure of the rate of breathing and a qualitative indication of its depth are recorded. A fall in the incidence of fetal breathing can be observed in high risk pregnancies.

If fetal growth retardation and placental malfunction is suspected on clinical assessment, other investigations can be performed (see below).

Hormonal excretion

HUMAN CHORIONIC GONADOTROPHIN

This is a protein hormone which is produced by the cytotrophoblast. It has a luteotrophic action and is responsible for prolongation of the activity of the corpus luteum during pregnancy especially the first trimester. Chorionic gonadotrophin appears in the urine as early as eight days after the first missed period. It reaches its peak concentration at fifty to sixty days, then falls rapidly to a low level at which it remains steady apart from a slight rise about thirty weeks gestation (Fig. 10.6). The hormone appears in the blood about ten days after ovulation.

Human chorionic gonadotrophin forms the basis of tests for pregnancy (see p. 20) and can be used in early pregnancy to determine the wellbeing of the pregnancy. If levels are low in cases of threatened abortion there is an increased chance the pregnancy will proceed to an inevitable abortion. In cases where the levels are normal for the period of gestation, the prognosis is good. Chorionic gonadotrophin is produced in large amounts in hydatidiform mole (see p. 176) and higher than normal levels may be associated with multiple pregnancy.

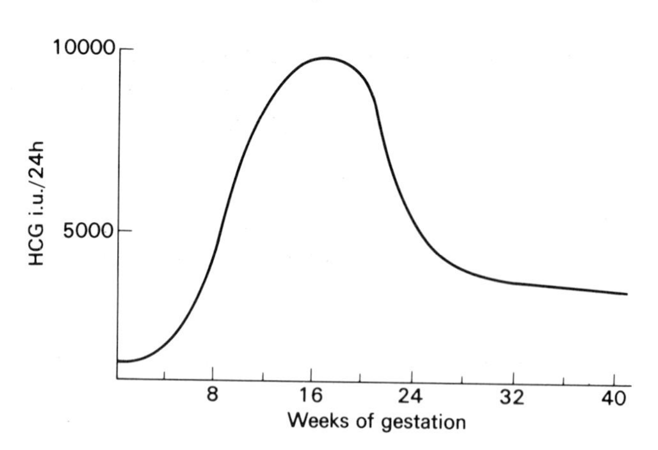

Fig. 10.6 Human chorionic gonadotrophin levels.

HUMAN PLACENTAL LACTOGEN (SOMATOMAMMOTROPHIN)

This is a protein hormone secreted by the syncitiotrophoblast. It is measured in maternal serum by means of a radioimmunoassay. It is detected at about six to eight weeks and is produced in progressively increasing quantities rising to 4–6 μg/ml at thirty-four to thirty-six weeks gestation (Fig. 10.7). Human placental lactogen is thought to facilitate maximum fetal growth and development because it has immunological and biological resemblance to human growth hormone. Its values correlate well with placental weight up to thirty-six weeks of pregnancy. Persistently low levels may indicate placental insufficiency.

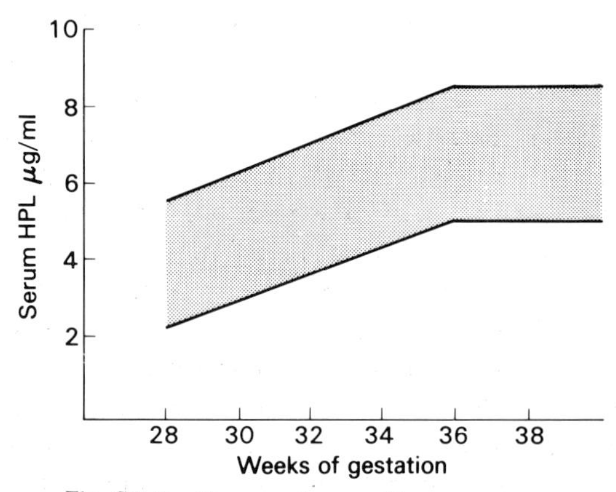

Fig. 10.7 Human placental lactogen levels.

OESTROGEN EXCRETION

Although many oestrogens have been identified, the three main ones used in clinical practice are oestrone (1 hydroxid), oestradiol (2 hydroxiol) and

Table 10.3 The conversion of androgen to oestriol.

Fetal adrenal enzymes ⟶	Dehydroepiandrosterone sulphate (DHAS)
	↓
	Fetal liver enzymes
	↓
	16α hydroxydehydroepiandrosterone sulphate (16α—OH DHAS)
	↓
	Placental enzymes
	↓
Oestriol ⟵	16α hydrodehydroepiandrosterone (16α—OH DHA)

oestriol (3 hydroxiol). Oestrogens are steroid hormones which can only be produced by the placenta in conjunction with the fetus, therefore, measurements of total oestrogens or oestriol levels assess not only placental function but also fetal wellbeing. Oestriol forms 90% of the total oestrogens found in pregnancy.

The placenta is able to convert androgens such as dehydroepiandrosterone and androstenedione to oestrone and oestradiol. The fetal adrenal glands metabolise pregnenolone to dehydroepiandrosterone sulphate (DHAS). This undergoes 16α hydroxylation in the fetal liver to form 16α hydroxydehydroepiandrosterone sulphate (16α-OH DHAS). This sulphate is hydrolysed by the placenta to the free steroid, 16α hydroxydehydroepiandrosterone (16α-OH DHA) which can then be aromatised to oestriol by the placenta (Table 10.3).

Measurement of total oestrogens or oestriol output are made on twenty-four hour urine collections because there is a 25% variable within twenty-four hours. If the levels are correlated to urinary creatinine excretion it helps to eliminate mistakes due to incomplete sample collection or impairment of renal function. Creatinine output is more or less constant in twenty-four hours and oestriol output can be expressed per gram of creatinine.

Low oestriol or total oestrogen excretion is associated with significant fetal growth retardation. The reason is unknown but may be due to lack of precursor steroids from fetal adrenal glands or deficiency of an enzyme such as placental sulphatase. In 10–20% of cases, fetal growth retardation can occur with normal oestriol output. In prolonged severe pre-eclampsia urinary oestriol levels are usually low, but mild pre-eclampsia is associated with a minimal reduction in urinary oestriol levels. Low levels prior to onset of labour predicts acute anoxia causing fetal distress in normal weight babies.

It has been shown that pre-eclampsia accompanied by proteinuria but with normal urinary oestriol levels, is associated with a perinatal mortality rate of 3.4%. This level rises to 31.7% if the urinary oestriol levels are low (Fig. 10.8).

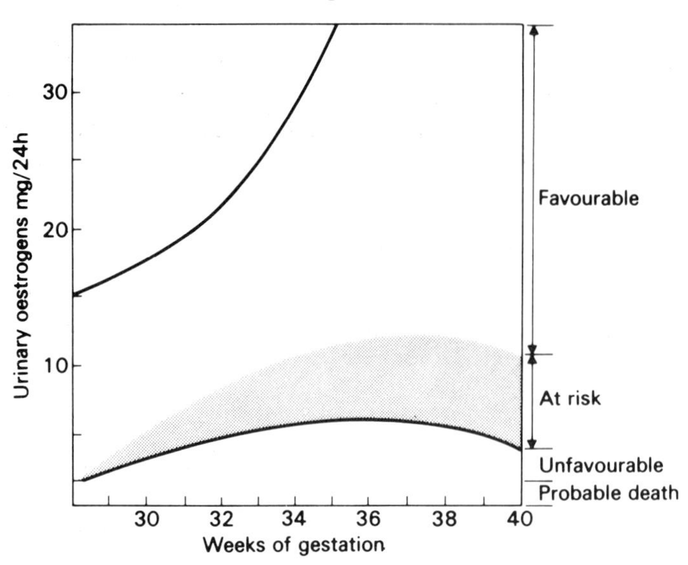

Fig. 10.8 Urinary oestriol levels.

Therefore, perinatal deaths are frequently associated with falling or low urinary oestriol levels.

Serum oestrogens show a close relationship to urinary oestriol excretion both in normal and abnormal pregnancy and because there is no diurnal variation, it is possible to reflect accurately the whole twenty-four hours from a single sample.

PROGESTERONE

This is a steroid hormone produced by the syncitiotrophoblast. The placenta synthesises progesterone from circulating precursors, acetate, cholesterol and pregnenalone from both maternal and fetal sources. Progesterone can be measured in the maternal serum and as pregnanediol in maternal urine in a twenty-four hour specimen, but due to the great variation in the excretion patterns urinary pregnanediol estimations are not now used to measure placental function.

PLACENTAL ENZYME PRODUCTION

Heat stable alkaline phosphatase

This is an enzyme which originates in the placental trophoblast and is distinguished from other non-placental phosphatase because it is heat stable other phosphatases being inactivated at 56 °C. Measurements are performed on samples of maternal serum. Levels of heat stable alkaline phosphatase are proportionate to per gram of placental tissue. Abnormally high and abnormally low levels are found in association with placental insufficiency.

Oxytocinase
This is a placental enzyme which inactivates oxytocin. Oxytocinase increases as pregnancy progresses. Rising levels indicate good prognosis for the fetus, whilst decreasing levels indicate intrauterine growth retardation and the likelihood of intrauterine death.

Fetal distress

Fetal distress is associated with intrauterine hypoxia (reduction in oxygen) and the resultant intrauterine hypercapnia (increase in carbon dioxide).

Aetiology

While it is convenient to consider the causes of fetal distress under the following headings, many of the causes of intrauterine hypoxia are interchangeable because of the close relationship between the mother, placenta and fetus.

MATERNAL
Hypertension. A rise in the maternal blood pressure to 140/90 mmHg or above is associated with interference to the blood flow to the placenta due to spasm of the blood vessels leading to the placenta.
Hypotension. A severe fall in the maternal blood pressure is accompanied by a reduction in a placental perfusion. Hypotension may occur due to vena caval occlusion, epidural analgesia and shock.
Diseases. Maternal diseases such as severe anaemia, cardiac and pulmonary diseases may lead to a reduction in oxygen uptake and transportation, whilst other diseases such as diabetes mellitus or syphilis have a direct effect on the placental tissue.
Smoking. Tobacco contains nicotine which reduces transport of oxygen and inhibits enzyme activity, and carbon monoxide which constricts the blood vessels.

PLACENTAL
Impairment of the placental function may occur due to the following reasons.
a Infarction may occur as the result of maternal hypertension and antepartum haemorrhage.
b Separation of the placenta may occur in early pregnancy when it presents as a threatened abortion, or after the twenty-eighth week of pregnancy causing antepartum haemorrhage which may be due to placental abruption or placenta praevia.
c Degenerative changes in the placenta occur towards the end of pregnancy and, if pregnancy is prolonged, placental insufficiency occurs.
d Diseases such as diabetes mellitus, syphilis and Rhesus haemolytic diseases adversely affect the placenta.

UMBILICAL CORD

Compression of the umbilical cord causing interference with the cord circulation may occur when there is a cord presentation or prolapse or when there is a true knot in the cord.

UTERINE

During uterine contraction there is interference with placental blood flow and oxygen and carbon dioxide exchange. If the contractions are excessively strong (hypertonic uterine action), the resting tone is high or of short duration or the uterine action is incoordinate, there is abnormal interference with the uterine blood flow.

FETAL

Various conditions of the fetus are associated with fetal distress and linked with placental efficiency. The postmature or small-for-dates fetus is at risk, as is the fetus with Rhesus haemolytic disease and a cardiac malformation.

Signs

Fetal hypoxia is associated with changes in the fetal heart and the presence of meconium in the amniotic fluid. During labour the fetal heart is auscultated at frequent intervals or continuously and the rate, rhythm, volume, response to uterine contractions and beat to beat variations are noted.

The normal baseline fetal heart is between 120 and 160 beats/min, the volume is good, there is little or no response to uterine contractions and the beat to beat variation is five or more. Baseline fetal heart is the fetal heart when the woman is not in labour, or in an interval between uterine contractions when the woman is in labour.

FETAL HEART CHANGES

Tachycardia. A fetal heart rate of above 160 beats/min. The term baseline tachycardia is used to describe the fetal heart that is persistently above 160 beats/min. Tachycardia occurs in response to oxygen deprivation, the heart beating faster in an attempt to maintain adequate oxygenation. Tachycardia may occur as a reflection of maternal tachycardia due to acidosis or infection. If oxygen deprivation continues bradycardia follows.

Bradycardia. A fetal heart rate of less than 120 beats/min. The term baseline bradycardia describes the fetal heart rate that is persistently below this level. Bradycardia may follow an episode of tachycardia where hypoxia continues or it may occur as the result of an acute episode, e.g. placental abruption. Bradycardia is more serious than tachycardia because it indicates a more severe degree of hypoxia where the heart muscle is affected.

Rhythm. Irregularities in the rhythm of the fetal heart may be noted.

Volume. The fetal heart may be difficult to hear due to the position of the fetus, polyhydramnios or if the woman is obese. These problems can be overcome by the use of the ultrasound detector. If the fetal heart is still weak this indicates an abnormality.
Response to uterine contractions. The fetal heart should return to its normal baseline as soon as the uterus has ceased to contract. Slow recovery may indicate placental insufficiency.

The changes in the fetal heart mentioned above may be detected by using the monaural stethoscope. The advantage of continuous monitoring of the fetal heart is that not only is there continuous record of the fetal heart rate as opposed to an intermittent one, but the response to uterine activity and the beat to beat variation can also be observed.
Type I dips (early decelerations). The heart rate decelerates in response to the contraction, reaching its lowest level at the height of the contraction and returning to the normal baseline by the end of the contraction (Fig. 10.9). This type of deceleration is thought to be due to compression of the head and, unless the dip is very deep, is not thought to be significant unless associated with other changes.
Type II dips (late decelerations). The fetal heart decelerates after the onset of the contraction and there is a time-lag between the height of the contraction and the lowest level of the heart rate (Fig. 10.10). Type II dips are indicative of uteroplacental insufficiency.
Variable deceleration. This may be associated with compression of the umbilical cord.
Loss of beat to beat variation. The variation between beats is normally greater than 5 beats/min. A reduction in this variation is referred to as loss of beat to beat variation and is associated with central depressant drugs such as diazepam (Valium) and pethidine.

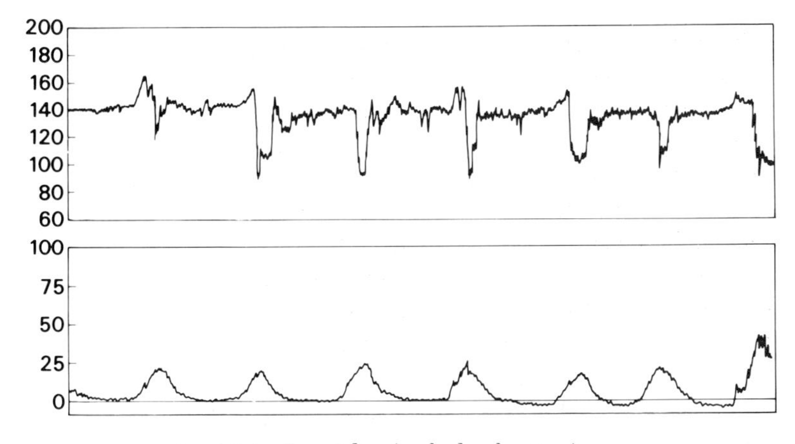

Fig. 10.9 Type I dips (early deceleration).

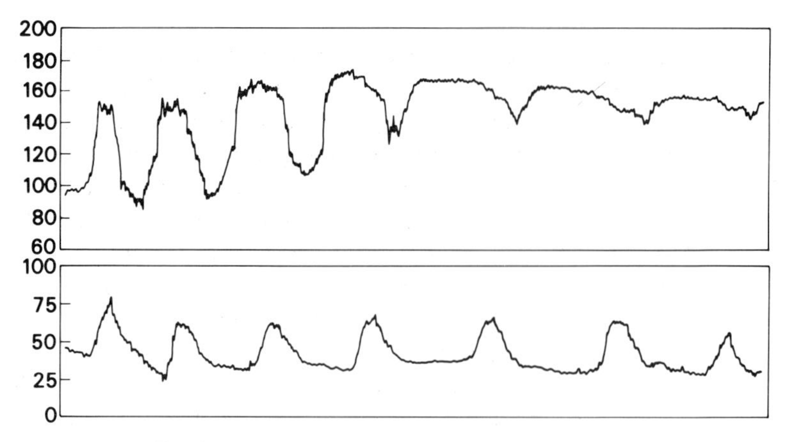

Fig. 10.10 Type II dips (late deceleration).

MECONIUM

The passage of meconium into the amniotic fluid is abnormal, except in the presence of a breech presentation, and is associated with fetal hypoxia.

MANAGEMENT

The management of fetal distress depends on the stage of labour at which it presents, its severity and other factors such as past obstetric history.

First stage of labour

If the midwife observes any abnormal change in the fetal heart, or the presence of meconium in the amniotic fluid, she must inform the doctor immediately. If there is fetal tachycardia, the maternal pulse rate should be checked and the urine tested to exclude maternal tachycardia or acidosis as the cause. Bradycardia may be due to compression of the cord which may be relieved by adjusting the woman's position.

The fetal heart should be monitored frequently and, if the apparatus is available, continuous monitoring should be commenced so that other aspects of the fetal heart can be observed, i.e. response to uterine activity and beat to beat variation.

Abdominal and vaginal examinations are performed to assess progress in labour and the length, strength and frequency of uterine contractions. If intact the membranes are usually ruptured so that the amniotic fluid can be observed for the presence of meconium.

If facilities are available, fetal blood sampling may be performed by the doctor to estimate the pH of the capillary blood.

FETAL BLOOD SAMPLING

The procedure is explained to the woman and if necessary she is transferred to the delivery room and placed in the lithotomy position. The vulval area is swabbed and a vaginal examination performed to determine the dilatation of the os uteri and the station of the presenting part. Depending on this a suitable endoscope is selected and passed into the vagina and placed against the fetal head ensuring a close application. The obturator is withdrawn, a light source is attached to the outer end of the endoscope and the fetal head visualised. If intact the membranes are ruptured and the scalp cleaned with a dry swab. The area is then sprayed with ethyl chloride to produce reflex hydraemia. A thin layer of silicone jelly is applied to the scalp to contain the blood and an incision is made into the scalp using a specially mounted blade to limit the depth of the incision. The blood is collected into a glass capillary tube either by capillary attraction or by sucking the blood from the scalp by means of a rubber tube connected to the glass tube. The blood in the tube is mixed by means of inserting a metal stirring rod which is inserted into the glass tube and moved up and down by a magnet. Following the procedure pressure is applied to the incision until the bleeding has almost stopped. The specimen of blood is taken to the analyser and the pH is estimated (Fig. 10.11).

COMPLICATIONS

Complications following fetal blood sampling are rare but there is a risk of haemorrhage from the incision site. There should be in all delivery rooms a test for differentiating between fetal and maternal blood. If vaginal bleeding is observed following fetal blood sampling or if vasa praevia is suspected, some of the blood is collected for testing.

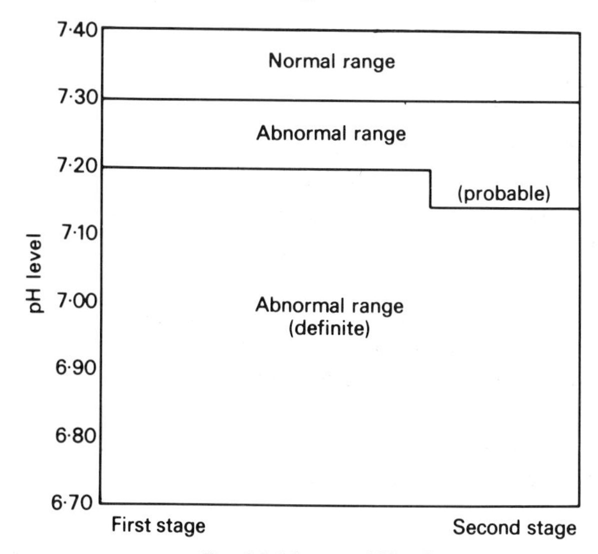

Fig. 10.11 Fetal blood sampling.

Singer test
The blood is mixed with 2 ml of 12th normal sodium hydroxide in a test tube. The specimen is thoroughly shaken and 4 ml of 50% saturated ammonium sulphate and 2 ml of 10th normal hydrochloric acid are added. Fetal haemoglobin (HbF) gives a pink colour, maternal haemoglobin a brown colour to the mixture.

The outcome of fetal distress in the first stage of labour will depend on the results of investigations and on other relevant factors, e.g. the woman's obstetric history, how far the first stage has advanced, and whether a multigravida or primigravida, in relation to the expected duration of labour.

Outcome
1 Conservative management may be used with continuous monitoring of the fetal heart and repeat blood samplings.
2 Ventouse extraction may be used if there is an indication to terminate labour but there is no immediate urgency.
3 Caesarean section is indicated where there is an indication to terminate the labour in the shortest time.

Second stage

If signs of fetal distress present in the second stage of labour and the fetal head is low in the pelvic cavity, the perineum is infiltrated and an episiotomy performed to accelerate delivery. If the head is too high to deliver following episiotomy, the doctor is informed and a forceps delivery performed.

If signs of fetal distress have been observed during labour an asphyxiated baby must be anticipated and the paediatrician called for the delivery.

Chapter 11
The Normal Neonate

The normal mature newborn weighs approximately 3.5 kg if a male and 3.4 kg if female. The length from vertex to heel is about 50 cm and the occipitofrontal head circumference between 34 and 36 cm. The baby's head appears large in comparison with the body, the arms are longer than the legs and the anteroposterior diameter of the chest is equal to the transverse diameter.

The baby's skin is pale pink and the skin creases are well defined. Lanugo if present will only be seen on the shoulders and vernix caseosa in the axilla and groin creases. The baby has rounded contours due to the presence of subcutaneous fat. The nails reach the tips of the fingers.

The liver is large and can be palpated 2.5 cm below the costal margin. The external genitalia are well developed; in the female infant the labia majora enclose the labia minora and the clitoris, and in the male infant the testes are descended into the scrotum, the skin of which has well defined rugae.

The baby's movements are irregular, jerky and asymmetrical and the reflexes are well developed. The muscle tone is good and the baby lies in a flexed attitude, and if disturbed may protest with a good strong cry.

Physiological changes at birth

The baby has to make considerable physiological changes to adjust to an extrauterine existence some of which take place immediately, others taking place within days, weeks or months of births.

Respiratory system

In utero, the fetus obtains oxygen from the gaseous exchange between the maternal and fetal blood in the placenta (see p. 99). At birth, the clamping of the umbilical cord instantly cuts off the placental oxygen so that the atmospheric oxygen must be utilised by the lungs within a relatively short space of time. The build up of carbon dioxide in the baby's blood immediately prior to delivery, stimulates the respiratory centre and initiates respirations. This is aided by external stimuli such as an alteration in environmental temperature, handling, noise and light.

The baby's respiratory rate is about 50/min at birth but decreases gradually, as respiration is established to about 40/min. The respirations are irregular and accompanied by short periods of apnoea.

Cardiovascular system

At birth, two important factors bring about changes in the cardiovascular system. First, the umbilical cord is clamped and the baby is separated from the placental circulation, and therefore, the blood no longer flows along the umbilical vein and into the inferior vena cava via the ductus venosus, nor through the hypogastric arteries to the umbilical arteries (see p. 312). Secondly, the baby breathes, the lungs expand and pulmonary respiration is established.

As a result of the clamping of the umbilical cord, the abdominal portion of the umbilical vein, and the ductus venosus close and are gradually transformed into fibrous cords, the ligamentum teres and the ligamentum venosum. When the lungs expand the blood flows into the pulmonary arteries instead of the ductus arteriosus which contracts and subsequently becomes the ligamentum arteriosum. The amount of blood returning to the left atrium via the pulmonary veins is greatly increased with the result that the pressure in the left atrium increases relatively to that in the right atrium, sufficiently to cause a cessation of the flow of blood through the foramen ovale and to close the flat-like valve, the septum primium, at its orifice (Fig. 10.3).

Changes in the blood

The fetus has a greater number of red blood cells than is required for an extrauterine existence, and those extra cells are haemolysed after birth with the result that the baby may develop a physiological jaundice which appears after twenty-four hours and reaches a peak on the fourth or fifth day (see p. 364).

The conversion from fetal haemoglobin (HbF) to adult haemoglobin (HbA) commences *in utero* and by birth the amount of fetal haemoglobin remaining is about 20–40%. Conversion to adult haemoglobin has taken place by two years of age.

The haemoglobin concentration is approximately 18–19 g/dl at birth and falls to 12 g/dl by about three months. The baby has a blood volume of 90 ml/kg body weight.

Hypoprothrombinaemia, due to lack of vitamin K, occurs between twelve hours and five days after delivery and may manifest as haemorrhagic disease of the newborn (see p. 371).

Renal tract

Since excretion *in utero* is mainly carried out by the placenta, the fetal kidneys are relatively immature at the time of birth. The medulla and medullary glomeruli are better developed than the cortex and the cortical glomeruli. The ability to filter and concentrate urine is relatively undeveloped. The infant therefore requires a proportionately larger volume of water to eliminate solids than an adult and passes relatively larger amounts of hypotonic urine. If the infant is given too little water or loses too much, the kidney retains urea and sodium chloride. The kidneys of the newborn are relatively inefficient and cannot deal effectively with more than minor variations in normal physiology. Therefore, the careful management of water and electrolyte balance in the treatment of infants who are ill is essential.

Temperature regulation

The newborn baby is not very efficient at regulating its body temperature. The baby's metabolism and heat production takes several days to function properly, and therefore, even the normal infant is prone to chilling (see p. 392).

Gastrointestinal tract

In utero, the fetus acquires nutrients from the maternal blood and to a lesser extent from swallowing amniotic fluid (see p. 99). Following birth, feeding is commenced along with digestion and absorption. The newborn infant has a full complement of digestive enzymes and the digestive process is essentially the same as in the adult except that the greater part of the digestive process takes place in the small intestine.

The intestinal bacteria necessary for the synthesis of vitamin K are not present in the baby's intestines at birth, and because this is required for the synthesis of prothrombin in the liver, hypothrombinaemia occurs. This is corrected when the infant starts feeding and acquires the bacteria necessary for the synthesis of vitamin K.

Meconium is formed in the intestines from the fourth month of fetal life and is the substance present at birth in the intestine of the newborn baby. It is dark green in colour due to the presence of bile pigments and in addition consists of epithelial cells, fatty acids and mucus. Meconium is passed for about two days after birth, followed by 'changing stools' which are brown in colour and last for two to three days and then normal stools are passed. The type and frequency of the subsequent stools depend on the method of feeding. The breast fed baby passes soft frequent stools whereas the bottle fed baby passes more formed stools at less frequent intervals.

Care of the Neonate

An important part of the midwife's role is the care of the baby from birth to the end of the neonatal period and teaching the mother how to care for her baby.

Care at birth

The immediate care of the baby is vitally important and can influence subsequent events.

ESTABLISHMENT AND MAINTENANCE OF RESPIRATIONS

As soon as the baby's head is born, and before the first inspiratory gasp, the nasopharynx should be cleared of mucus and amniotic fluid to avoid inhalation of these substances. The baby must be observed carefully as more mucus may collect and the procedure may need to be repeated.

APGAR SCORE

The baby's condition is assessed by means of the Apgar score at one and five minutes after birth (see p. 344).

CARE OF THE UMBILICAL CORD

The umbilical cord is clamped in two places and cut between the two forceps. Subsequent care involves shortening the cord to 4 cm in length and replacing the forceps with a cord clamp or latex rubber band to prevent bleeding. The cord must be inspected frequently to ensure there is no oozing.

MAINTENANCE OF TEMPERATURE

As soon as the cord is clamped and cut, the baby's skin is gently dried and the baby wrapped in a warm blanket and given to the mother to hold or placed in a pre-heated cot under a heat lamp. The baby's temperature is recorded rectally using a low-reading thermometer.

IDENTIFICATION

Identification labels are completed with details of the delivery and these are checked with the mother before being placed on the baby's wrists.

WEIGHT AND MEASUREMENTS

The baby is weighed and the vertex-heel length and occipitofrontal head circumference measured and compared with the period of gestation.

EXAMINATION

An examination is performed soon after delivery to exclude congenital malformations and birth injury. The baby is examined in a warm room and in a good light. A note is made of the baby's colour which should be pink with the possible exception of the hands and feet which may be slightly blue. The baby's posture and movements are also noted.

A systematic head to toe examination is then performed and throughout the procedure a note is made of the texture of the skin, the amount of subcutaneous tissue and any birth marks such as strawberry naevi or haemangiomata.

Head. The size of the head is noted in comparison with the rest of the body. The shape of the head is observed and the presence of moulding and caput succedaneum noted. The finger is used to trace the suture lines and fontanelles. The suture lines may be felt to overlap due to moulding but may be separated or closed when examined later. The anterior fontanelle is easily palpated but the posterior fontanelle may be closed or just palpable.

Eyes. The eyelids are separated and the eyes carefully examined for conjunctival haemorrhages and cataract. The angle of the eyes is noted to exclude one of the features of Down's syndrome (see p. 390).

Face. Symmetry of the face is noted and the shape, size and position of facial features observed.

Mouth. A cleft lip is an obvious feature but the palate must be clearly visualised or felt to exclude a cleft. The size and shape of the mouth are noted and the lower jaw seen in profile to exclude a receding chin. Epstein's pearls, white spots in the midline at the junction of the hard and soft palates, are normal. Teeth are rarely present at birth.

Ears. The position of the ears is noted and the upper border should be level with the eyebrows. Low-set ears are associated with renal abnormalities and Down's syndrome. The shape and size of the ears are observed and accessory auricles looked for.

Neck. The thyroid gland is observed for enlargement and the head rotated and extended laterally in both directions to outline the sternomastoid muscle in order that haematoma or sternomastoid 'tumour' may be observed (see p. 350). The clavicles are examined to exclude fractures and the length of the neck observed.

Chest. The shape and size of the chest are noted and the type and rate of the respiratory movements observed. The baby uses the abdominal muscles and, therefore, there is little movement of the chest. The apex beat is felt and its position is noted. The development of the nipples is noted.

Abdomen. The abdomen is usually slightly distended and moves with respirations. The umbilicus is inspected and cord noted to ensure that it is securely clamped.

External genitalia. In females, the labia are separated and the genitalia examined. In males, the testes should be felt in the scrotum and opening of the urethra noted in the centre of the tip of the penis.
Anus. If the baby has passed meconium, the anus is usually patent, if not, it is inspected and a thermometer inserted.
Limbs. The length of the arms and legs is noted and the hands and feet examined for accessory digits, webbing and palmar and plantar markings. The ankles are examined to exclude talipes (see p. 383).
Hips. The baby's hips are examined to exclude congenital dislocation. Barlow's test, which is a modification of the test described by Ortalani, is normally used. The baby is placed on his back and the examiner grasps the baby's legs around the knee joints. The thumbs are placed on the lesser trochanter and the index fingers on the greater trochanter. The legs and hips are gently flexed and the hips first abducted and then adducted. Limitation of abduction and a palpable and sometimes audible click indicates the replacement of the head of the femur into the acetabulum of the dislocated hip (see p. 382).
Spine. The baby is placed face downwards and a finger is run down the spine to exclude spinal defects. A 'Mongolian' blue spot may be noted over the sacrum in coloured babies.
Central nervous system. The integrity of the central nervous system can be assessed by observing certain reflexes which are present in the normal newborn. These can be noted as the baby is being examined or following the physical examination.

1 The sucking and swallowing reflexes are tested by placing a clean finger or teat in the baby's mouth. A first feed of sterile water may be given to test the integrity of the oesophagus.
2 The rooting or searching reflex is tested by touching the angle of the baby's mouth with the finger or teat. The baby will turn his head towards it and search for it.
3 The grasp reflex is demonstrated by stroking the back of the baby's fingers so that they extend, and on placing a finger in the palm the baby takes a firm grasp. Similar reflexes can be also noted in the toes.
4 The moro reflex is tested by dropping the baby's head a short distance from one hand to the other or making a loud noise near the baby. When startled the baby first throws out his arms and then brings them together in an embracing movement.
5 The primitive walking reflex is demonstrated by holding the baby so that his feet are touching a firm surface. He will raise one leg and take a large hesitating stride forward.

This examination will be repeated by the doctor within twenty-four hours of birth and in addition the baby's heart and lungs will be auscultated and femoral pulses felt.

PREVENTION OF HAEMORRHAGIC DISEASE OF THE NEWBORN

An injection of vitamin K_1 phytomendadione (Konakion) (1 mg intramuscularly) is given to prevent hypoprothrombinaemia (see p. 371).

URINE AND MECONIUM

The baby may pass urine and meconium shortly after birth. These functions indicate the presence of kidneys and a patent anus. The staff of the postnatal ward must be informed in order to avoid concern if there is a delay before urine and meconium are passed again.

FEEDING

If the mother wishes to breast feed her baby and if her condition is satisfactory, this is an ideal time to introduce the baby to the breast. Babies are often alert and eager to suck following delivery and this can be a good initial step in establishing successful breast feeding and a normal mother-baby relationship. If the mother has elected to bottle feed she should be given the opportunity to offer the baby a feed.

The details of the delivery and the immediate postnatal care and observations are recorded in the neonatal records and the birth notification completed and sent to the District Medical Officer within thirty-six hours of birth. The baby is transferred to the postnatal ward with his mother approximately one hour following delivery.

Care during first ten days

On admission to the nursery the baby's labels and cot card should be checked by the midwife receiving the baby with the midwife who has taken the baby to the ward. The baby's temperature is checked, he is re-examined, dressed and warmly wrapped. A feed of sterile water may be given to check the integrity of the oesophagus. If the baby's temperature is satisfactory he is taken to the mother's bedside.

OBSERVATIONS AND RECORDINGS

Temperature. The temperature is recorded four-hourly for twenty-four hours and then daily using a low-reading thermometer. The baby's temperature should not fall below 36.6 °C.

Respiration. The baby uses its abdominal muscles and breathes irregularly at about 40/min.

Colour. The baby's colour is observed and although there may be slight cyanosis of the hands and feet initially this soon disappears. Slight jaundice may be noted after twenty-four hours and reaching a peak about the fifth to sixth day. This is physiological jaundice (see p. 364).

Skin. The skin is inspected daily for rashes and septic spots and the eyes observed for stickiness or discharge.
Mouth. The mouth is inspected daily to exclude infection.
Urinary output. A note is made of the frequency of the passage of urine and the odour.
Stools. A note is made of the number of stools passed, the colour, texture and odour.
Weight. The baby is weighed on alternate days. There is usually an initial weight loss which should not be more than 0.25 kg. The baby should regain his birth weight by the end of the first week and then gain about 30 g/day.

CARE OF THE SKIN

The baby's buttocks are washed and dried carefully at each napkin change. Zinc and castor-oil cream or Vaseline is applied when meconium is being passed to prevent it adhering to the baby's buttocks and to make it easier to remove. A complete toilet is carried out daily during which the observations are made and the identification labels checked. The timing of the first bath is very variable, and ranges from soon after birth until after the cord stump has separated.

CARE OF THE CORD

The cord is inspected each time the napkin is changed and the base of the cord cleaned with a spirit swab and powdered with an antibacterial powder during the daily toilet. The cord should separate between the fourth and sixth days, although it may take longer.

EXAMINATION

The baby should be examined by a doctor within twenty-four hours of birth and again prior to discharge from hospital or from the care of the domiciliary midwife.

SCREENING FOR PHENYLKETONURIA AND HYPOTHYROIDISM

Blood is taken from a heel prick for the test to exclude phenylketonuria and congenital hypothyroidism. This is usually taken on the seventh day after six days of milk feeds which are necessary to detect raised levels of phenylalanine (see p. 397).

BREAST FEEDING

Unless it is contraindicated the mother should be encouraged to breast feed her baby especially in the immediate postnatal period. However, there will always be mothers who cannot or who prefer not to breast feed their baby.

If possible the baby should be put to breast soon after delivery and then at approximately four-hourly intervals for the first four days. During this time the baby should be allowed to suckle for three minutes at each breast for the first day, five minutes on the second day, seven minutes on the third and ten minutes on the fourth day. This regime ensures the necessary stimulus that is required to initiate lactation without allowing the baby to suckle at an empty breast or for too long which might result in sore nipples. By the fourth day, the milk should be established and demand feeding should be commenced. Some mothers may prefer to demand feed from the beginning while others may prefer to continue a timed regime. The length of time at each breast will vary from one baby to another and from one feed to another, but should be approximately ten minutes (see p. 166).

Complementary feeds

If the baby is not satisfied following breast feeding, which may occur in the first three days before the milk comes in, a drink of water should be offered. A complementary feed of milk is only recommended after the fourth day if the mother's lactation is inadequate to meet the baby's needs, although this problem may be overcome by more frequent feeds.

Advantages of breast feeding

The composition of breast milk is ideal for normal growth and development. The breast fed baby has more resistance to infections and to allergic illness of all kinds.

The risk of microbial contamination which can occur in both the preparation and in the giving of bottle feeds is avoided. Gastroenteritis is much less common in breast fed babies. Evidence suggests that the breast fed baby's resistance to gastroenteritis may be associated with a higher acidity and a different bacterial flora of the large intestines.

The breast fed baby derives antibodies from the mother, e.g. protection against the poliomyelitis virus is conferred in this way.

The proteins and fats in breast milk are more easily digested and consequently calcium absorption is not reduced and hypocalcaemia does not occur (see p. 396).

The low sodium content of breast milk gives the baby an extra reserve of water which keeps him well hydrated. This maintains the plasma-electrolyte balance at normal levels even during fever and diarrhoea.

Fat laid down by the mother during pregnancy is normally metabolised during lactation and the mother who breast feeds is more likely to return to her normal pre-pregnancy weight.

Breast feeding is important in promoting maternal-infant attachment and providing a foundation for normal emotional development of the infant.

Breast milk is free and requires no preparation.

Contraindications to breast feeding

The mother who finds the idea of breast feeding repulsive or embarrassing should not be persuaded to breast feed.

Medical conditions such as severe cardiac disease, diabetes mellitus that is difficult to stabilise and pulmonary tuberculosis are contraindications to breast feeding.

The unmarried mother who is planning to have her baby adopted should not breast feed her baby unless she elects to do so.

Congenital malformation of the baby such as cleft lip and palate, Pierre Robin syndrome and Down's syndrome makes breast feeding difficult if not impossible. A baby with a cardiac abnormality may tire too easily for breast feeding to be successful.

BOTTLE FEEDING

The baby is offered 30 ml/kg body weight in the first twenty-four hours, this is increased by 20 ml/kg body weight/day until a maximum of 150/kg body weight/day is reached by the seventh day (Table 11.1). The daily requirement is divided into six feeds.

This is only an example and it must be remembered that babies are individuals and some will need more and some less than the recommended amount, and the baby's requirements may vary from one feed to another.

In hot weather the baby may be thirsty rather than hungry and should be given a drink of sterile water.

Table 11.1 Example of requirements for a baby weighing 3 kg.

Day	*Daily requirement (ml)*	*Amount per feed (ml)*
1	90	15
2	150	25
3	210	35
4	270	45
5	330	55
6	390	65
7	450	75

Hazards associated with bottle feeding

There are important differences between human and cows' milk. Fat is not well absorbed and the unabsorbed fatty acids combine with calcium and absorption of calcium is reduced. As a result of this, hypocalcaemia may occur in the second half of the first week of life. Convulsions may occur if the serum calcium level is below 1.8 mmol/l.

There is the risk of microbial contamination both in the preparation and in the giving of bottle feeds. There is also low acidity of the stools of babies fed on cows' milk and a different bacterial flora of the large intestines which does not provide resistance to bacterial growth. Gastroenteritis is, therefore, much more common among bottle fed babies.

There are difficulties associated with the preparation of feeds which usually result in an overconcentrated feed being prepared.

The baby who is bottle fed is exposed to allergens which may be present in cows' milk (see p. 395).

The early introduction of solids is more likely to occur in babies who are bottle fed.

Promotion of maternal-infant attachment may be more difficult to achieve as it is possible for other people to feed the baby.

ADVICE REGARDING PREPARATION AND GIVING OF ARTIFICIAL FEEDS

All mothers, including those who are breast feeding, should be shown how to prepare a bottle feed and how to clean and sterilise the utensils. Attention to detail reduces the risks associated with bottle feeding and therefore midwives have an important role in educating mothers in this aspect of care.

Preparation of feed

1 Close any windows near the working area and clean the working surface.
2 Wash hands and set out all the items required; remove lid from sterilising unit and open packet containing milk.
3 Wash hands again and using hands, remove utensils from sterilising unit and shake off excess liquid. *Do not rinse.*
4 Carefully following the instructions on the packet, measure the required amount of water. This is boiled water that has been allowed to cool.
5 Using the scoop supplied, measure the required amount of powder. The instructions will vary, some manufacturers require the scoop to be lightly packed before levelling, others do not. The other variable is whether the water is put into the bottle before or after the powder. These points must be carefully followed otherwise the concentration of the feed will be altered. You are replacing the water that was removed during manufacture and therefore the amount used in reconstituting the milk is crucial. The bottle is covered and shaken to mix the powder and water.
6 If several feeds are prepared they must be stored in a refrigerator until required.

Feeding the baby

1 The feed is removed from the refrigerator and left at room temperature for about half an hour or placed in a jug of hot water.
2 The mother washes her hands before putting the teat on the bottle, taking care not to touch the part which goes into the baby's mouth. A cover is placed over the teat when it is not being used.

3 The temperature of the feed is tested by allowing a few drops of milk to drop on to the inner aspect of the arm. This also checks the patency of the teat and ensures the hole is not too large.
4 The baby is held in the arms against the mother's body with the upper part of the body raised.
5 The bottle is held at an angle to ensure that the teat is filled with milk at all times to avoid the baby sucking in air.
6 The baby should be winded at least halfway through the feed and at the end although some babies need to be winded more often.
7 Any milk left at the end of the feed must be discarded.

Sterilisation of utensils

1 All equipment used is rinsed in cold water and then thoroughly washed in warm soapy water. A bottle brush is used to ensure that the inside of the bottle is thoroughly cleaned.
2 The outside of the teat is rubbed with salt and the teat turned inside out and the procedure repeated. Water is flushed through the hole.
3 All the utensils are rinsed under a running water tap and the excess water shaken off before they are placed into the sterilising unit.
4 All utensils must be completely immersed and all air bubbles excluded.
5 The utensils must remain in the sterilising fluid for at least one hour or according to the instructions on the packet.
6 The fluid in the sterilising unit must be replaced every twenty-four hours following the instructions on the packet.

It is important to point out to the mothers that the introduction of solids before the baby is four to six months old is not necessary and in some circumstances may be harmful. Normal growth and development occur if the child is given milk alone up to six months of age. The mother should also be told to use only low solute preparations during the first six months of life.

Care from the eleventh to twenty-eighth day

The care of the baby is transferred from the midwife to the health visitor during this period. The health visitor usually makes a home visit to introduce herself to the mother if she is not already known to her and to discuss problems that may have arisen since the midwife's last visit. The mother is advised to take her baby to the Child Health Centre or to her general practitioner to be weighed, to obtain vaccinations and to enable periodic developmental assessments to be carried out (see p. 426).

Chapter 12
Neonatal Complications

Asphyxia neonatorum

Failure of the newborn infant to establish respiration within one minute of birth is referred to as asphyxia neonatorum. Various internal and external stimuli assist in bringing about spontaneous onset of respiration.

1 A moderate degree of hypoxia will stimulate the respiratory centre.
2 The infant is exposed to a dramatic change in environmental temperature.
3 Handling, noise and light all act as stimuli.
4 The use of suction apparatus to clear the nasopharynx.

Asphyxia in the newborn should be anticipated if there have been signs of intrauterine hypoxia at any time during labour, and if there is to be an instrumental delivery. In these circumstances facilities for resuscitation should be immediately available and a paedriatrician present at the delivery. However, asphyxia may present without warning and therefore the midwife must be proficient in dealing with the situation until a paediatrician arrives so that there is no delay in establishing respirations, which may lead to cerebral damage.

Causes

BIOCHEMICAL DEPRESSION

Intrauterine hypoxia. The causes of intrauterine hypoxia have already been described (see p. 325).

Extrauterine hypoxia. Obstruction of the airway with mucus, amniotic fluid, blood or meconium may occur if the baby inhales before the nasopharynx is cleared. This can occur during any delivery but is most likely in a breech delivery. In this situation, the baby's trunk is born while the head is still in the birth canal and therefore exposure to temperature change and handling is taking place. Also the placenta will start to separate. These factors stimulate premature respiratory efforts while the baby's head is in the vagina.

DYSFUNCTION OF THE RESPIRATORY CENTRE

Pharmacological depression. Drugs such as pethidine and anaesthetic agents cause depression of the respiratory centre and if administered within two to three hours of birth may be the cause of asphyxia.

Cerebral damage. This may occur due to haemorrhage or as a result of hypoxic changes.

IMMATURITY

The immature newborn is more susceptible to pharmacological depression, the risk of cerebral damage is increased due to fragility of blood vessels, and the immaturity of lung tissue may cause primary atelectasis.

Types of asphyxia

There are two degrees of asphyxia; mild and severe.

Mild asphyxia. The baby is in a stage of primary apnoea and mild shock. Signs of fetal distress are unlikely to have been apparent unless these were noted immediately prior to delivery.

Severe asphyxia. The infant is in a state of secondary apnoea and severe shock. This may be present at birth as a result of intrauterine hypoxia, or it may occur if a baby, born in a state of mild asphyxia fails to respond to treatment or receives inadequate treatment.

Apgar score

The baby's condition is assessed at one and five minutes after birth by means of the Apgar score. This system of assessing the baby's condition observes five signs for which a score of nought, one or two is awarded for each sign (Table 12.1).

Table 12.1 Apgar score.

Sign	0	1	2
Heart rate	Absent	Less than 100	More than 100
Respiratory effort	Absent	Weak cry	Good cry
Muscle tone	Limp	Some flexion of extremities	Well flexed
Reflex irritability	No response	Some motion	Cry
Colour	Blue/pale	Body pink with blue extremities	Completely pink

You will notice that the higher the score the better the baby's condition. A maximum score of nine is usually scored because a newborn baby is rarely completely pink within five minutes of birth. A baby with an Apgar score of five to eight at one minute would be described as being in a state of mild asphyxia, less than five as being severely asphyxiated, although when you are familiar with the scoring system you will realise that there are degrees within the two types, e.g. a baby with an Apgar score of one is more severely asphyxiated than a baby with an Apgar score of four.

Management

It must always be remembered that an asphyxiated baby is in a state of shock and must be handled gently. It is also important to keep the baby warm as chilling increases the demand for oxygen and glycogen and will, therefore, place additional stress on the baby.

It is routine to clear the baby's airway immediately after birth, before the baby breathes in order to avoid secretions in the nasopharynx being inhaled and causing obstruction. If the baby fails to breathe spontaneously, the cord is clamped and cut, and skin dried and the baby wrapped in a warm dry towel. The baby is placed supine on a resuscitation table with the head lower than the trunk.

Resuscitation of the newborn

Maintain a clear airway. It is often necessary to repeat mucus extraction and great care must be taken to avoid traumatisation of the delicate mucous membrane.
Administration of oxygen. A positive pressure face mask is used to administer oxygen if the respiratory effort is poor or a face mask if the baby is making respiratory efforts.
Antidote. If the mother has received pethidine within two to three hours of delivery, a narcotic antagonist such as neonatal naloxone hydrochloride (Narcan) neonatal (0.01 mg/kg intramuscularly) will be given to the baby.

The mildly asphyxiated baby should respond quickly to this treatment and the Apgar should be normal within five minutes.

Severe asphyxia

If the baby is severely asphyxiated at birth or if a baby with mild asphyxia fails to respond to treatment the paediatrician should be summoned immediately as endotracheal intubation is required. Midwives should be capable of undertaking intubation so that there is no delay if a doctor is not immediately available. Experience in intubating can be gained by practice on an intubation model or a stillborn infant.

ENDOTRACHEAL INTUBATION

A laryngoscope with a short blade is held in the left hand and the blade placed over the infant's tongue as far as the epiglottis and then advanced over the epiglottis. This presses the epiglottis against the root of the tongue and reveals the opening of the trachea, the glottis. Secretions are aspirated under direct vision. A size 12 (occasionally 10) endotracheal tube, held in the right hand, is guided through the larynx into the trachea ensuring the tube is not inserted beyond the bifurcation and into one bronchus as this would result in stimulation of only one lung. A fine catheter FG 5 can be used to aspirate secretions in the endotracheal tube. The oxygen source is connected to the endotracheal tube and intermittent positive pressure is applied at a rate of 15 times/min. The pressure must not exceed 30 cmH_2O otherwise there is a danger of pneumothorax. These low pressures are adequate to induce reflex respiratory movements.

An increase in the heart rate is a good sign that resuscitation is satisfactory. The chest movements are noted to ensure they are equal on each side, unequal movements indicates the endotracheal tube is beyond the bifurcation of the trachea and needs to be withdrawn slightly. The positive pressure should be stopped for fifteen seconds every three minutes to see whether spontaneous respiratory movements will start. An antidote is used if indicated.

Correction of acidosis with 8.4% sodium bicarbonate and hypoglycaemia with 2–4 ml of 20% glucose solution intravenously may be necessary in very severe cases. Because of the risk of hypothermia the infant's rectal temperature is recorded using a low-reading thermometer.

This is a very anxious time for the parents who will be aware that something is wrong but are often too afraid to ask any questions. Anyone who has been involved in this situation realises how easy it is to concentrate on the baby to the exclusion of the parents; however as soon as possible the parents should be informed and given the opportunity to see and touch or hold their baby before it is transferred to the Special Care Baby Unit.

This is an 'at risk' infant whose name is placed in the 'At Risk' (Observation) Register' to ensure periodic developmental assessment in order to detect early any failure to develop normally. The Apgar score at five minutes is significant when considering the long-term prognosis.

Birth trauma

Improved standards of obstetric care have reduced the risk of birth trauma but it is still a major cause of perinatal death and is, therefore, an important subject. In addition, trauma is associated with an increased risk of infection which in itself is a cause of mortality and morbidity.

EXTRACRANIAL

Cephalhaematoma. This is bleeding between the bone and the periosteum, and is caused by friction between the fetal skull and the maternal pelvis. It is not

observed at birth but appears within twenty-four hours. The pericranium is bound down at the bone edges and therefore the bleeding and consequently the swelling is confined to one bone and cannot cross a suture line. The swelling does not pit on pressure, an important factor in distinguishing a cephalhaematoma from a caput succedaneum (see p. 125), as is the time of appearance, duration and limitation by suture line. A double cephalhaematoma is usually bilateral. The cephalhaematoma persists for several weeks but is usually resolved by approximately six weeks. Treatment is rarely necessary but occasionally a large or bilateral haematoma may cause anaemia and a blood transfusion may be required. It is thought that in the majority of cases there is a hairline fracture of the underlying bone, but this is not significant. Occasionally a depressed fracture may occur. An intramuscular injection of vitamin K_1 phytomendadione (Konakion) 1 mg may be given if not used routinely. Jaundice may be more marked in babies with cephalhaematoma.
'*Chignon.*' Vacuum extraction is associated with the formation of an oedematous swelling known as a 'chignon', where the suction cup has been applied. This is very marked at delivery but resolves within a few days leaving a discolouration of the skin which persists for several days. Very occasionally the skin becomes necrotic but healing is usually rapid.
Forceps marks. The baby born by forceps may have the marks of the blades on the side of the face. These usually heal without any difficulty.
Fracture of the skull. Hairline fractures are usually associated with severe trauma but usually go unnoticed as it is the cerebral injury which is the cause of the symptoms. Depressed fractures are rare and usually benign.

INTRACRANIAL

Causes

Injury may occur due to:
Hypoxia/anoxia. Congestion leading to oedema, petechial, subarachnoid or intracerebral haemorrhage or rupture of sinuses may occur as the result of severe hypoxia or anoxia.
Tentorial tear. Laceration of the tentorium cerebelli at its junction with the falx cerebri involves the cerebral vein.

Predisposing causes

1 Prolonged labour leading to intrauterine hypoxia.
2 Cephalopelvic disproportion leading to excessive moulding of the fetal skull bones.
3 Rapid moulding may occur in a precipitate labour or of the aftercoming head in a breech delivery.
4 Rapid decompression occurs if the delivery of the head occurs rapidly. This is the danger in a precipitate delivery or in a breech delivery.

5 Prematurity. The immature infant is more prone to cerebral injury due to the compressibility of the soft skull bones and the fragility of blood vessels.

Signs of cerebral irritation

There are degrees of cerebral irritation which may be subdivided into mild, moderate and severe. It is important to recognise and treat the mild form in order to prevent progression.

MILD

These babies lie awake between feeds and usually resent handling. They should be allowed to rest, and sedation may be necessary.
unusually wakeful,

MODERATE

a The infant usually lies awake.
b Resents handling.
c Cries when touched—usually high pitched.
d Muscle tone is increased.
e Appears to feed but is unable to suck.

Sleep is essential to these babies and they will require sedation, Chloral Hydrate being the drug of choice. Feeds should be given via an intragastric tube.

SEVERE

a The infant may present with severe asphyxia at birth and may be difficult to resuscitate.
b Pallor may be noted.
c Apnoeic attacks.
d Anxious wide awake expression. ^ wrinkled brow.
e Muscle tone may be poor or increased tone with hyperextension of the spine may be evident.
f Difficulty with feeding. M. convulsions if handled or disturbed.
g Vomiting may occur.
h Irritability.
i High pitched crying. ^ shrill cry.
j Lethargy.
k Temperature lability. ^ hypothermic
l fontanelle is tense

Management

The baby is nursed in an incubator to facilitate observation and the temperature adjusted according to the baby's temperature and its size. The baby is handled as little as possible and every available aid used to observe him without disturbing him.

Observations are made of the baby's temperature, respirations and apex beat, also muscle tone, reflex irritability and cry. The blood glucose level is estimated by Dextrostix to exclude hypoglycaemia.

The feeding regime is determined by the baby's condition, and feeding via a nasogastric tube may be necessary if the baby is lethargic or difficult to feed.

If convulsions occur, intramuscular paraldehyde is given (using a glass syringe); or phenobarbitone 3–4 mg/kg/dose or phenytoin (Epanutin) 3 mg/kg/dose intramuscularly or 5 mg/kg/dose orally (six-hourly).

Nerve injury

FACIAL PALSY

Damage to the facial (7th cranial) nerve due to direct pressure by obstetric forceps may cause transitory facial palsy lasting one to two weeks. There is asymmetry of the face, the eye on the affected side remains open and the mouth is drawn towards the unaffected side. A baby with facial palsy is able to suckle at the breast.

BRACHIAL PLEXUS

Three types of injuries to the brachial plexus (5th, 6th, 7th and 8th cervical nerves and part of the 1st thoracic nerve) are recognised.

Erbs palsy. This is caused by pressure of the fingers at the root of the neck or by pulling on the neck during delivery of the aftercoming head in a breech presentation or by excessive traction on the neck in the delivery of the shoulders in a cephalic presentation. There is hyperextension of the arm which is rotated medially with the hand flexed.

Klumpke palsy. This is caused by traction on the arm in delivering the shoulders. There is extension of the hand with failure of the wrist to flex.

Erbs and Klumpke palsy. A combination of the two types of palsy.

The infant is referred to an orthopaedic surgeon.

Skeletal injury

FRACTURE OF THE CLAVICLE AND HUMERUS

The infant's clavicle or humerus may be fractured during delivery of a breech presentation. There is lack of spontaneous movements and absent Moro reflex on the affected side. X-ray examination should be performed if fractures are suspected.

Fracture of the humerus is treated by splinting the infant's arm to the chest using a crepe bandage.

Fracture of the clavicle requires no treatment.

Muscular injury

STERNOMASTOID 'TUMOUR'

Traction on the neck of the fetus either during delivery of the shoulders or of the aftercoming head may cause injury to the sternomastoid muscles and cause a haematoma. A firm mass may be felt anywhere along the length of the muscles, but more usually in the middle or lower third. Physiotherapy is performed to avoid torticollis.

Injury to the skin

Bruising. Contusion of the skin is a common feature of a malpresentation. In a breech presentation the external genitalia are bruised and oedematous as is the face in a face presentation.
Abrasions. These may occur to the face due to poor application of the forceps blades.
Fat necrosis. This is a firm subcutaneous swelling at the site of pressure which is painful when touched. Treatment is not usually required but the baby should be positioned to avoid pressure to the area.
Petechiae. Tiny haemorrhages may appear on the skin of the head and neck and because the baby appears cyanosed, the term traumatic 'asphyxia' is used. No treatment is required.

Injury to the eyes

Subconjunctival haemorrhages are common in the newborn and have no significance.

LOW BIRTH WEIGHT INFANTS

A low birth weight infant is one weighing less than 2.5 kg at birth and a baby weighing less than 1.5 kg is referred to as being of very low birth weight.

A breakdown of the 1980 statistics shows that babies weighing under 2.5 kg accounted for over 55% of all stillbirths and deaths in the first year of life, while only forming 6.9% of all live and stillbirths. The highest mortality rates were in babies weighing less than 1.5 kg—over 50% of all births in this group resulted in a stillbirth or infant death. Mortality rates fell dramatically with increasing birth rate, reaching a low of 0.6% of all live and stillbirths in babies weighing between 3.5 and 4 kg.

Classification

Pre-term. A baby born before thirty-seven completed weeks of pregnancy.

Light-for-dates. A baby whose weight is below the tenth percentile for gestational age. This may be as the result of:

a Intrauterine growth retardation due to placental insufficiency.

b Hypoplasia due to intrauterine infection or chromosomal abnormality.

c Genetic, the baby is small because of genetic factors, e.g. familial or racial.

Some infants are of low birth weight due to more than one factor, e.g. the baby may be pre-term and also light-for-dates.

The pre-term infant

Immaturity is a major cause of perinatal mortality and it is therefore an important subject.

Causes

A pre-term infant may be born following spontaneous onset of labour or where a complication of pregnancy has necessitated premature intervention.

Spontaneous: cause unknown (50%); multiple pregnancy (10%); fetal abnormality (5%); polyhydramnios.

Contributory causes: age and parity; smoking; alcohol; hyperpyrexia; low socioeconomic group; unmarried mother; emotional stress.

Induced: pre-eclampsia (20%); antepartum haemorrhage; Rhesus haemolytic disease.

Characteristics

The appearance and behaviour of the infant will vary according to the period of gestation. This is calculated from the date of the mother's last normal menstrual period and can be confirmed by a neurological examination, as the development of the central nervous system is related to gestational age of the infant, and by observation of external features.

Weight. The baby's weight will range from 1.4 kg at twenty-eight weeks to 2.5 kg at thirty-four weeks and 3 kg at thirty-seven weeks gestation (Fig. 12.1).

Length. This ranges from 38 cm at twenty-eight weeks to 45 cm at thirty-four weeks and 48 cm at thirty-seven weeks gestation (Fig. 12.2).

Head circumference. The occipitofrontal head circumference is approximately 26 cm at twenty-eight weeks, 31.5 cm at thirty-four weeks and 33.5 cm at thirty-seven weeks gestation (Fig. 12.3).

Head. The baby's head appears large in proportion to the body. The bones of

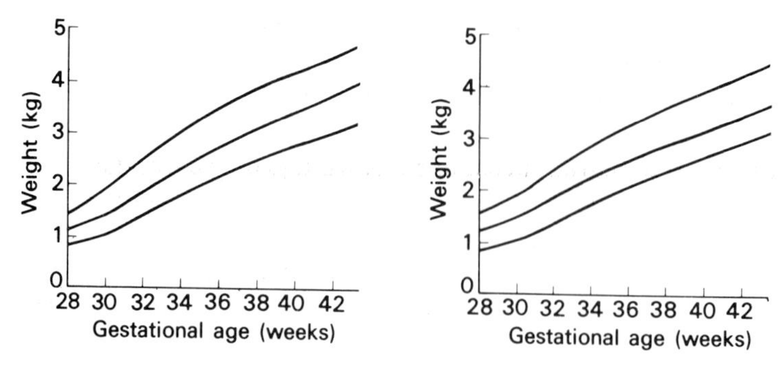

Fig. 12.1 Weight charts for newborn babies, 10th, 50th and 90th centiles; boys (left), girls (right).

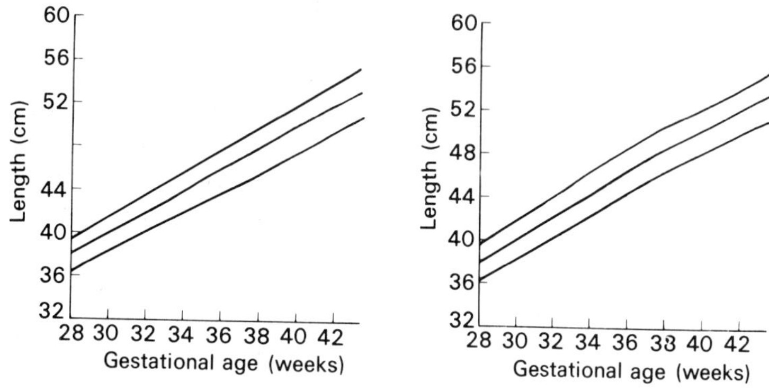

Fig. 12.2 Length charts for newborn babies, 10th, 50th and 90th centiles; boys (left), girls (right).

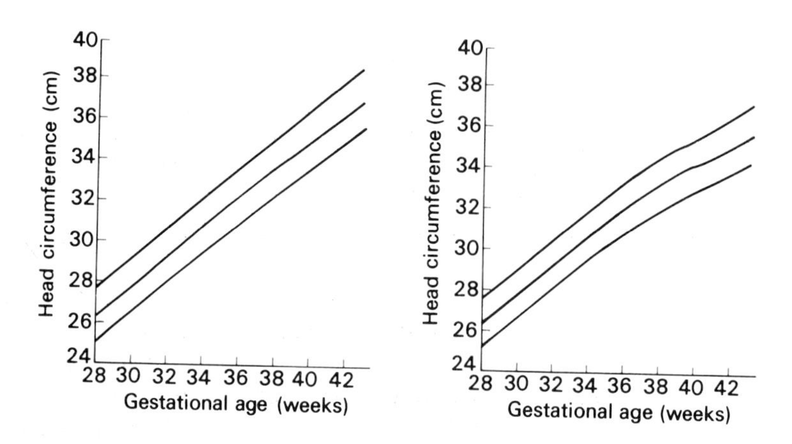

Fig. 12.3 Head circumference charts for newborn babies, 10th, 50th and 90th centiles; boys (left), girls (right).

the skull are soft and the sutures and fontanelles are wide. The ear is flat and shapeless, the cartilage is soft and the pinna stays folded prior to thirty-four weeks gestation but after this time there is incurving of the periphery of the pinna and it returns slowly from folding.
Skin. The skin is thin, translucent and red. Lanugo may cover the entire body or be present on the shoulders only. Vernix caseosa will be seen to cover the whole of the body. The sole creases appear about thirty-two weeks gestation but will not be well defined in an immature baby. There is obvious oedema of the hands and feet with pitting over the tibia in the very immature baby.
Chest. The chest is narrow, breast tissue is not present before thirty-five weeks gestation and the nipples are barely visible before thirty-two weeks gestation but after this time the areola is well defined.
Abdomen. The abdomen is distended and appears large in comparison with the narrow chest.
Genitalia. In the male infant the testes are undescended and the scrotum smooth prior to thirty weeks gestation, by thirty-six weeks gestation there are a few rugae on the scrotum and the testes are high in the canal. In the female infant the labia majora are widely separated and the clitoris prominent until about thirty-six weeks gestation by which time the labia majora almost cover the labia minora.
Reflexes. The reflexes are absent or poorly developed in the immature baby.
Muscle tone. The muscle tone is poor and the very immature baby lies with arms and legs extended. The baby adopts a more flexed attitude with increasing maturity.

Complications

Prematurity is a major cause of perinatal mortality and for every day less *in utero* the mortality rate increases by 1.5%.
Asphyxia neonatorum. The baby has an immature respiratory centre which is easily depressed by drugs used in labour. The lung tissue may fail to expand—primary atelectasis (see p. 343).
Respiratory distress syndrome. This may occur due to lack of surfactant in the immature baby's lungs (see p. 360).
Hypothermia. The immature baby has a large surface area in relation to its body weight and there is lack of subcutaneous fat, especially brown fat which is metabolised rapidly to produce heat. The baby's thin skin results in loss of heat and the immature heat regulating centre produces thermolability.
Hypoglycaemia. This may occur due to low glycogen and is aggravated by asphyxia and hypothermia.
Jaundice. There is a deficiency in the liver enzyme glucuronyl transferase which is required for conjugation of bilirubin (see p. 364). The reduced rate of conjugation results in a build up of unconjugated bilirubin causing

jaundice which appears about the third day and may, in an immature baby, last for about two weeks. The danger of this is damage to the brain cells of the basal ganglia and brain stem resulting in kernicterus (see p. 370).

Infection. The immature baby has a low immunity and a less effective immunoglobulin and white cell reaction. It is also more prone to chilling which predisposes to infection.

Anaemia. This may be primary due to haemolysis of red blood cells or secondary due to low iron stores.

Intraventricular or subarachnoid haemorrhage. The immature baby has fragile blood vessels which can easily rupture due to trauma or anoxia.

Inhalation. The baby's cough and swallowing reflexes may be absent or poor and this can lead to inhalation if oral feeding is commenced.

Additional complications

Retrolental fibroplasia. This is due to the toxic effect of high concentrations of oxygen in the arterioles of the retina. An opaque membrane forms behind the lens causing blindness.

Congenital malformations. The incidence of congenital malformations is higher in babies born prematurely.

Management

The principles of care of the immature baby are:

ESTABLISHMENT AND MAINTENANCE OF RESPIRATIONS

The management of the immature baby at birth with regards to establishing respirations is as for the mature newborn (see p. 334), but if this baby is asphyxiated and resuscitation is required, even greater care needs to be taken to prevent chilling. The baby is transferred to the Special Care Baby Unit in a transport incubator as soon as possible and placed in an incubator on an apnoea monitor. The baby's colour and respirations are observed at frequent intervals. Any signs of cyanosis may indicate the need to clear the mouth, nose and nasopharynx.

OBSERVATIONS AND RECORDINGS

The baby's respiratory movements are recorded continuously by an apnoea monitor which will give a signal if movements cease for longer than ten seconds.

The frequency of observations will depend on the condition of the baby.

Temperature. This is checked on admission and at half-hourly to hourly intervals until the baby's temperature is 36.8 °C then two to four-hourly as indicated. An electric thermometer with skin probe is used for ill babies and the skin temperature kept at 36.5 °C.

Incubator temperature. The temperature of the incubator is checked at each feed prior to opening the portals.
Respirations and apex beat. These are recorded half-hourly for at least six hours and then as indicated.
Colour. This is observed at the same frequency as the respirations and apex beat.
Oxygen concentration. This is checked hourly using an oxygen analyser.
Dextrostix test. The blood glucose level is estimated using the Dextrostix test every three hours for forty-eight hours or as ordered by the doctor.
Blood test. Blood is taken to exclude phenylketonuria on the seventh day. Immature babies may have a transitory rise in blood phenylalanine due to immaturity of the liver, therefore the test may need to be repeated later.

REGULATION OF TEMPERATURE

Because of the risk of hypothermia, temperature control is an important aspect of the care of the immature newborn. A high environmental temperature is required to prevent heat loss, and this is obtained by nursing the baby in an incubator under a Perspex hemicylindrical shield to reduce heat loss by radiation. The incubator temperature is determined initially on the size of the baby and the room temperature, e.g. if the room temperature is 27 °C, a baby weighing 2 kg will need to be nursed in an incubator with the temperature set at 34 °C to maintain a body temperature of 37 °C.

It is of vital importance to maintain the baby's temperature in the thermoneutral range, i.e. a temperature at which the infant has to use less energy and the oxygen demand is at its lowest level. Every effort should be made to prevent heat loss at delivery, and resuscitation if necessary should be performed under a radiant heater. The baby is placed in a pre-heated incubator and transferred to a Special Care Baby Unit as soon as possible. Transport incubators are available for transferring babies from one hospital to another although ideally the mother should be transferred at the onset of premature labour or before if labour is to be induced.

PREVENTION OF INFECTION

The risk of infection is high in all newborn babies but this is especially so in the immature infant, therefore special precautions must be taken to reduce the risk. The use of gowns, masks and separate shoes or overshoes will depend on the preference of the paediatrician but in many units the use of gowns and masks has been discontinued.

Measures to prevent infection can be considered in three ways.
Personnel. All staff should wash their hands thoroughly before and after handling each baby, ensuring the correct use of elbow taps and pedal bins. The soap or solution used for handwashing will vary from unit to unit but a bacteriocidal solution such as chlorhexidine is recommended. Disposable

gloves may be worn for changing the baby's napkin and carrying out the daily toilet. No member of staff with a cold, diarrhoea or vomiting or any form of septic lesion is allowed in the unit.

Incubator and other equipment. The inside and outside of the incubator is cleaned daily with a solution of chlorhexidine by the nurse caring for the baby. The portals at the top end of the incubator are used for introducing feeds and clean equipment and the portals at the foot end of the incubator are used for removal of soiled linen. Each baby's equipment is stored in the incubator or cot cupboard and used only for that baby. On discharge any unused equipment is discarded and linen although clean sent to the laundry.

Domestic cleaning. Cleaning equipment is used only in the unit and not in other working areas. Damp dusting of ledges and wet mopping of floor surfaces is carried out.

NUTRITION

The method of feeding the immature baby will depend on the preference of the paediatrician and the regime described is intended as a general guide. Early feeding is usually advised to prevent hypoglycaemia, dehydration and jaundice. The size and activity of the baby will determine whether tube or bottle feeding is undertaken but infants of less than thirty-four weeks gestation lack the neuromuscular ability to suck and swallow, so even the healthiest baby will need nasogastric feeding to ensure the required fluid intake and reduce the risk of aspiration. Babies of more than thirty-four weeks gestation may suck well but require half the feed, or alternate feeds by tube to avoid tiring.

Tube feeding

A 3.5–6.0 FG nasogastric tube is used, the size depending on the baby's weight. The tube is measured from the bridge of the nose round the front of the ear to the tip of the sternum. The required length is marked with a piece of clear tape. The tube is passed and its position checked by using a stethoscope over the stomach, injecting 2 ml of air into the tube and listening for air in the stomach. The stomach is washed out with Dextrose water until the aspirate is clear. An initial feed of 5 ml of 5% Dextrose is given and milk feeds commenced at two hours.

Intermittent tube feeding. Expressed breast milk or a low solute cows' milk preparation is used and 60 ml/kg is given in the first twenty-four hours and increased by 30 ml/kg daily to a maximum of 180 ml/kg a day. The feeds may be given at three-hourly intervals or more often and in some cases as frequently as every half an hour.

An infusion pump may be used during the first few days when volumes are small. The amount of feed given in the twenty-four hours is as for intermittent tube feeding but to a maximum of 300 ml/kg a day if this is tolerated by the baby. The bottle of milk is changed every four hours and the giving set every twenty-four hours. Alternate bottle feeding may be introduced when the baby weighs 2 kg.

Intravenous feeding

Total parental feeding is recommended by some paediatricians for very low birth weight babies. It is thought that their enzymes are not able to cope with milk feeds, not even expressed breast milk. Amino acid, lipid and electrolyte solutions can be infused into the right atrium of the heart via a fine silastic catheter. The mixture provides balanced nutrition during a period which is vital for brain growth.

Supplements

An iron supplement in the form of Sytron is commenced at two weeks of age and continued until the baby is six months old. Multivitamins in the form of Abidec is also commenced at two weeks and continued until the baby is a year old.

MOTHER-INFANT RELATIONSHIP

The baby who is nursed in a Special Care Baby Unit is separated from its mother and, if born by Caesarean section under a general anaesthesia, the mother may not have seen the baby at birth. It is important that the staff from the Special Care Baby Unit visit the mother to inform her of the baby's condition and as soon as possible the mother should visit the unit. A photograph of the baby may be taken and given to the mother. If the baby is nursed in an incubator this creates a barrier between the mother and her baby and this can be partially overcome by allowing the mother to put her hands through the port and touch the baby. Both parents are encouraged to visit the unit as often as possible and allowed to do things for the baby as soon as they can. If the mother wishes to breast feed she is encouraged to express the milk using the humolactor. This is then sterilised and given to the baby.

When the baby is ready to go home the mother is encouraged to spend at least a day, or longer of this can be arranged, in the mother and baby unit so that she can get used to handling her baby before taking him home.

Other members of the family should not be excluded and a viewing corridor provides a means by which they can see the baby. Some units are now permitting other children and grandparents to enter the nursery.

The light-for-dates infant

The majority of infants in this category are those whose low birth weight in relation to their gestational age is the result of intrauterine malnutrition, the fetus being deprived of those substances necessary for its full growth. In some cases, however, it is associated with an intrauterine injection or a congenital malformation.

Causes

Placental insufficiency: hypertension— pre-eclampsia, essential hypertension; threatened abortion; antepartum haemorrhage; multiple pregnancy; smoking; alcohol.
Intrauterine infection: rubella; toxoplasmosis; cytomegalovirus; syphilis.
Congenital malformation: Down's syndrome.
Maternal disease: respiratory and renal diseases.
Low socioeconomic status, age, parity, marital status.
No obvious cause: this type tends to be repetitive.

Characteristics

As with the immature infant the appearance and behaviour of these babies depends on the gestational age but the majority of these babies are born after thirty-seven completed weeks and are, therefore, mature infants.
Weight. The baby's birth weight is below the tenth percentile for gestational age due to lack of subcutaneous fat (see p. 351, Fig. 12.1).
Length. This is usually normal for gestational age but may be marginally reduced.
Head circumference. As with the length this is usually normal for gestational age but may be reduced if intrauterine malnutrition is very severe or the baby is small as the result of intrauterine infections causing microcephally. Because of the lack of subcutaneous fat, the head usually appears disproportionately large.
Skin. In the postmature light-for-dates baby the skin is dry and loose due to lack of subcutaneous fat. In severe cases the skin is flaking and cracked and the skin, umbilical cord and nails may be stained with meconium.
Expression. The baby's face may be small and wizened with an anxious, wide awake expression.
Reflexes. The baby is often jittery and hypertonic with exaggerated reflexes. The baby is hungry and sucks ravenously at his hands.

The baby's appearance and behaviour will depend on the severity of the intrauterine deprivation and mild cases may be missed at birth if the midwife is not alert to this problem.

Complications

Intrauterine hypoxia. Signs of fetal distress may have presented during labour.
Birth asphyxia. This may occur as a result of intrauterine hypoxia or due to meconium aspiration.
Hypothermia. Due to lack of subcutaneous fat this baby is very prone to heat loss. This risk would be increased if the baby was asphyxiated at birth.
Hypoglycaemia. The baby's glycogen stores are low and rapidly depleted if the baby was asphyxiated at birth or becomes hypothermic.
Hypocalcaemia.
Infection. Aspiration pneumonia or skin infections may occur.
Pulmonary haemorrhages.

Management

The care of this baby is aimed at preventing the complications or treating them if they occur.

Asphyxia neonatorum is anticipated if the fetus is known to be small-for-dates and the paediatrician is called for delivery so that resuscitation can be undertaken without delay (see p. 343).

Hypothermia is avoided by preventing heat loss at delivery and transferring the baby to the Special Care Baby Unit without delay. The baby is then nursed in an incubator under a Perspex shield to prevent heat loss due to radiation.

Hypoglycaemia and hypocalcaemia are prevented by early feeding. Blood glucose levels are estimated three-hourly using Dextrostix test. If the level is below 1.4 mmol/l (25 mg/dl) a specimen of blood is sent for laboratory testing. If asymptomatic, the hypoglycaemia is treated by giving a milk feed and the Dextrostix test repeated an hour later. Hypoglycaemia is indicated by a plasma glucose level below 1.1 mmol/l (20 mg/dl) and if this is accompanied by convulsive movements, 2–4 ml of 20% Dextrose/kg body weight may be given intravenously. A nasogastric tube is passed and a full strength milk is given as a continuous drip at 60 ml/kg body weight in twenty-four hours.

Infection is prevented by attention to personal hygiene and to the environment (see p. 355).

Sequelae

The light-for-dates baby usually responds well to treatment and gains weight rapidly. However, there are often long-term problems and many of these babies fail to reach their potential. The baby's name is entered on the Observation Register to ensure periodic recall for developmental assessment.

Idiopathic respiratory distress syndrome

Respiratory failure is a common cause of perinatal mortality and morbidity. In babies born after a short gestation or to a mother with diabetes mellitus or following Caesarean section the respiratory distress may take the form of a complex syndrome which is known as idiopathic respiratory distress syndrome or hyaline membrane disease.

Diagnosis

The baby's condition is usually reasonably good at birth but within a few hours of birth difficulty in breathing develops and progresses. The respiratory rate rises to more than 60/min and difficulty in breathing is shown by flaring of the nares, intercostal and substernal recession on inspiration and grunting on expiration. Cyanosis occurs which may be relieved by 40% oxygen but later may become unresponsive to very high levels of oxygen.

Auscultation of the lungs reveals reduced breath sounds and X-ray examination the characteristic fine 'ground glass' mottling distributed fairly evenly through the lung fields. As the disease progresses this mottling may coarsen, and in fatal cases a uniform opacity may ensue. The X-ray examination not only gives confirmatory evidence of the disease but excludes other causes of respiratory distress such as pneumothorax, diaphragmatic hernia, atelectasis, pneumonia, meconium aspiration and emphysema.

Cause

The cause of respiratory distress syndrome is thought to be a deficiency of pulmonary surfactant, a substance usually present in the alveolar walls. This lowers the surface tension in the alveoli so that, whatever their size, the same pressure is required to inflate them, therefore ensuring uniform inflation of all the alveoli. Surfactant also prevents collapse of the alveolar walls during expiration. If surfactant is deficient, the surface tension in the smaller alveoli is very great, causing them to collapse. The larger alveoli continue to expand resulting in uneven expansion with progressive alveolar collapse.

Autopsy examination reveals atelectasis, oedema, interstitial haemorrhages and hyaline membrane which consists of protein rich fibrin derived from the plasma of the pulmonary vessels.

Prognosis

The baby's condition deteriorates progressively but by the age of twenty-four to forty-eight hours the signs of respiratory distress may decrease and recovery occurs. In many babies the signs worsen and cyanosis becomes more profound or a greyish pallor indicative of peripheral circulatory collapse occurs. Increasingly frequent apnoeic attacks occur accompanied by slowing of the heart beat and death ensues. If the baby survives for seventy-two hours he has a good chance of recovery.

The incidence of idiopathic respiratory distress is approximately 10–15% of babies weighing 2.5 kg or less due to short gestation. It is unusual in low birth weight babies of more than thirty-seven weeks gestation. The incidence is higher in babies of mothers with diabetes mellitus and weighing more than 2.5 kg and born after thirty-six weeks gestation. Conversely, there is a lower incidence in babies of short gestation born where the pregnancy was complicated by pre-eclampsia and premature rupture of membranes. It is thought that certain complications of pregnancy that are stressful to the fetus are associated with accelerated development of pulmonary surfactant and therefore protect the baby of short gestation against the development of the idiopathic respiratory distress syndrome.

The mortality rate associated with the idiopathic respiratory distress syndrome varies according to the gestational age of the baby but the overall mortality is between 20 and 40%.

Management

The management of babies suffering from the idiopathic respiratory distress syndrome is general supportive measures supplemented by corrective measures.

General care

The nursing care and general supervision of these infants requires to be performed by trained, experienced nurses who are not only skilful in observing and handling these babies but also skilled in the technical aspects involved in the care. The infant should be handled as little as possible and every available aid used to observe the baby without disturbing him.

TEMPERATURE CONTROL

The inability of these infants to maintain control of body temperature may lead to additional complications. To avoid the necessity of frequently recording the baby's rectal temperature, the skin temperature of the exposed abdominal surface is recorded using a surface mounted probe. Heat loss by radiation is reduced by placing a Perspex shield over the baby. The aim is to maintain the baby's skin temperature between 36.5 and 37 °C which is the level at which the metabolic cost to the baby is minimal.

OXYGEN THERAPY

This is an important aspect in the care of these babies but oxygen therapy does have its dangers and may cause retrolental fibroplasia (see p. 354), direct damage to the alveoli and cerebral vasoconstriction. However, hypoxia is equally dangerous and may result in acidosis, delay in closure of the ductus arteriosus and cerebral damage or death.

The most reliable way to control oxygen therapy is to measure arterial oxygen tensions directly, and to adjust the inspired oxygen concentrations so that the arterial oxygen tension is between 60 mmHg and 80 mmHg. A continuous measurement can be made by a P_{O_2} and P_{CO_2} monitor but if this is not available samples of blood are obtained four-hourly through an indwelling umbilical artery catheter. If facilities are not available for monitoring arterial oxygen tensions the concentration of oxygen in the incubator is gradually increased until central cyanosis is relieved but this carries the risk of hyperoxaemia or hypoxaemia.

The oxygen concentration in the incubator near the baby's nose should be measured every hour using an oxygen analyser. If oxygen concentrations above 30% are required, a Perspex (Gairdner) headbox is used.

Correction of acidosis

Acidosis is a common complication of idiopathic respiratory distress syndrome and blood is taken via the umbilical catheter to estimate the pH at regular intervals. Corrective measures are taken to maintain the pH above 7.25. Sodium bicarbonate is one base used to correct the acidosis, the amount depending on the pH, e.g. if pH is less than 7.8 milliequivalents per kilogram (mEq/kg) is recommended. An 8.4% solution of sodium bicarbonate contains just under 1 mEq/ml. The pH is remeasured an hour later and further adjustments made if necessary.

VENTILATION

Indications for using ventilation include:

1 Rising arterial carbon dioxide tension (Pa_{CO_2}).

2 Falling arterial oxygen tension (Pa_{O_2}) despite increased concentrations of inspired oxygen, i.e. more than 70% oxygen is needed to maintain Pa_{O_2} greater than 50–60 mmHg.

3 Increasing acidosis, i.e. falling pH partly respiratory due to high Pa_{CO_2} and partly due to hypoxaemia.

4 Fall in respiratory rate or apnoea.

5 Cyanosis unrelieved by high concentrations of inspired oxygen.

6 Falling blood pressure and tachycardia progressing to pallor, evidence of peripheral circulatory failure and bradycardia.

Methods

Continuous positive airway pressure (CPAP). This is the first method used. It prevents the alveoli from closing by maintaining a continuous positive transpulmonary pressure throughout the pulmonary cycle. A pressure of approximately 2–7 cmH_2O is used but higher levels may be needed if these levels fail to produce an improvement. Oxygen concentrations are usually high, 80% initially but are reduced by 5% decrements until reaching 40%. The level of continuous positive airway pressure is reduced 1 cmH_2O at a time taking several days to discontinue ventilation.

Intermittent positive pressure ventilation (IPPV). Indications for changing to mechanical ventilation include a Pa_{O_2} of less than 40 mmHg in 100% oxygen and apnoea not responding to resuscitative measures. An endotracheal tube is passed and connected to a ventilator. The ventilator is set on inspiratory time, e.g. 1.5 seconds, to expiratory time, e.g. 1 second, a peak pressure, e.g. 24 cmH_2O, and end pressure, e.g. 5 cmH_2O and a respiration rate, e.g. 32/min. The inspiratory:expiratory ratio is adjusted according to the Pa_{CO_2}, if low the inspiratory time is increased.

The endotracheal tube is aspirated hourly following introduction of 0.5 ml of normal saline to loosen secretions.

An intra-arterial infusion of 5% or 10% Dextrose and 0.18% sodium chloride is maintained to provide nutrition and the amount given each day calculated according to the age and weight of the baby. Calcium supplements of 5–10 ml of 10% calcium gluconate are added to the infusion fluid over twenty-four hours. As the baby's condition improves, oral feeding via a nasogastric tube is introduced and gradually increased and the intra-arterial infusion reduced accordingly.

Frequent measuring of the arterial oxygen tensions and other estimations involves removing over a period of days a comparatively large quantity of blood and a replacement blood transfusion may be necessary.

Neonatal jaundice

Approximately 11% of all babies become clinically jaundiced within the first week of life with a higher incidence in pre-term and sick babies. Jaundice is a sign of a disease causing yellow pigmentation of the skin and is due to raised levels of serum bilirubin. Jaundice is not detectable until the level of serum bilirubin rises to 75 µmol/l and may vary from mild to severe.

Degrees of jaundice. Mild 75–175 µmol/l; moderate 175–250 µmol/l; severe 250 µmol/l or more.

Conjugation of bilirubin

Unconjugated (fat soluble) bilirubin is produced due to the haemolysis of red blood cells. The bilirubin binds with albumen in the plasma and is transported to the liver for conjugation. The bilirubin is conjugated, i.e. made water soluble, by the action of the liver enzyme, glucuronyl transferase. The water soluble bilirubin does not bind with protein and is excreted in the stools and urine.

The fetus copes with only 1% of its bilirubin, the remainder is excreted to the mother via the placenta. It is thought that steroid hormones from the placenta suppress the fetal liver enzyme activity.

Causes of jaundice

The commonest causes of jaundice in the newborn.

Hepatic immaturity. This is also known as 'physiological' jaundice because, although it is unphysiological to become jaundiced, this type is due to a normal physiological process, namely, the haemolysis of the red blood cells. Following delivery there is a delay in the function of the liver enzyme activity, glucuronyl transferase being only about 1% efficient at birth but becoming more efficient within the first week of life. This process is slower in the immature baby who is, therefore, more likely to develop jaundice. In addition, the extra red blood cells necessary for an intrauterine existence are no longer required and excessive haemolysis takes place. In the mature infant the jaundice appears after twenty-four hours and reaches a peak on the fourth or fifth day, but in the immature infant it usually begins forty-eight hours after birth and may last up to two weeks.

Haemolytic disease of the newborn. The excessive breakdown of red blood cells is due to antibodies resulting from incompatibility between the maternal and fetal blood groups.

a Rhesus haemolytic disease. There is incompatibility between the Rhesus negative mother and the Rhesus positive fetus. The Rhesus system is composed of several different antigens, the six main Rhesus antigens are classified as C, D, E, c, d, e. Rhesus positive refers to the presence of the D antigen and Rhesus negative to the absence of the D antigen. The D antigen is present in red blood cells of 83% of Europeans but is higher in other ethnic groups, and is responsible for Rhesus isoimmunisation in 90% of cases. Other groups that have been identified include Lutheran, Kell, Lewis, Duffy, MNS and Kidd.

The disease is characterised by varying degrees of jaundice, anaemia and oedema. Three degrees are described.

1 Haemolytic anaemia. The baby is anaemic at birth but not severely so.

2 Icterus gravis neonatorum. The baby is severely anaemic and there is enlargement of the liver and spleen, hepatosplenomegaly.
3 Hydrops fetalis. The baby is severely anaemic, grossly oedematous and in heart failure. Hepatosplenomegaly is present.
b ABO incompatibility. The mother is blood group O and the fetus A, B or AB. This form of haemolytic disease is more common than Rhesus haemolytic disease and more complex in that the mother can be isoimmunised in a variety of ways not just through exposure to an incompatible blood group. The disease is usually mild in character.
Toxic. The haemolysis is due to an infection.
1 Septicaemia. This may be the cause of late onset jaundice, i.e. occurring after the fourth day and may follow an exchange transfusion.
2 Urinary tract infection.
3 Prenatal infections such as rubella, cytomegalic inclusion disease, toxoplasmosis and syphilis cause jaundice in the newborn infant.
Rare causes of jaundice in the newborn
1 Obstruction due to atresia or absence of the bile duct.
2 Galactosaemia, an inborn error of metabolism resulting in deficiency of an enzyme required for the transformation of galactose to glucose. Clinitest on the urine is positive but the Clinistix test is negative (see p. 380).
3 Glucose-6-phosphate dehydrogenase is an enzyme essential for normal metabolism of glucose in the red blood cells. Lack of the enzyme results in excessive breakdown of red blood cells, and prolonged, severe jaundice. It is a sex-linked disorder usually affecting male infants of Eastern Mediterranean, African and Chinese origins.
4 Steroid inhibitors present in the breast milk of some mothers may lead to prolonged jaundice in the baby. If breast feeding is stopped for two or three days the infant's serum bilirubin level falls. This excludes other causes and the mother can then continue to breast feed having maintained lactation by expressing her milk.
5 Drugs. Certain drugs compete with unconjugated bilirubin for plasma proteins and the bilirubin is displaced.
6 Cretinism. Prolonged physiological jaundice may occur in association with this condition.

Rhesus haemolytic disease

As previously mentioned the mother's blood does not contain the Rhesus antigen but the fetus's blood does. This incompatibility can occur in one of the following ways.

In Fig. 12.4, the father of the child is Rhesus positive homozygous, i.e. he has acquired the Rhesus antigen from both parents and can, therefore,

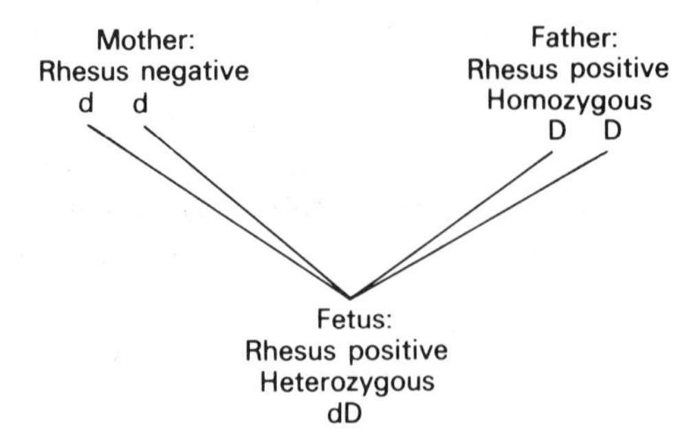

Fig. 12.4 Rhesus incompatibility 1.

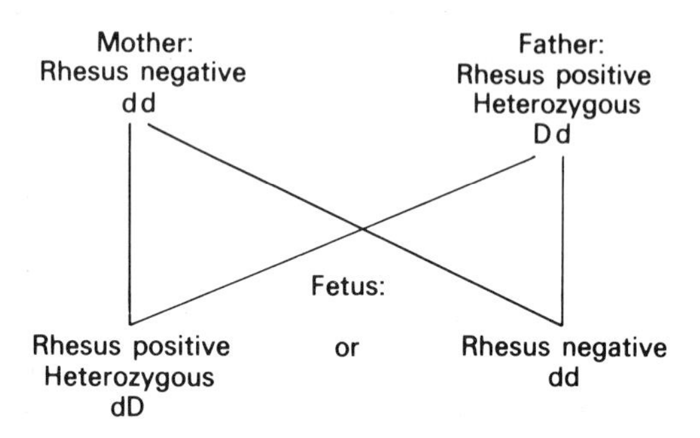

Fig. 12.5 Rhesus incompatibility 2.

only pass on the Rhesus antigen to the fetus who is, therefore, incompatible with the mother.

In 12.5, the father of the child is Rhesus positive heterozygous, i.e. he has acquired the Rhesus antigen from one parent but not the other and can, therefore, either pass on the Rhesus antigen causing the fetus to be Rhesus positive heterozygous and, therefore, incompatible with the mother, or not pass on the Rhesus antigen, and therefore, the fetus will be Rhesus negative and compatible with the mother. The Rhesus antigen is the dominant factor and therefore the person is always Rhesus positive; heterozygous and homozygous determines whether the person carries the antigen in one or both genes.

RHESUS ISOIMMUNISATION

If a Rhesus negative woman receives into her circulation Rhesus positive red blood cells these will act as a foreign antigen and the woman may form antibodies against them, i.e. become Rhesus isoimmunised. If the mother's blood group is O and the fetal blood is of an incompatible group, i.e. A, B or AB this will protect against the formation of Rhesus antibodies because of more rapid formation of anti-A or anti-B antibodies which destroy the cells before Rhesus antibodies can be produced.

Isoimmunisation of the Rhesus negative woman may occur if she is given an incompatible blood transfusion or, more usually during her first pregnancy particularly at the time of placental separation. This means that the first fetus is usually unaffected because the time when the fetal cells are most likely to enter the maternal circulation is in the third stage of labour. Less commonly fetal cells may enter the maternal circulation following amniocentesis, placental abruption or in hypertensive conditions. Rhesus antibodies take some months to form and for this reason even if the fetal leak occurs during pregnancy that fetus is not usually affected.

MANAGEMENT OF RHESUS INCOMPATIBILITY

The expectant mother's blood is taken at booking to determine, amongst other things, the Rhesus factor and if she has Rhesus negative blood it must be screened for antibodies at booking, twenty-eight and thirty-four weeks gestation. If no antibodies are detected the pregnancy is allowed to progress.

At delivery, a specimen of cord blood is obtained and the baby's Rhesus and ABO groups ascertained. An 8 ml sample of the mother's blood is taken at least one hour following delivery and the Kleihauer test performed to estimate whether or not there has been a leak of fetal blood into the maternal circulation and if so, the size of the fetal leak. The Kleihauer test is an acid elusion test and is based on the fact that fetal haemoglobin is more resistant to treatment with acid than maternal haemoglobin. The acid removes the haemoglobin from the maternal cells, they appear pale and are called 'ghost' cells. The fetal cells stand out clearly against this background.

If the test on the cord blood shows the fetus to be Rhesus positive the mother is given an intramuscular injection of anti-D immunoglobulin within sixty hours of delivery. The standard dose is 100 μg but this is increased if the fetal leak is higher than two fetal cells per low power field. Further daily blood samples may be requested, to check that all fetal cells have been eliminated.

It is recommended that Rhesus negative women having a spontaneous or induced abortion should be given 50 μg of anti-D immunoglobulin within sixty hours of delivery if the duration of pregnancy is twenty weeks or less and 100 μg if the duration of pregnancy is more than twenty weeks.

Transplacental haemorrhage occurring during pregnancy may be caused by trauma to the placenta from amniocentesis, threatened abortion, placental abruption or external cephalic version. The unsensitised Rhesus negative woman should be given a dose of 50–100 μg of anti-D immunoglobulin. This is not harmful to the fetus.

Anti-D immunoglobulin provides the mother with antibodies which destroy the fetal cells, but will themselves eventually be eliminated. If this is not given, or given too late or the dose is inadequate, the mother forms antibodies to destroy the foreign antigen on the fetal cells, and the naturally formed antibodies remain in her circulation. If in a subsequent pregnancy she is carrying a Rhesus positive fetus the antibodies, which are capable of crossing the placenta, destroy the fetal red blood cells causing anaemia of varying degrees of severity (see p. 364).

The management of pregnancy in a woman with Rhesus antibodies depends on the level of antibodies, the mother's past history, and the genotype of the husband, i.e. is he Rhesus positive homozygous or heterozygous. If the level is high, i.e. 7 i.u./ml, an amniocentesis is performed and the liquor bilirubin level estimated. The subsequent management depends on the severity of the disease and the period of gestation. If there is a need to intervene before thirty-three weeks gestation an intrauterine transfusion is indicated and involves injecting small quantities of Rhesus negative blood into the fetal peritoneal cavity to maintain the haemoglobulin until the fetus is mature enough to have a chance of surviving an extrauterine existence. In some centres a transfusion directly into the umbilical vein is performed using the technique of fetoscopy (see p. 475). The advantages of an intravascular transfusion is that the transfused blood is immediately available to the fetus and is not dependent on absorption which may be poor if the fetus is oedematous, and fetal haemoglobin estimation enables the degree of anaemia to be determined. After thirty-three weeks of gestation induction of labour and postnatal management may be more appropriate.

MANAGEMENT AT DELIVERY

The Rhesus and ABO groups of the cord blood are estimated and also the Coombs' test, haemoglobin and serum bilirubin levels. The Coombs' test is a direct antihuman globulin test and indicates the presence of maternal antibodies on the baby's red blood cells. A cord blood result showing a strongly positive Coombs' test, a haemoglobin level of below 11 g/dl and a serum bilirubin level above 50 μmol/litre indicates a severely affected infant requiring immediate treatment.

MANAGEMENT OF RHESUS HAEMOLYTIC DISEASE OF THE NEWBORN

Jaundice appears within minutes or hours of birth depending on the severity of the disease. The baby may appear pale or normal at birth and the progress of the disease is monitored by observing the baby for the onset of jaundice. Phototherapy may be used to control the level of bilirubin. The serum bilirubin level is estimated at five to eight-hourly intervals and the rate of the rise is noted as well as the actual level. If the level rises to 340 μmol/litre or is rising rapidly and will reach that level before the next estimation, an exchange transfusion is arranged.

Extra fluids are encouraged by giving the baby plain water following breast feeding or added to the bottle feed. Increasing the fluid intake is thought to reduce the rate at which the serum bilirubin level rises.

EXCHANGE TRANSFUSION

This procedure was first used in the management of haemolytic disease of the newborn in 1949 and involves replacing the baby's blood with Rhesus negative donor blood which is of the same ABO group. Twice the baby's blood volume is exchanged, i.e. 180 ml/kg body weight. The aim of the exchange transfusion is to remove the maternal antibodies, lower the serum bilirubin level and increase the haemoglobin concentration.

Procedure

The procedure is carried out under strict aseptic conditions with the baby in an incubator or on a specially prepared table. During the procedure the baby's colour, respirations, apex beat and temperature are recorded to monitor the baby's reaction to the exchange transfusion. The umbilical vein is catheterised and the catheter secured at the umbilicus with a suture. A syringe and a three-way tap is used to withdraw blood from the baby, the tap is turned and this blood is discarded apart from a sample collected for haemoglobin and serum bilirubin estimation. The tap is turned to draw up donor blood and returned to the first position to inject the blood slowly through the umbilical catheter. The volume removed and replaced at a time is approximately 20–30 ml depending on the size of the baby. The procedure takes approximately two hours to complete. After the transfusion a sample of blood is taken from the catheter for haemoglobin and serum bilirubin estimations. The exchange transfusion may need to be repeated on one or more occasions in severe cases.

Complications of exchange transfusion

Infection. There is a risk of septicaemia occurring and antibiotics may be used if the procedure is repeated or involved a great deal of manipulation.

Ischaemic lesions. These lesions of the large and occasionally the small intestines, sometimes complicated by perforation may occur following catheterisation of the umbilical vein. This is characterised by abdominal distention and vomiting of bile-stained fluid on the day following the catheterisation.

Sequelae

Maternal antibodies can remain in the baby's circulation for about six weeks following delivery.

The baby's bone marrow will take seven to eight weeks to compensate for the haemolysis, therefore the anaemia persists for several weeks. If the haemoglobin is very low, a top-up transfusion may be given but this can delay the natural mechanism for making good the deficiency.

Management of jaundice due to other causes

Jaundice due to causes other than Rhesus haemolytic disease rarely requires exchange transfusion especially in units where phototherapy is used. Jaundice usually presents on the second or third day reaching a peak on the fourth or fifth day. An icterometer can be used to give an indication of the approximate serum bilirubin level and if this indicates a level of 250 μmol/litre in a full-term or 175 μmol/litre in a baby of low birth weight, blood is taken for a serum bilirubin estimation. As the serum bilirubin level rises the baby becomes lethargic and reluctant to feed, making an increase in the fluid intake difficult to achieve.

PHOTOTHERAPY

If the laboratory test confirms the levels mentioned above, phototherapy may be used. The baby's eyes are protected by eye pads and all articles of clothing removed. The phototherapy unit is placed over the cot or incubator; if the baby is being nursed in an incubator, the temperature needs to be adjusted to prevent overheating but if in a cot he may need to be nursed on an electric blanket to maintain a normal temperature. The baby's temperature is recorded three-hourly during phototherapy and extra fluids given to prevent dehydration. Babies under phototherapy pass loose greenish stools.

The phototherapy unit provides daylight which converts bilirubin into biliverdin which does not cause damage to the brain cells. Serum bilirubin levels must be estimated by laboratory test during phototherapy, because the fading of the jaundice makes the icterometer readings unreliable.

Dangers

The risk to the baby of high levels of unconjugated bilirubin is kernicterus due to damage to brain cells of the basal ganglia and brain stem. The baby can cope with a serum bilirubin level of 340 μmol/litre provided the serum globulin level is normal, i.e. 4 g, as there is sufficient protein to bind the bilirubin for excretion. It is when the level of serum bilirubin rises above 340 μmol/litre that there is the risk of kernicterus.

Clinical features of kernicterus

The baby is severely jaundiced, very drowsy and appears gravely ill. The anterior fontanelle may be tense, the eyes are turned down and rolling and twitching may be noted as well as neck retraction and opisthotonus. The infant may die and a high percentage of those who survive develop mental retardation and cerebral palsy.

Haemorrhagic disease of the newborn

This is a temporary coagulation defect associated with spontaneous haemorrhage between the second and fifth days of life.

Aetiology

HYPOPROTHROMBINAEMIA

Prothrombin is not stored in fetal tissues and vitamin K which is essential for the synthesis of prothrombin in the liver is not present in the fetal intestines. Therefore prothrombin levels are low from twelve hours after birth until the baby is about five days old. Hypoprothrombinaemia is corrected when normal infants start feeding and acquire the intestinal bacteria necessary for the synthesis of vitamin K.

Haemorrhagic disease occurs more commonly in pre-term infants.

Clinical manifestations

Bleeding may occur into the alimentary tract resulting in haematemesis or melaena. Swallowed blood during delivery or from a cracked nipple in a baby who is being breast fed must not be overlooked as a differential diagnosis. Bleeding may occur from the umbilical cord or into the skin (purpura).

Pallor may become apparent if there is a significant loss of blood. An increase in the heart rate may also be noted.

Prevention

The incidence of haemorrhagic disease of the newborn can be reduced by giving every infant 1 mg of vitamin K_1 in the form of phytomendadione (Konakion) intramuscularly or orally.

Treatment

Phytomendadione 1 mg intramuscularly is given immediately. A transfusion of blood may be necessary if bleeding has been severe.

NEONATAL INFECTIONS

Infections presenting in the infant may be the result of intrauterine infections occurring during pregnancy or in labour or as the result of postnatal contact.

Prenatal

Intrauterine infections may occur in one of three ways.

1 Organisms reach the fetus through the bloodstream therefore maternal viraemia will result in fetal viraemia, e.g. rubella.

2 Via the genital tract, e.g. *Herpesvirushominis* type II.
3 Direct entry, e.g. amniocentesis or intrauterine transfusion, and following rupture of membranes if there is a delayed rupture-delivery interval.

Effects
Intrauterine infection may result in a spontaneous abortion, intrauterine death or an obvious congenital defect at birth.

Viral causes

RUBELLA
The infection persists through fetal life and for weeks, months and possibly years after birth. The fetus is at risk if the expectant mother is exposed to a primary infection during pregnancy. The gestational age of the fetus determines the types of defect. The risk of multiple damage is about 60–70% if the gestational age is six to eight weeks, whereas a single defect is more likely if the gestational age is between eight and sixteen weeks. The most common single defect is deafness. The incidence of congenital deafness is 1:1000 live births. Congenital rubella accounts for between 20–24% of known causes of severe congenital deafness in children. There is still some risk to the fetus between sixteen and twenty-four weeks.

In addition to congenital deafness which may not be diagnosed until the infant is several weeks old, the following may present.
1 Congenital heart defect. Patent ductus arteriosus is the commonest defect but pulmonary stenosis and ventricular septal defects may occur.
2 Cataract. This is usually present at birth but may appear later. Microphthalmia and retinitis may also be present.
3 Microcephaly and mental retardation.
4 Thrombocytopoenic purpura may occur as a result of a temporary reduction in the number of platelets.
5 Hepatosplenomegaly with or without jaundice.
6 Light-for-dates. Growth retardation occurs due to the direct action of the virus in slowing down the normal process of cell division.
7 Fatal encephalitis has been reported in the second decade of life as a result of intrauterine exposure to the rubella virus.
8 Failure to grow, probably as a result of hormonal disorders, has been recognised.

Prevention
Vaccination of all schoolgirls between the ages of eleven and fourteen or women in the postnatal period if rubella antibodies were not present on an antenatal screening test is the most effective means of prevention. The vaccine must not be given during pregnancy because of the risk to the fetus, and the

woman is advised not to conceive for at least eight weeks following vaccination.

CYTOMEGALOVIRUS

This virus usually results in a mild illness with minor symptoms that often go undiagnosed. However, it is now recognised that this causes intrauterine infection more commonly than rubella. The effects on the fetus are very similar to those of rubella and include hepatosplenomegaly with or without jaundice, thrombocytopoenic purpura and low birth weight. Neural lesions may occur resulting in encephalitis which is usually fatal.

VARICELLA

Although less common than infections caused by the cytomegalovirus and rubella virus, this may also result in fetal defects and may be fatal if the infection occurs less than five days prior to delivery, probably because the baby is not protected by maternal antibodies.

Diagnosis

The virus is cultured in the baby's urine and pharangeal secretions. Antibody levels and specific immunoglobulin test may also be performed.

Treatment

There is no specific treatment but it must be remembered that these babies are infectious and must be isolated from other babies and not handled by members of staff who are themselves pregnant.

Bacterial causes

SYPHILIS

This may result in abortion, intrauterine death, premature onset of labour or congenital syphilis. At birth, the baby may present with a purulent nasal discharge which may be bloodstained. Hepatosplenomegaly with jaundice may also occur.

TUBERCULOSIS

This is a rare cause of intrauterine infection and only occurs when the placental tissue is infected.

AMNIONITIS

This may occur as the result of infection occurring during amniocentesis, intrauterine transfusion and following rupture of the membranes.

Protozoal causes

TOXOPLASMOSIS

This causes signs and symptoms similar to glandular fever and causes signs in the baby similar to the cytomegalovirus. Hydrocephaly and mental retardation may also occur.

Postnatal

It is often difficult to differentiate between infections occurring during labour and those occurring in the early neonatal period and they will therefore be considered collectively.

Causative organisms

Staphylococcus aureus; Escherichia coli; Bacillus proteus; Pseudomonas aeruginosa; Streptococcus; Listeria monocytogenes; Gonoccocus.

SIGNS

1 Temperature. The ill baby is unable to maintain its body temperature and hypothermia may occur, but the temperature may be normal or raised.
2 Lethargy. The baby is drowsy and difficult to feed.
3 Vomiting and/or diarrhoea and abdominal distension.
4 Weight loss. Due to poor feeding and vomiting there is loss of weight and failure to thrive.
5 Jaundice.
6 Cyanosis, apnoea and convulsions.

Prevention

Newborn infants are prone to infection although they are protected by some antibodies from the mother which last for about six months. Babies who are breast fed acquire antibodies, and therefore immunity via the breast milk.

Special measures must be taken to prevent infection in maternity departments and to prevent cross-infection.

PERSONNEL

The use of gowns and masks has been discontinued in many units, but if gowns are used, a separate one is kept for each baby. Masks must be put on and removed touching only the straps and not handled during use. They must be disposed of by placing in a bin. Handwashing using an antibacterial soap or solution and drying on a paper towel is essential. The hands are washed under running water and the flow controlled by the elbow. Hands must be washed before and after handling the baby and after changing the napkin. If a member of staff has an infection she/he is not permitted to work with babies until free of infection.

ENVIRONMENT

Rooming-in overcomes many of the problems relating to cross-infection. If nurseries are used they should be small and newly delivered babies separated from older babies and the cots should be placed well apart to avoid overcrowding. Damp dusting and wet mopping or vacuum cleaning are used for cleaning the ward. Early transfer home following delivery is another effective way of avoiding cross-infection.

MOTHERCRAFT

As soon as she is able to do so the mother is taught to look after her own baby. This reduces to a minimum the number of people handling the baby and also going from one baby to another. It is essential that the mother is taught the importance of handwashing and disposal of linen and napkins and that she is supervised to ensure that she is scrupulous in her attention to these details.

SKIN CARE

Bacterial colonisation of the neonate begins shortly after birth, and within a few days *Staphylococcus aureus* can often be isolated from the skin and around the base of the cord with no evidence of infection of those sites.

Antibacterial soap or solution is used for bathing the baby and powder for applying to the umbilical area.

EQUIPMENT

There should be an adequate supply of clean linen available and other equipment used, such as thermometers, should be kept in a cot locker and used only for that baby. Cots should be of a type that can easily be cleaned. Pedal bins should be available for the disposal of paper towels following handwashings and soiled linen and napkins. Prepacked feeds reduce the risk of contamination of milk during preparation.

ISOLATION AND BARRIER NURSING

Isolation units should be available so that any baby who has an infection can be effectively barrier nursed.

Sites of infection

SKIN

Infections of the skin are usually due to the *Staphylococcus aureus*.
Pustules. These may appear singularly or in groups.
Pemphigus neonatorum. Skin eruptions characterised by the formation of watery vesicles or bullae.
Paronychia. Infection of the nailfold.
Umbilicus. Localised redness and discharge occurs.
Mastitis. Breast engorgement due to maternal hormones may occur and requires no treatment unless a superimposed infection occurs.

EYES

Conjunctivitis. Inflammation of the conjunctiva may be slight and result in a watery discharge causing stickiness of the eyelids. This can be managed by swabbing the affected eye with a sterile solution of normal saline. The baby is nursed on the affected side to prevent infecting the unaffected eye.
Ophthalmia neonatorum. A purulent discharge from the eyes of the infant commencing within twenty-one days of birth. It is a notifiable disease.

Causative organisms are the *Staphylococcus aureus* and *Bacillus proteus* in the majority of cases but may be due to the *Streptococcus*, *Pneumonococcus* or the *Gonococcus*. Gonococcal ophthalmia may lead to blindness and intensive therapy with penicillin eye drops and systematic penicillin is required to avoid this danger. Infection with *Staphylococcus aureus* is treated with chloramphenicol eye drops.

GASTROINTESTINAL TRACT

Thrush. This is due to the *Candida albicans* and is characterised by white patches in the mouth. This can spread to involve the entire gastrointestinal tract, causing oesophagitis and enteritis, and may also affect the buttocks. This infection may be contracted during delivery if the mother has vaginal thrush. Nystatin suspension (100 000 units) is given after each feed for one week.
Gastroenteritis. This infection is found more commonly in babies who are bottle fed. *Escherichia coli* is the commonest cause but other organisms such as *Salmonella* and *Shigella* may be the cause. In addition to treating the infection, dehydration and electrolyte imbalance usually require to be managed by intravenous fluids.
Necrotising enterocolitis. This is a serious disease of the newborn of unknown aetiology and characterised by necrosis of the intestines. It occurs most commonly in babies of low birth weight with the highest incidence among babies weighing less than 1500 g, but it may also occur in term, normal weight infants.

Onset is usually in the first two weeks of life but can be as late as two months of age. Meconium is passed normally.

Some form of perinatal stress such as asphyxia or hypothermia, is thought to predispose the infant to ischaemia of the intestines. A factor that may contribute to mucosal injury and subsequent infection leading to bowel necrosis is umbilical catheterisation.

The first sign is abdominal distension; there may be vomiting and blood in the stools. The onset is often insidious and sepsis may occur before an intestinal lesion is suspected. Once affected the baby usually deteriorates rapidly becoming lethargic and acidotic; shock and disseminated intravascular coagulation may develop.

Diagnosis is confirmed on radiographic evidence of pneumatosis intestinalis; protal vein gas is an ominous sign of severe disease and pneumoperitoneum indicates a performation.

Management involves intensive care. Oral feeding is discontinued and intravenous fluids given with careful attention to acid-base and electrolyte balance. A nasogastric tube is placed *in situ*. Cultures are taken of blood, urine and cerebrospinal fluid and systemic antibiotics given. If an umbilical catheter is *in situ*, this is removed. Resection of the necrotic bowel is performed or peritoneal drainage if the baby is too ill to withstand surgery.

The prognosis is poor if pneumatosis intestinalis is present but in babies who survive there is no long-term sequelae unless massive bowel resection is necessary.

URINARY TRACT

Infections of the urinary tract are not uncommon in the neonate and they are often difficult to diagnose because they do not present in a specific way. Acquiring an uncontaminated specimen of urine is difficult in a baby and suprapubic aspiration may be performed. *Escherichia coli* is the commonest causative organism.

RESPIRATORY TRACT

Pneumonia may present following prolonged rupture of membranes or inhalation of stomach contents. The signs include rapid respirations, apnoea and respiratory distress. The baby should be transferred to a Special Care Baby Unit for specialised nursing care and oxygen therapy.

SEPTICAEMIA

In addition to the signs associated with other infections, this baby appears gravely ill, has a greyish pallor and peripheral cyanosis. Jaundice may occur giving the skin a greenish discolouration. Vomiting, diarrhoea and abdominal distension occur and there is a tachycardia. *Escherichia coli, Staphylococcus aureus* and beta haemolytic *Streptococcus* are the commonest causative organisms.

MENINGITIS

The signs of meningitis are non-specific in the early stages but late signs include irritability, high pitched cry, hypertonicity of limbs, tense fontanelle and convulsions. *Escherichia coli* is the commonest cause.

Investigations

Because in many cases of infection the early signs are non-specific, investigations usually involve taking many specimens in order to isolate the causative organism. If the site of the infection is obvious then this would not be necessary. Swabs may be taken from the nose, throat, umbilicus, rectum and any site of local infection. A specimen of urine and blood may be obtained and in some cases a lumbar puncture performed and the cerebrospinal fluid sent for culture. A chest X-ray would only be performed if pneumonia is suspected.

Treatment

In addition to the specific treatments mentioned, where applicable under each heading, systemic antibiotic therapy may be required to control the infection. Drugs used include gentamicin and penicillin which may be given until the causative organism is known.

GROUP-B STREPTOCOCCI

The incidence of group-B streptococcal infection in the newborn has risen sharply in recent years.

There are two ways in which the group-B infection presents.

1 The early form presents with acute respiratory distress, apnoea, shock, septicaemia and meningitis. The onset is usually within twenty-four hours of delivery, though it may be as late as ten days. Organisms may be cultured from many sites, including blood, umbilicus, skin and nasopharynx. The condition may closely resemble hyaline membrane disease; and the fact that the strains from the baby are usually identical with those from the mother suggests that the infection is transmitted from mother to infant during delivery.

2 The second type of infection presents, usually after the tenth day of life, as meningitis. The route of this infection is uncertain.

Management

The baby is transferred to the Special Care Baby Unit and isolated. Swabs are taken from the ear, throat, skin, umbilicus and rectum, and the blood is cultured. Intramuscular injections of gentamicin and penicillin are given.

The mortality rate for the early form of group-B streptococcal infection is high (60–75%) but for the second type of infection it is lower (14–18%).

Inborn errors of metabolism

There have been considerable advances made in the understanding and diagnosis of inborn errors of metabolism since the term was originally used in 1908. To date about 100 inborn errors have been defined but since the majority are extremely rare only three will be dealt with. These are phenylketonuria, because all babies are routinely screened for this disorder which if diagnosed and treated early can prevent mental retardation; glactosaemia, because it may be the cause of jaundice in the early neonatal period; and cystic fibrosis, because screening tests are being used in some centres.

Phenylketonuria

This inborn error of metabolism was discovered in 1934 and is an autosomal recessive disease. The incidence is 1 in 10000.

CAUSE

Disturbances occur in the function of an enzyme phenylalanine hydroxylase in the liver, resulting in an inability to convert phenylalanine into tyrosine. This, in turn, results in an accumulation of phenylalanine in the bloodstream. Normal concentrations are 1–2 mg/dl but levels of 20–30 mg/dl may occur in untreated cases. Metabolites of phenylalanine are formed and phenylpyruvic acid is excreted in the urine.

DIAGNOSIS

Urine test

The presence of phenylpyruvic acid in the urine may be detected by use of the Phenistix test or aqueous ferric chloride solution. Urine tests have been replaced by more accurate blood test.

Blood test

Blood is collected by heel prick and four drops of blood, each forming a spot 0.5 cm in diameter, are formed on a specially designed card.

This test can be modified to screen for other inborn errors of metabolism such as galactosaemia, homocystinuria, histidinaemia, tyrosinaemia and maple syrup urine disease.

The test is not performed before the baby is six days old because there is a normal level of phenylalanine at birth, rising two to three days following feeding. Antibiotics can interfere with the assay. If the baby or mother of the breast fed baby is receiving systemic antibiotics, forty-eight hours should be allowed to elapse after the therapy is finished before taking blood sample. If long-term antibiotic therapy is being given, the specimen is taken as usual and the antibiotic and dose displayed on the specimen.

Immature babies may have a transitory rise in blood phenylalanine due to an immature liver, therefore, the test may need to be rechecked later.

MANAGEMENT

The management involves giving a low protein diet to maintain the blood phenylalanine below 5 mg/dl. Small amounts of protein require to be given to avoid protein deficiency and growth retardation.

Special products are available on prescription and include Minafen for babies and Cymogran, Aminograin food supplements and mineral mixture and Pk Aid 1, a metabolic mineral mixture for older children. Low phenylalanine foods such as bread, biscuits, cakes and pasta can also be obtained on National Health Service prescription.

CLINICAL FEATURES IN AN UNTREATED CHILD

Early features include vomiting and feeding problems and irritability. The high level of phenylalanine in the blood inhibits the production of melanin which is necessary for pigmentation, therefore, these children have blonde hair and blue eyes. Slowing of milestone development becomes apparent towards the second half of the first year of life. Older children show lack of concentration, psychosis and mental retardation. A feature of this disease is that, for reasons that are not known, some affected children who have not received treatment develop normally.

Galactosaemia

An autosomal recessive inborn error of metabolism resulting in the deficiency of an enzyme galactose-1-phosphate uridyl-transferase required for the transformation of galactose to glucose. Lactose, the carbohydrate of milk, is a disaccharide and is split into two components, glucose and galactose for utilisation. Galactose must then be converted to glucose by an enzyme.

DIAGNOSIS

Urine test. When the urine is tested with Clinitest the result is positive but the Clinistix test is negative.

MANAGEMENT
A lactose-free milk substitute preparation is used (see p. 00).

CLINICAL FEATURES
Galactosaemia is one of the rare causes of neonatal jaundice and enlarged liver. The baby may present with vomiting, loss of weight, lethargy and irritability. More serious complications involving the heart, kidneys and eyes can occur in untreated cases.

Cystic fibrosis

This is the commonest Mendelian recessive disorder with an incidence of 1 in 2000 infants. It was originally thought to be a pancreatic disorder but is now known to be a disease affecting all the exocrine glands of the body including the liver and sweat glands.

CLINICAL FEATURES
This disorder is characterised by recurrent and severe chest infections, malabsorption and growth failure. Intestinal obstruction may develop in the neonatal period.

The prognosis is serious and many children die of progressive respiratory disease.

DIAGNOSIS
Cystic fibrosis can be recognised in 80% of affected infants in the newborn period by screening meconium for increased albumin content, i.e. more than 20 mg%.

TREATMENT
Early treatment of respiratory infections and pancreatic supplements with dietary adjustments is improving the prognosis.

Congenital abnormalities

In 1900, the infant mortality rate was 154 per 1000 live births in England and Wales, in 1970 it was 18 per 1000. In this period the deaths from congenital malformations have shown only a small reduction so that their relative importance is much greater today. In 1900, congenital malformations accounted for 1 in 30 infant deaths, in 1970 1 in 5 infant deaths were due to congenital malformations. There is also a higher proportion of infants with genetically determined diseases and congenital disorders who reach adult life.

AETIOLOGICAL FACTORS

1 Maternal age is associated with Down's syndrome.
2 Genetics—dominant, recessive and sex-linked conditions.
3 Infections such as rubella, cytomegalovirus, toxoplasmosis and syphilis.
4 Geographical—some abnormalities have a higher incidence in certain parts of the country and world.
5 Irradiation—X-rays if undertaken in early pregnancy.
6 Drugs may have a teratogenic effect on the fetus if given in early pregnancy, i.e. thalidomide.

Abnormalities of the musculoskeletal system

CONGENITAL DISLOCATION OF THE HIP

An anomaly of the hip joint, present at birth, in which the head of the femur is partially or wholly displaced from the acetabulum.

Incidence: 1 in 800 live births. Approximately 1 in 200 infants have unstable hips at birth. Most recover spontaneously by the time they are two months old.

Aetiology

1 The incidence is commoner in girls than in boys.
2 The left hip is more commonly affected than the right although both hips may be affected.
3 It is associated with an extended breech presentation.
4 A family history should alert those responsible to the possibility of its occurrence.

Diagnosis

The importance of diagnosis cannot be overemphasised as congenital dislocation of the hip is a treatable abnormality but if allowed to persist, is a progressive condition. Secondary structural changes develop and in time the growth of the joint is impaired.

Neonatal screening for congenital dislocation of the hip should be carried out on all infants using Barlow's modification of Ortolanis's test. The examination is performed by the midwife shortly after birth and repeated by the doctor during his initial examination of the infant.

Barlow's modification of Ortolanis's test. The infant is placed on his back with legs towards the examiner and hips and knees flexed. The examiner grasps the infant's legs placing the middle finger of each hand over the greater trochanter and the thumbs on the inner aspect of the thighs over the lesser trochanter. With the legs held at 45° of abduction, the middle finger applies pressure upon the greater trochanter. If the hip is dislocated a click is heard or a movement felt as the head of the femur is replaced in the acetabulum.

Backward pressure is then applied with the thumbs and, in some cases, the head of the femur can be felt to slide backwards on to the posterior aspect of the acetabulum. This hip is described as dislocatable, it is not dislocated.

Management

Early diagnosis enables early and effective treatment to be carried out. An orthopaedic surgeon is asked to see the infant. A Von Rosen or Barlow splint is applied to keep the hips flexed and abducted. This remains in place for three months with periodical adjustment to allow for the infant's growth. This method of treatment is effective in the majority of cases of dislocated and dislocatable hips.

Late diagnosis

If congenital dislocation of the hip is missed in the neonatal period it may not present until the infant attempts to walk, by which time retarded ossification of the affected joint will have occurred and long-term treatment, often involving surgery, may be required.

TALIPES

This is a deformity of the feet due to contraction of muscles and is commonly caused by the posture of the fetus *in utero*. Incidence: 1 in 1000. There are three types of talipes.

Talipes equinovarus. This is the commonest form of club-foot with hyper-extension and incurving of the entire foot.

Talipes calcaneovalgus. This foot is flat or slightly convex. The heel is turned downwards and inwards.

Talipes metatarsovarus. The heel and posterior part of the foot appear normal, but the fore-foot angulates sharply inwards.

Management

Postural talipes is corrected by manipulation of the foot through the whole range of movements although it will usually return to normal within a few weeks without treatment. The mother is taught how to manipulate the foot after each feed.

In structural talipes the range of passive movements is limited and manipulation and strapping or a plaster cast is required.

EXTRA DIGITS

Careful examination of the hands and feet is required to exclude extra digits which may range from no more than a skin tag to a complete digit known as polydactyly. The skin tag is tied off with a linen thread and separates by aseptic necrosis. In the case of polydactyly the advice of a plastic surgeon is needed.

SYNDACTYLY

In this condition the fingers or toes are webbed and are held together by skin or due to fusion of bone. The advice of a plastic surgeon is required in this case.

ABSENCE OR DEFORMITY OF LIMBS

Amelia is the term used to describe the absence of one or more limbs, ectromelia is the absence of part of a limb and phocomelia the absence of the long bones of a limb so that a rudimentary or well developed hand or foot is positioned at the shoulder or hip.

Abnormalities of the skin

Naevi. A naevus is localised malformation of the skin. Naevi are either vascular or pigmented; vascular naevi are caused by overgrown blood vessels, either capillaries or larger vessels or both. Pigmented naevi are due to localised proliferation of pigment-bearing cells.
Mongolian blue spot. This is an accumulation of pigment usually found over the sacral area in infants of races in whom pigmentation of the skin occurs. Therefore, they are common in babies of Mongolian and African races but may also be seen in babies of Mediterranean races. They become less obvious as the skin darkens.

Abnormalities of the cardiovascular system

A cardiovascular malformation is suspected when a heart murmur is discovered, if there is an abnormal rate or rhythm, cyanosis is present or there are signs of heart failure. Incidence: 1 in 100.

PATIENT DUCTUS ARTERIOSUS

Closure of the ductus arteriosus normally occurs soon after birth. If the ductus remains patent, the direction of blood flow is reversed by the higher pressure in the aorta.

VENTRICULAR SEPTAL DEFECT

An abnormal opening between the right and left ventricle. The defects vary in size and may occur in either the membranous or muscular part of the ventricular septum. A shunting of blood from left to right occurs during systole due to higher pressure in the left ventricle.

ATRIAL SEPTAL DEFECT

An abnormal opening between the right and left atria. An incompetent foramen ovale is the most common defect. In general, left to right shunting of blood occurs in all atrial septal defects.

COARCTATION OF THE AORTA

This is characterised by a narrowing of the aorta which may be a preductal or postductal obstruction, depending on the position of the narrowing in relation to the ductus arteriosus. There is an obstruction to the blood flow through the aorta causing increasing left ventricular pressure.

TRANSPOSITION OF THE GREAT VESSELS

In this malformation the aorta originates from the right ventricle and the pulmonary artery from the left ventricle.

TETROLOGY OF FALLOT

This malformation is characterised by the combination of four defects, pulmonary stenosis, ventricular septal defect, overriding aorta and hypertrophy of right ventricle.

General signs of congenital cardiovascular malformations

The signs are similar with the exception of cyanosis which is not present in some malformations, e.g. ventricular septal defect. Dyspnoea on feeding; feeding difficulties; failure to gain weight; tachycardia; heart murmurs; liver enlargement—an early sign of heart failure in babies and rarely oedema.

Investigations

Chest X-ray. This will reveal the size of the heart, the size of the pulmonary vessels and the presence of pulmonary oedema.

Electrocardiogram.

Cardiac catheterisation. This measures the pressure and oxygen concentration in each chamber. Dye is added at the end of the procedure and an angiograph is performed to demonstrate the septum. This procedure is not usually performed unless surgery is to be undertaken.

Treatment

Medical treatment of heart failure includes nursing the baby in an upright position and tube feeding to prevent exhausting the baby. Digoxin and a diuretic are used and antibiotics in the case of an infection.

Surgical treatment is undertaken in the case of transposition of the great vessels, coarctation of the aorta, patent ductus arteriosus and ventricular septal defect.

Abnormalities of respiratory system

CHOANAL ATRESIA

This is an obstruction at the conjunction of the posterior terminus of the nasal airway and the nasopharynx, namely the posterior naris or choana. An oropharangeal airway is inserted and produces an immediate improvement.

Surgery is required if there is a bony obstruction, but not until the infant is older.

DIAPHRAGMATIC HERNIA

Although this is not as such part of the respiratory system, it is included under this heading as it is characterised by the presence of the abdominal viscera in the thoracic cavity. Herniation usually occurs through the left diaphragm.

The condition of the baby depends on the volume of abdominal viscera in the thoracic cavity. The baby may be seriously ill from the moment of birth or becomes ill later. An endotracheal tube is passed to relieve dyspnoea and is kept in place until an emergency operation can be undertaken.

Abnormalities of the gastrointestinal tract

Abnormalities of the gastrointestinal tract are amongst the most common congenital abnormalities. They are often highly dangerous to life but at the same time many are readily amenable to surgical or medical correction.

CLEFT LIP AND CLEFT PALATE

These abnormalities are frequently associated and have a combined incidence of 1 in 1000.

Cleft lip. This may be unilateral or bilateral and although it is often associated with cleft palate, it may occur on its own. This is visually a distressing abnormality for the parents and photographs of a similar case taken before and after surgical repair should be available.

Cleft palate. This should be detected in routine examination but because it is not easily visualised it may be overlooked if great care is not taken. Like cleft lip, with which it is often associated, it may be unilateral or bilateral and involves the soft or hard palate or both.

Feeding difficulties may occur and a flanged teat may be used to overcome these problems. Surgical repair to the lip is undertaken when the baby is three months old and to the palate at one year.

OESOPHAGEAL ATRESIA

In this malformation the upper end of the oesophagus is blind. It is often associated with a tracheo-oesophageal fistula which is usually between the upper end of the oesophagus and the trachea but may occur at the lower end. In rare cases a double fistula may occur in association with oesophageal atresia or a fistula in the absence of atresia.

This condition is suspected if there was polyhydramnios present during pregnancy or if at birth the baby produces excessive amounts of frothy mucus. An attempt should be made to pass a tube into the stomach to exclude or confirm the diagnosis of oesophageal atresia. If the diagnosis is not made at birth, choking and cyanosis will occur when the baby is fed and for this reason a first feed of sterile water should be given, if it is not the usual practice to pass a tube into the stomach as part of the initial examination.

Immediate surgery is necessary and may be life-saving in some cases.

HIATUS HERNIA

In this condition a pouch of stomach slides up into the thoracic cavity through a lax oesophageal hiatus in the diaphragm. The cardia is situated above instead of below the diaphragm and the oesophagus is shortened.

Vomiting may be projectile, and the vomit is occasionally blood-stained. The diagnosis is confirmed by barium swallow. The infant is nursed prone on a firm surface at an angle of 30–45°.

PYLORIC STENOSIS

Congenital hypertyrophy of muscles of the pylorus has an incidence of 3 in 1000.

Clinical features manifest in the second or third week of life and include projectile vomiting occurring shortly after feeds, visible gastric peristalsis during feeding, constipation and weight loss.

Medical treatment includes giving atropine methonitrate (Eumydrin) drops prior to the feeds, to relax the pyloric sphincter.

Ramstedt's operation may be performed and involves division of the hypertrophic muscles.

DUODENAL ATRESIA

Duodenal obstruction may occur due to atresia. If the obstruction is proximal to the entrance of the common bile duct into the duodenum vomiting of milk occurs, if distal to that point the vomit characteristically is bile-stained and white 'meconium' may be passed. Plain abdominal X-rays in the erect, supine and lateral positions are taken immediately to confirm the diagnosis, and surgery is then undertaken.

MECONIUM ILEUS

In this condition, which is due to cystic fibrosis, intestinal obstruction occurs due to blockage with abnormally thick tenacious meconium.

HIRSCHSPRUNG'S DISEASE

In this condition there is a congenital absence of ganglion cells of the plexus of Auerbach in a segment of the large bowel. It is also known as congenital megacolon or congenital aganglionosis.

Vomiting, distension and constipation usually present due to intestinal obstruction.

IMPERFORATE ANUS

Testing patency of the anus is part of routine examination of every infant at birth. If the diagnosis is not made at birth failure to pass meconium within twelve hours of birth should make the midwife suspicious. There are many types of abnormalities associated with this condition. In females the imperforate anus is frequently associated with a rectovaginal fistula and in males with a fistula to the bladder or urethra. Surgical treatment is undertaken.

Abnormalities of the genitourinary tract

HYPOSPADIAS

The urethral orifice is on the under surface of the glans penis. Treatment is not usually required.

EPISPADIAS

The urethral orifice is on the anterior shaft of the penis. This is less common than hypospadias and is generally associated with other major defects.

PSEUDOHERMAPHRODITISM

Problems of sex determination may occur when the clitoris is enlarged or the penis small and a bifid scrotum resembles the labia majora. The doctor is informed and if a diagnosis cannot be made on clinical examination, chromosomal studies will be undertaken. Hermaphroditism is very rare.

RENAL AGENESIS

Congenital absence of the kidneys is a rare and fatal condition. Certain clinical characteristics have been recognised. The infants are usually male, oligohydramnios or complete absence of amniotic fluid may have presented in pregnancy, the ears are low-set and the eyes are widely separated with prominent epicanthal folds. The presence of only two umbilical cord vessels is associated with this condition.

Abdominal wall

EXOMPHALOS

A herniation of the intra-abdominal viscera through the umbilical ring. There may be an intact sac or it may rupture before, during or after birth.

UMBILICAL HERNIA

This is a small type of exomphalos. An operation to replace the viscera and repair the hernia is performed.

GASTROSCHISIS

This is a defect in the abdominal wall separate from the umbilicus, usually to the right, with evisceration of stomach and large and small intestines and with no covering membrane.

The combined incidence of these abnormalities is 1 in 5000.

'PRUNE BELLY' SYNDROME

Absence of abdominal muscles causing a wrinkled appearance of the abdominal wall.

Abnormalities of the central nervous system

ANENCEPHALY

An absence of the vault of the skull and the major portion of the brain. This is a gross malformation that is incompatible with life. Incidence 2 in 1000.

MICROCEPHALY

This is a small head which may be due to failure of the brain to grow as may occur in association with intrauterine infections such as rubella, cytomegalovirus and toxoplasmosis. The cause may be due to premature ossification of the sutures constricting the growth of the brain. It is invariably associated with mental retardation.

HYDROCEPHALY

The head is enlarged due to an excess of fluid within the ventricular system. The head feels soft, the fontanelles are large and the sutures are wide. A catheter with a valve is inserted from the brain to the right side of the heart to reduce the cerebrospinal fluid pressure.

SPINA BIFIDA

This is due to an abnormality of the dorsal laminae and dorsal spinous processes of one or more vertebrae. There are four varieties of spina bifida.
Spina bifida occulta. This is a mild form and no tumour occurs except in some cases a lipoma or dermoid cyst with discolouration of the skin and long hair at the site of the lesions.
Meningocele. This is a moderate form. A tumour is present and is formed of spinal membrane, dura and arachnoid. The spinal cord tissue is not affected.
Myelomeningocele. This is a severe form of spina bifida. A tumour is present and is formed of spinal membrane with spinal cord and nerves attached. This form is most common and most debilitating.
Syringomyelocele. A very severe form of spina bifida which is usually

associated with other congenital defects and is not usually compatible with life.

The only therapy possible is surgery and the advisability of this depends on whether or not there is an associated hydrocephalus and the degree of neurological involvement.

Chromosomal abnormalities

Since 1956, when the correct number of chromosomes in man was discovered, there has been significant advances in the study of chromosomes and their abnormalities. A karotype can be prepared from blood, bone marrow or skin cells and the number and structure of the chromosomes noted.

Abnormalities may result from an alteration in the number or structure of the chromosomes. Structural changes may be the result of the loss of a part of the chromosome which is referred to as deletion, or from translocation where chromosomal material from one chromosome breaks off and becomes attached to an adjacent chromosome.

Numerical changes occur when there are three chromosomes instead of two and the term trisomy is used to describe this alteration (see below). Theoretically it is possible for any of the autosomes to have three chromosomes, but in practice numbers 21, 18 and 13 are the ones most usually affected. Additional sex chromosomes also occur, the most common being Klinefelters Syndrome in which the male has an extra X-chromosome.

Autosomes comprise essential genetic material and loss of any one of the forty-four autosomes appears to be incompatible with life. However, Turners Syndrome is the result of a single X chromosome which is referred to as monosomy-X (see p. 391).

DOWN'S SYNDROME (TRISOMY 21)

This is due to the presence of an extra chromosome attached to chromosome number twenty-one. Down's syndrome is an association of congenital anomalies which causes a marked similarity in appearance. The head is small with a flattened occiput, the eyes slant upwards and there are prominent epicanthic folds. The iris may be speckled with white spots known as Brushfield's spots. The nose is short and flat-bridged. The mouth is small and the tongue tends to protrude.

The fingers are short and the hands appear square. The thumb is low-set and separated more than usual from the index finger. There is a single deep palmar crease. The large toe is separated from the second toe and there is a deep dorsal crease. Muscular hypotonia is present. A common associated malformation is an interventricular septal defect. There is reduced intellectual capacity to a variable degree. The baby is usually of low birth weight.

Down's syndrome has an incidence of 1.5 per 1000 births, but the overall incidence is higher as chromosomal anomalies are associated with spontaneous abortion. The incidence of Down's syndrome increases with maternal age, with women over forty years of age at greatest risk (1:4). It can be diagnosed during the antenatal period by performing chromosomal studies of the fetal cells found in the amniotic fluid (see p. 475).

EDWARD'S SYNDROME (TRISOMY 18)

This is a syndrome caused by an extra chromosome attached to chromosome number eighteen. The baby is of low birth weight, has low-set abnormal ears, micrognathia and characteristically flexed fingers with flexion contraction of the two middle digits which are overlapped by the flexed thumb and index and little fingers. A congenital heart defect, usually ventricular septal defect, often with patent ductus arteriosus is present. The infant also has prominent heels and rocker-bottom feet. Mental retardation occurs.

PATAU'S SYNDROME (TRISOMY 13)

This is due to an extra chromosome attached to chromosome number thirteen. This syndrome has several defects in common with Edward's syndrome such as mental retardation, malformed ears, flexion deformities of wrist, hand and fingers, congenital heart defects and prominent heels with rocker-bottom feet. In addition they manifest abnormalities not commonly associated with Edward's syndrome such as microphthalmia, cataracts, a broad flattened nose, cleft lip and cleft palate.

CRI DU CHAT SYNDROME

This is due to deletion of the short arms of chromosome number five. The infant has microcephaly, micrognathia, epicanthus, oblique palpebral fissures, low-set ears, mental retardation and a peculiar cry resembling that of a cat which gives the syndrome its name.

TURNER'S SYNDROME (XO)

This syndrome is due to the absence of an X chromosome. The infant has webbing of the neck, oedema of the hands and feet and coarctation of the aorta.

Mental retardation to a variable degree is common to most chromosomal abnormalities and therefore as the child gets older the parents may need assistance in providing care in the home or the child may need to be taken into care (see p. 430).

A major congenital malformation is found in 2.1% of all deliveries, 32% of stillbirths, 1.6% of live births, 18% of first week deaths and 1.3% of survivors over one month of age. Most abnormalities arise from defects of organogenesis in the first trimester and as such they are true malformations.

Genetic counselling should be available to couples who are at risk of having an abnormal child, and consists in giving as accurate information as possible in the risks of transmission of inherited or partially inherited conditions (see p. 469).

Neonatal cold injury

A syndrome developed by babies due to accidental exposure to cold. The neonate is very susceptible to heat loss because there is a large surface area in relation to weight. The skin of the body is wet at birth and if drying by evaporation occurs, heat will be lost. The baby's metabolism and heat production takes several weeks to function properly. The neonate is unable to shiver and therefore is lacking one of the body mechanisms for maintaining or raising body temperature. The skin of the neonate is thin and, especially in immature or light-for-dates infants, the layer of subcutaneous fat may be so deficient as to allow heat loss. The inactivity of the newborn makes them susceptible to cold injury.

Babies more prone to chilling even in a warm environment: low birth weight babies, immature and light-for-dates; following asphyxia neonatorum; when suffering from an infection or hypoglycaemia; as a result of maternal drugs, e.g. diazepam (Valium).

PREVENTION OF CHILLING

The room in which the baby is delivered and nursed must be kept at a temperature of approximately 21 °C day and night for at least four weeks after birth.

The baby's skin should be dried as soon as possible after birth and the baby wrapped in a dry warm wrapper and placed in a warm cot under a heater if this is available.

If the baby is asphyxiated at birth, time should still be taken to dry the baby's skin before placing him on the Resuscitaire under a heat lamp. Although a certain amount of exposure is necessary to facilitate observation this must be kept to a minimum and heat loss prevented by use of a radiant heater.

All newly born babies should have their temperatures recorded with a low-reading thermometer after delivery, four-hourly for at least twenty-four hours and then daily until the tenth day.

Babies more prone to chilling, e.g. low birth weight should be nursed in a Special Care Baby Unit.

The baby should not be bathed unless the room temperature is at least 21 °C.

RESULTS OF CHILLING

If the baby is exposed to cold its body temperature may fall to a dangerously low level, 32 °C or lower. The baby becomes lethargic and difficult to feed and consequently fails to thrive.

The baby feels cold to touch and there may be oedema of the hands, feet and eyelids.

A condition known as sclerema, diffuse hardening of the subcutaneous tissue may occur. The affected area feels solid and the skin cannot be picked up separately from the muscle. The absence of pitting, on pressure, is characteristic of sclerema. It usually starts on the thighs and buttocks but may spread to involve the whole body.

The majority of the babies develop a redness of the face and extremities due to vasodilatation and haemoglobin trapped in the capillaries. This feature gives the baby a deceptively healthy appearance which may delay the recognition that something is wrong.

Hypoglycaemia is common and there may be raised levels of urea, potassium and phosphate.

MANAGEMENT

The baby must be transferred to an Intensive Care Baby Unit without delay and placed in an incubator under a Perspex shield. The baby's temperature is allowed to rise gradually over a period of several hours, otherwise the superficial tissues warm up but the deep vital organs remain hypothermic and unable to cope with the increased demands upon them as toxins from the periphery enter the general circulation. The hypoglycaemia and electrolyte imbalance are corrected and antibiotic therapy commenced because of the increased risk of infection.

The baby of the diabetic mother

The effects of maternal diabetes on the fetus (see p. 213) and, therefore, on the condition of the infant depends on the degree of control achieved during pregnancy and whether or not any other complication occurred, e.g. pre-eclampsia.

High blood glucose levels cause islet cell hyperplasia and deposition of excessive amounts of subcutaneous fat. The infant's weight may be above the ninetieth percentile (see Fig. 12.1) and he appears oedematous and plethoric. In addition, despite being of high birth weight, the baby may be immature.

If the maternal diabetes has been well controlled throughout pregnancy the infant's weight will be normal, but if the pregnancy has been complicated by severe pre-eclampsia the infant may be light-for-dates.

Hypoglycaemia is a common problem and is the result of increased secretions of insulin rapidly utilising the glycogen. Early feeding helps to prevent this condition and a Dextrostix test performed every three hours will indicate a falling blood glucose level and the need for laboratory estimations (see p. 396).

Idiopathic respiratory distress may occur in the baby born to the mother with diabetes mellitus even after thirty-six weeks gestation (see p. 360).

Congenital malformations are more common in babies born to women who have diabetes mellitus.

Neonatal diabetes

This is a very rare condition which has its onset at or soon after birth.

CLINICAL FEATURES

1 Rapid weight loss in the absence of diarrhoea and vomiting.
2 Dehydration despite a good intake of fluids and calories.
3 Glycosuria.
4 Hyperglycaemia.

Complete recovery from the diabetic syndrome occurs if the baby can be kept alive. There is a high risk of cerebral damage resulting from hyperglycaemia.

In some babies the glycosuria and hyperglycaemia are very sensitive to insulin. A further group of neonatal diabetics is less responsive to insulin and die within a few days.

Neonatal problems

This section will consider some of the problems that may occur during the neonatal period and look at their possible causes. Most of these problems have been mentioned under other headings but need to be dealt with in more detail.

Vomiting

The majority of babies regurgitate at one time or another during the first ten days of life and usually this is mild and of no significance. But it is important for the midwife to distinguish between regurgitation and vomiting and to recognise the different types of vomiting as there may be a serious cause.

OBSERVATIONS

The following are observations that should be made and reported to the doctor.

1 Colour of the vomitus.
2 Amount.
3 Relation of vomiting to feeding.

4 Frequency and force of vomiting.
5 General condition of the baby.

TYPES AND CAUSES

Mucus. Irritation of the gastric mucosa.
Frothy mucoid. Oesophageal atresia with or without a tracheo-oesophageal fistula. Copious amounts may be vomited (see p. 386).
Milk. Feeding problems including inadequate 'winding' or hole in the teat too small. Infections such as gastroenteritis and urinary tract infection. Drugs such as cloxacillin. Cerebral trauma.
Bloodstained. Swallowed maternal blood at delivery or from a cracked nipple. Haemorrhagic disease of the newborn (see p. 371). Specks of blood may occur due to trauma. Intestinal obstruction.
Bile-stained. Intestinal obstruction due to atresia or stenosis, volvulus or Hirschsprung's disease (see p. 387).

Diarrhoea

The more frequent passage of looser than normal stools may be due to:
Breast fed babies. Frequent loose stools are not unusual during the early stages of breast feeding, but the frequency may be increased and the stools become abnormally loose if the baby is being overfed or the mother has included foods such as grapes in her diet or taken an aperient such as cascara.
Bottle fed babies. Gastroenteritis (see p. 376).

Allergy to cow's milk

An adverse reaction to cow's milk may be the cause of a baby failing to thrive. The baby may either be sensitive to the cow's milk protein or lactose.

In the first few months of life the gastro-intestinal mucosa is more permeable, and incompletely digested proteins are absorbed. The antigens in the proteins produce an antibody response, and, in some babies, an allergic reaction.

Lactose intolerance is the result of an enzyme deficiency resulting in an inability to metabolise lactose. See also galactosaemia (p. 380).

Feeding with cow's milk preparations should be discontinued and replaced with a lactose-free soya protein based milk substitute, e.g. Cow and Gate Formula S or Wysoy.

Sore buttocks

CAUSES

1 Frequent loose stools.
2 Inadequate washing of buttocks.

3 Concentrated urine.
4 Infection—*Candida albicans*.
5 Rough napkin.
6 Unsuitable soap, powder, or creams.

Dyspnoea

Difficulty with breathing may be due to pulmonary factors or other disorders.
Respiratory distress syndrome. Hyaline membrane disease; pneumonia; pneumothorax; diaphragmatic hernia, choanal atresia or stenosis; transient tachypnoea.
Cerebral. Respiratory depressant drugs given to the mother shortly before delivery; trauma; hypoxaemia.
Cardiac conditions.

Convulsions

Irregular movements of the limbs or body due to involuntary contraction of muscles.
Causes. Hypoglycaemia, hypocalcaemia; cerebral anoxia or haemorrhage; meningitis.

Hypoglycaemia

A blood glucose level below 20 mg/dl. Infants particularly at risk of developing hypoglycaemia are light-for-dates and immature babies and babies born to the diabetic mother (see p. 393). It may also occur in babies who are asphyxiated at birth or who become hypothermic. A Dextrostix reading of below 45 mg/dl is an indication for sending a specimen of blood for laboratory testing.

Hypocalcaemia

A plasma calcium level of 7 mg/dl or less. Infants receiving cows' milk preparations are liable to develop hypocalcaemia particularly in the second half of the first week of life, due to loss of calcium with ingested unabsorbed fat, and also due to the high phosphate content of the feed when the infant's parathyroid function is likely to be impaired.

Hypernatraemia

The greater solute load of cows' milk preparations and the inaccuracies in measurement and reconstitution of the powder result in an excessive dietary solute intake. Therefore, only minimal water loss by sweating, vomiting or diarrhoea may precipitate a dangerous situation where the immature kidneys are no longer able to maintain osmotic homeostasis.

Low solute cows' milk preparations now on the market are recommended for babies under six months of age, and meticulous attention to detail in reconstituting the milk (see p. 341).

The 'at risk' infant

An infant 'at risk' is any infant who during pregnancy, labour or the neonatal period is exposed to risk. The baby's name should be notified to the District Health Authority and entered in an 'At Risk' or Observation Register. In this way staff responsible for the subsequent care of the child are alerted to those children who are likely to develop an abnormality, so that they can be recognised and treated early.

Categories of risk

FAMILY HISTORY

1 Deafness.

2 Blindness.

3 Genetic factors: inborn errors of metabolism, e.g. phenylketonuria; chromosomal disorders, e.g. Down's syndrome.

PRENATAL

1 Infections: rubella, toxoplasmosis, cytomegalic inclusion disease, syphilis.

2 Medical disorders: diabetes mellitus, hypertension.

3 Complications: hyperemesis gravidarum, threatened abortion, antepartum haemorrhage, pre-eclampsia, eclampsia, polyhydramnios.

4 Blood group incompatibilities.

5 Miscellaneous: drugs, smoking, alcohol, X-rays.

LABOUR

1 Prolonged or precipitate labour.

2 Fetal distress.

3 Multiple birth.

4 Instrumental delivery.

5 Ruptured membranes for more than twenty-four hours.

NEONATAL

1 Pre-term infant (immature): gestational age less than thirty-seven completed weeks.

2 Postmature infant: gestational age more than forty-two completed weeks.

3 Light-for-dates infant: birth weight below the tenth percentile for gestational age.

4 Birth asphyxia.
5 Respiratory distress syndrome.
6 Jaundice.
7 Haemorrhagic disease of the newborn.
8 Infection.
9 Congenital abnormalities.
10 Convulsions.
11 Cold injury.
12 Failure to thrive.
13 Inborn errors of metabolism, i.e. phenylketonuria.

The midwife has a duty to ensure that any condition which has exposed the fetus to risk during pregnancy and labour, or any condition present at birth is recorded on the birth notification which is sent to the District Medical Officer within thirty-six hours of birth. Any condition occurring during the early neonatal period when the baby is in the care of the midwife should be notified on a discharge form.

The health visitor is notified of an infant at risk in her area and arrangements made for the infant to be followed up at frequent intervals. Developmental assessment includes observing milestones and muscular development, testing hearing and sight and, when the child is older observing social behaviour. The number of infants on the 'At Risk' Register decreases as the infants get older and normal development is observed.

Handicap register

In some cases a handicap is detected and the infant's name is transferred to a Handicap Register.

CATEGORIES OF HANDICAP

The blind or partially blind; deaf or partially deaf; educationally subnormal; physically handicapped; speech defect; maladjusted; delicate; epileptic.

Further reading

Barson A.J. (1981) *Laboratory Investigation of Fetal Disease*. John Wright & Sons Ltd.

Davies P.A., Robinson R.J., Scopes J.W., Tizzard J.P.M. & Wigglesworth J.S. (1972) *Medical Care of Newborn Babies*. Spastics International Medical Publications, London.

Klaus M.H. & Fanaroff A.A. (1973) *Care of the High-Risk Neonate*. W.B. Saunders, London.

SECTION IV
ASSOCIATED SUBJECTS

Chapter 13
Sociological Aspects in Relation to Childbearing

The study of human society and social problems is an important part of the midwife's education, for her practice brings her into contact with people from all walks of life during one of the most important events in their lives.

The family in society

The family is a microcosm of society and if we study the family unit, we see changes that reflect those in society as a whole. If we define society as an association of persons with common aim, interest and principle; a state of living in association with other individuals, it is easy to see the relationship of the one to the other, and how the customs and organisation of an ordered society are reflected in family life and vice versa. Therefore, anything that undermines the structure of society has implications for the fabric of family life.

The family is a social group, a single economic unit that has worldwide recognition, although what constitutes a family varies from one culture to another. In our own society considerable changes have taken place in our concept of a family, and although we still recognise and accept as normal the traditional family unit, we are also aware of other social groupings.

The traditional family structures and relationships are those based on the nuclear and extended family. The nuclear family comprises a mother, father and children; the extended family refers to the immediate relatives such as grandparents, aunts, uncles and cousins.

The socio-economic factors that have influenced family life in this century range from the emancipation of women to more liberal divorce laws. At the beginning of the century the family unit would have had the father as the head of the family—the economic supporter, and the mother as the homemaker; the average family size was six and the parents could expect the death of at least one child before adulthood. Marriages were often arranged and were for the procreation and legitimisation of children.

The contribution of women to war work during the Great War, and women's suffrage in 1918, began the changing role of women in society where they were beginning to be recognised as individuals in their own right rather than a chattel of their husband and second class citizens. But it was probably the Second World War that made the greatest impact as women replaced men in factories and in the fields.

The changed role of women has had an effect on the role of men in the family and in society. In many families the man is no longer the only financial provider and in some may not be the major money earner. In others, the roles may have been reversed; and the father remains at home and cares for the children while the mother goes out to work. Marriage is more a partnership of equals with both parents sharing important decisions within the family. In some cases the changed role of women has resulted in a loss of identity for some men and subsequent insecurity.

The development of contraception has enabled couples to plan the size and spacing of their family and in some cases to decide against having children. This has not only given greater freedom to women, but has also reduced the average family size to less than two in the 1980s.

Attitudes to marriage and divorce have, in recent years, brought a change in the traditional idea of a family, and the term 'one-parent families' is now taken for granted. But even in this connection ideas have changed. Originally the term was applied to the unmarried or unsupported mother but more and more this has come to include separated and divorced women and, in more recent years, the lone-father bringing up children as more fathers receive custody of their children in the divorce courts.

As a result of their parents' remarriage children are now being brought up with, in some cases, four 'parents'; two natural parents and a step-father and mother; and siblings may be their natural brothers and sisters, or step or half brothers and sisters. The trauma associated with the break-up of their parent's marriage, and subsequent divorce and in some cases remarriage, and the difficulty in adjusting to a new family unit, is one of the problems facing the professionals whose work brings them into contact with young children. The long-term consequences of this social problem is difficult to envisage, but it is likely to influence the role of the midwife in the future.

The breakdown in communication between the generations, and the rejection of established practices has resulted in some couples deciding against marriage and living and raising children in a stable environment. Communal living is not new, although it is alien to present-day practices; however, this is another change that has affected our attitudes to traditional family life. In communal living the responsibility for childrearing, as with other tasks, is shared, and children growing up in this environment may not identify with one couple as their parents.

Advances in travel has resulted in many cases in the dissemination of families and the break up of the extended family. Even if families live in close contact, the fact that the grandmother has employment outside the home means she is not as available as in the past to provide support in times of need. Therefore many families with young children no longer have the support of an extended family, or friends and neighbours and feel a sense of isolation.

As well as the changes that have taken place in our society, we have in recent years become a multiracial society with peoples from different cultural backgrounds and speaking different languages, making their homes in this country.

The main ethnic groups that have immigrated to this country are the Negroes from West India and Africa; Asians from Pakistan, India and Bangladesh; Chinese; and Europeans, particularly from the Mediterranean countries, such as Italy, Greece and Cyprus, and Eastern Europe, such as Poland and Hungary.

People leave their country of origin because of political unrest, wars, religious persecution and unemployment, and they are seeking from the new country political stability, peace, freedom to practise their religion and employment.

Immigrant groups tend to concentrate in urban areas and group together in small communities according to the country of origin for social and economic reasons. This practice places considerable strains on the health and social services in these areas.

The extent to which these different ethnic groups have adapted to and integrated with the indigenous population, has varied from one group to another and according to their cultural background and the length of time they have settled in this country. But for all groups a period of adjustment is needed and the problems associated with this are not appreciated or are underestimated by the host nation. Immigrants are expected to adapt to the countries' culture, to respond in the same way as the indigenous population and to share common aims, interests and customs.

The culture and social structure of the African and West Indian groups have the same origins but those of the West Indians have been influenced and changed by slavery and Europeans. The main immigration from the West Indies took place in the 1950s; the majority of the immigrants came from Jamaica, were poorly educated and from a rural background. They had the advantage of speaking the language but had problems in adjusting to the climate and, because of their lack of education and qualifications, were employed in the least well paid jobs with limited prospects of advancement. The immigrants from Barbados were more urbanised and better educated and had less problems in adjusting.

The European immigrants have integrated into this country without major difficulties. The Chinese have come mainly from Hong Kong, Singapore and Malaysia, they have strong family and community ties and are mostly self-employed or employed in the catering trade as are the Mediterranean European groups.

It is the newest immigrants—the Asians—that are experiencing most difficulties, and when we consider that there are twelve major languages and many dialects spoken by the Asians it indicates the magnitude of the problem. Add to that eight major religions, four major castes and hundreds of sub-castes and the problems multiply. The differences in language, culture, religion and social structure create problems that are difficult to overcome. Many Asians come predominantly from small villages and rural areas in their country of origin and this background does not prepare them for living in the urban areas where they tend to concentrate.

It is important for the midwife to have some knowledge of the religious laws and local customs so that she has the essential information to ensure that the advice she gives is personally and culturally acceptable. The traditional role of women in the family varies in different cultures, and it is important to have an insight into the differences to understand the attitudes to childbearing and childrearing.

The Asian family is based on the extended structure where elders exert a great influence. Marriages are arranged, and on marriage the woman becomes part of her husband's family with no separate identity. It is a male-orientated society and women are often exploited and subjugated: the degree of emancipation being related to the level of education and urbanisation. Muslim women are secluded from social contact outside the family and their religion encourages modesty and marital fidelity.

The agricultural basis of the economy results in the need for many children, especially sons to work in the fields and also to provide security for old age. Therefore fertility and the birth of sons is of great importance to an Asian woman and the inability to have children and the birth of daughters, especially if she does not already have sons, is seen within the family as a failure. There is high maternal and infant mortality, and a short life expectancy among women.

Traditional attitudes may still exist even in immigrant families, or there may be conflict between the traditional role and the role of women in Britain. Many women are still isolated from contact outside their family, and the inability of many others to speak and write English discourages integration and creates difficulties in communication which may result in feelings of alienation.

The basis of effective care and health education is communication and understanding expectations. The barriers created by language and cultural differences hinder effective communication and prevents the provision of a high standard of care. Recognising the problems is one thing, how to overcome them is more difficult.

Various approaches are being made including the use of interpreters, English lessons at antenatal clinics, language cards and leaflets, and tape-slide programmes. These are not without problems; an interpreter may speak the same language but differences in dialect may hinder effective communication and with so many languages and dialects it is not possible to meet all needs; the woman may be illiterate in her own language, and therefore unable to learn English or read the leaflets provided.

Unfamiliarity with or lack of acceptance of the health services provided during pregnancy may prevent the woman from presenting for care until the pregnancy is well advanced. In the villages and rural districts traditional healers—hakims and vaids—provide health care and also act as counsellors in marital and other difficulties. Although these healers are not recognised in this country, the immigrants have brought with them the traditional systems of medicine—Unani and Ayurvedic. They use herbal medicines which often contain minerals and metals such as lead and arsenic.

The subdivision of conditions, diseases and foods into 'hot' and 'cold' has important implications in caring for Asian women during pregnancy and the puerperium. Pregnancy is a 'hot' condition and 'cold' foods such as milk products and citrus fruits are prohibited. These dietary restrictions could lead to a deficiency of vital nutrients during pregnancy. Failure to take iron and vitamin supplements may contribute to anaemia which is a common problem among Asian women (see p. 215). Conversely, lactation is a 'cold' condition and the prohibition of 'hot' foods such as legumes and pulses, which are important sources of protein in a vegetarian diet, may lead to dietary deficiencies.

Modesty among Asian women is important; immodesty affects not only the woman's reputation, but also that of her family. They may not find it acceptable to be examined by a male obstetrician or general practitioner and if there is no female doctor available the midwife should examine the woman.

The Asian woman's social and cultural background can result in a higher incidence of diseases such as anaemia, rickets, osteomalacia and dietary deficiency which can adversely affect pregnancy and labour.

An Asian woman in labour expects the women in her family to gather round and support her, and men are dissuaded from becoming involved. Therefore, we should adapt our practice of encouraging husbands to be present during labour to take account of this cultural difference. It may be more appropriate to suggest a female relative or relatives be present instead to avoid unnecessary anxiety.

In Asian families grandmothers frequently take over the care of the baby and expect to give advice and guide the young mother. Therefore it may not achieve anything to teach the mother alone and may cause conflict within the family if the young mother tries to put into practise what she has been taught. To overcome the difficulty the grandmother should be included in teaching sessions, and modern methods based on an understanding of the traditional customs, providing a balance between what is culturally acceptable and safe. For example, the application of Surma, a cosmetic paste, to the conjunctival margins of the baby's eyes from the fourteenth day is done in the belief that it will strengthen the eyes and ward off evil spirits. This is obviously very important to the family but, because the preparation is made from lead sulphide which can cause toxicity, it is a potential hazard. Lead has a cumulative effect and levels of 80 mcg are thought to be dangerous and may affect the nervous system causing inflammation of the peripheral nerves, convulsions and mental retardation, and the blood causing anaemia and bone marrow depression.

Traditionally it was natural for the Asian mother to breast feed her baby but the promotion of alternative methods in Third World countries in recent years, and the influence of seeing British women bottle feeding has resulted in some of these mothers thinking artificial feeding is superior. The lack of hygiene in the home, and the difficulties of teaching good preparation (see p. 341) are accentuated in immigrant mothers because of their inability to understand and read English, or their own language in some cases.

The tradition of milk feeding babies for the first two years of life and the unavailability of cereal preparations with added vitamins in the country of origin has resulted in a high incidence of iron deficiency anaemia in young Asian children. Therefore breast feeding should be actively encouraged and advice given not only about earlier weaning but also suitable foods to introduce.

Naming of children is another area of difference that if not understood may lead to confusion in recording babies names. The father's or mother's name and the family name are an integral part of the child's name; therefore the child has a given name, its father's or mother's name dependant on sex, and the family name—the equivalent of our surname. In some cases there is a lack of the use of a surname, and words such as Singh and Kaur are used which indicate male and female.

The average size family among Asian immigrants is four which is twice that of the indigenous population. The cultural and religious background of these people means there is a lack of knowledge about contraception and a natural inhibition about discussing sexual matters creates a barrier to family planning advice.

In contrast to the problems associated with the more recent immigrants, it is interesting to make a comparison with another major group that has settled in this country and has, over the years, adapted and changed and become well integrated.

Unlike their Asian counterparts, West Indian women play a dominant role in their culture with equal rights including education. The effect of slavery in discouraging marriage, but encouraging childbearing, resulted in a loose bond between parents with the main responsibility for children placed on the mother and along the maternal side of the family.

Procreation was seen as a sign of virility in the men and womanhood in women—something to be proved before marriage. Therefore there was no social stigma associated with having illegitimate children.

In the early days of West Indian immigration, children were often left at home with the maternal grandmother or aunt and children born in this country were also taken home. The male partner changed frequently therefore the father was not a central, stable figure but had a secondary role both socially and economically.

The lack of a warm, intimate, continuous relationship of the West Indian mother to her child was just one of the destructive effects of slavery; maternal deprivation can have an adverse effect on the child's development of speech, identity and emotional maturity.

A change of attitude and the influence of the culture of this country mean that West Indians are now forming more stable family units. However, the illegitimate birth rate is still higher among West Indian women and the placement of children with childminders is also more common.

The underprivileged status and predominance of Social Classes IV and V in all ethnic groups, but in particular among the Asians, can result in special needs and a higher incidence of problems than experienced by the community as a whole. To treat everyone equally fails to recognise unequal need. However, there is a limit to how far we can go in accommodating the needs of minority groups and that to do so to a high level may only limit further the tendency of these groups to make an effort to integrate more fully into British society.

Language problems and different cultural backgrounds and the feeling of alienation that result, and health problems do however create special needs and unfamiliarity with the system results in a low take up. Helping people to be aware of the availability and importance of the health service is vital, and voluntary organisations and local community groups are vital parts of the range of support and service which can be made available.

The employment of women during pregnancy and following childbirth

In the past, women who went out to work were expected to either give up employment when they became pregnant if they were not capable of doing the work or it was unsafe for them to do it, or they would resign at the end of the twenty-eighth week of pregnancy. There were incidences of women being dismissed solely on the grounds of pregnancy. If a woman wished to recommence employment following the birth of her baby she would not have been entitled to return to her previous employment and place of work.

The Employment Act 1975, included rights relating to the employment of women during pregnancy and following childbirth, and these rights were incorporated in the Employment Protection (Consolidation) Act 1978. The Employment Act 1980 which was implemented in November 1980 amended these rights.

It is important for the midwife to have some knowledge of the rights of women during pregnancy and following childbirth, under this Act, because her contact with women during this time makes her an ideal person to give guidance and advice.

The Employment Act 1980 provides four basic rights which apply equally to married and single women.

1 Dismissal of a woman from a job solely or mainly on the grounds of pregnancy constitutes unfair dismissal. However, dismissal is fair if the pregnancy has made the woman incapable of adequately doing the work, e.g. if it involved heavy lifting, or if it is illegal or usually dangerous for a job to be done by a woman during pregnancy, e.g. involving nuclear matter or the emission of ionising radiation (see p. 481).

The employer is, however, obliged to offer a suitable alternative job if there is one available and it must be on terms and conditions not substantially less favourable than her previous one.

The woman who is fairly dismissed does not lose her right to reinstatement (see below).

2 A woman has the right to be reinstated in her job, or a similar job, for up to twenty-nine weeks after the birth of her baby unless she is employed in a workplace with five or fewer employees when this right does not apply. To be entitled to the right to be reinstated, the woman must satisfy certain conditions. Firstly, she must have worked continuously for the same employer for at least two years at the end of the twenty-eighth week of pregnancy; she must therefore continue to work until that time. She must also inform her employer in writing at least twenty-one days before she leaves that she is taking maternity leave and intends to exercise her right of return. Finally, she must inform her employer in writing twenty-one days before the date of return; this condition also applies if she was fairly dismissed.

The twenty-nine week limit may be extended by four weeks if the woman is ill. The illness does not have to be related to childbirth but she must produce a medical certificate and notify the employer before the end of the twenty-ninth week.

The employer may delay the woman's return up to four weeks if he notifies the intention by the twenty-ninth week giving reasons and a new date for return. Industrial action may cause an extension of the twenty-nine week limit until work resumes.

The woman may not get the same job back when she resumes work but she must be given suitable alternative employment.

Maternity leave breaks continuity of employment in terms of rights under an individual contract, e.g. promotion prospects, access to pension schemes, but rights accumulated before taking leave are not lost and the leave counts regarding statutory rights such as redundancy pay.

3 A woman has the right to six weeks maternity pay if she satisfies certain conditions. She must have been employed continuously by the employer for

at least two years at the end of the twenty-eighth week of pregnancy and must continue to be employed until that time. She must give her employer twenty-one days notice. A Certificate of Confinement signed by a doctor or a midwife and giving the estimated date of delivery must be provided on request.

Maternity pay is 90% of the basic pay minus the flat rate maternity allowance (see p. 439).

To qualify for these three rights the woman must be employed for at least sixteen hours a week unless she has been employed for at least eight hours a week and has been with the same employer for at least five years.

4 This right applies to all women regardless of the hours of work, the size of the work force, or the length of time they have been employed. A pregnant woman has the right to time off work without loss of pay to receive antenatal care. After the first visit the woman may need to produce a Certificate of Confinement and her appointment card.

Although it is important for a midwife to have some knowledge and understanding about the employment of women during pregnancy and following childbirth so that they can give advice on these matters, the intricacies of the Employment Act require expert knowledge. Therefore the midwife should refer the woman to a personnel officer or a professional or union representative who will be able to advise her about her individual rights.

CLASSIFICATION OF SOCIAL CLASS

The classification of social class is based on the occupation of the family's chief economic supporter. The classifications provide data which can be used in research and surveys.

Class 1. Professions: dentists, doctors, pharmacists, lawyers, civil and electrical engineers, metallurgists, physical and biological scientists, accountants and company secretaries.

Class 2. Creative artists, painters, radio and radar supervisory mechanics, aircraft pilots, navigators and flight engineers, finance and insurance keepers, radiographers and occupational therapists.

Class 3. Skilled workers: restaurateurs, cooks, beauticians, glass blowers and decorators, furnacemen, plumbers and heating engineers, watchmakers and repairers, goldsmiths and jewellery makers, bakers and pastry cooks, butchers and meat cutters, printing press operators and compositors, bricklayers and lorry drivers.

Class 4. Semi-skilled workers: warehousemen, storekeepers, firemen, fibre preparers and spinners, deck and engine-room ratings, street vendors and hawkers.

Class 5. Unskilled workers: labourers, ticket collectors, lorry drivers' mates, charwomen and chimney sweeps.

Three-quarters of families fall into the upper three classes, with the majority in classes 2 and 3. The details used to determine the five socioeconomic groupings or classes have been taken from the 1981 census.

THE NATIONAL HEALTH SERVICE

To enable the student to see the present health services in perspective, I have listed below relevant events prior to 1982.

Historical background

1834 The Poor Laws—established that the parish workhouses should have sick wards.

1837 A medical statistician, William Farr, was appointed. Laid the foundation for the Registrar General's Department.

1843 A Royal Commission to enquire into the Health of Towns was set up.

1848 The Public Health Act—created General Board of Health.

1851 First links between workhouses and voluntary bodies.

1858 Privy Council took over functions of General Board of Health.

1867 The Metropolitan Poor Law Act—required local authorities within London to provide separate institutional care for tuberculosis, smallpox, fevers and insanity.

1868 The Poor Law Amendment Act—established same provision in the provinces.

1871 Local Government Board was created and took over health functions of the Privy Council and became responsible for the national functions of the Poor Law.

1872 Sanitary Districts were created and it became obligatory for each to appoint a Medical Officer of Health.

1875 The Public Health Act—laid down a national minimum standard of hygiene.

1886 Local Authorities were created and consisted of County Councils and County Borough Councils.

1894 Urban and Rural District Councils were instituted.

1902 The Midwives Act—made it illegal for unqualified persons to attend women in childbirth.

1907 School Medical Service established.

1911 The National Insurance Act, established a general practitioner service for insured persons, and most 'private' practitioners acted as panel doctors in the scheme.

1915 Notification of birth became compulsory.

1918 Maternity and Child Welfare Act.

1919 Ministry of Health was established.

1929 The Local Government Act transferred the Poor Laws locally to local authorities.

1936 A domiciliary midwifery service was introduced under local authority administration.

1942 A large-scale scheme for diphtheria immunisation was started.

1943 Beveridge Report on social security.

1945 Family Allowances were introduced.

1946 The National Health Service Act passed.
The National Insurance Act passed.

1948 The National Health Service Act implemented. The services were divided into three parts:

1 The hospital and specialist services run by twenty Regional Hospital Boards.

2 The general practitioner services run by Local Executive Councils and including the pharmaceutical, dental and ophthalmic services.

3 The community health services run by the local authorities. Their responsibilities included health centres; maternal and child welfare; domiciliary maternity services; health visiting; home nursing; ambulances; immunisation and vaccination; home-help service; preventative medicine including health education.

1948 The Children Act—set up an independent child care service under the central control of the Home Office and locally run by the local authority.

1956 The Clean Air Act—set up to reduce the problem of atmospheric pollution.

1959 The Mental Health Act—obliged local authorities to provide a full range of community services for the mentally handicapped, including residential homes and hostels, special schools and training centres, sheltered workshops and social support.

1967 The National Health Service (Family Planning) Act—extended the power of Local Authorities to help in cases of medical and social need.

1967 The Abortion Act—introduced legal abortion—implemented 1968.

1968 Health Services and Public Health Act—extended the law regarding the provision of home nurses and care of the elderly.

1970 The Chronically Sick and Disabled Persons Act—emphasised and extended the responsibility of local authority in relation to disabled persons.

1971 Education of the mentally handicapped was transferred from health to education department and junior training centres became special schools.

1972 National Health Service (Family Planning Amendment Act)—placed vasectomy on the same basis as other contraceptive services.

1973 The National Health Service Reorganisation Act—implemented in 1974.

1980 The National Health Service Act—implemented in 1982.

Reorganisation of the National Health Service

Since 1948, health care has been provided under the National Health Service by Local Authority Health Departments, the Hospital Services and the Family Practitioner Service including general practitioners, dentists, pharmacists and opticians. The three parts of the service were separately managed and financed.

The National Health Service Reorganisation Act 1973, which was implemented on 1st April 1974, integrated the three parts of the service under a single management and brought the health services into line with the reorganised local government structure. Social services were not brought into the unified Health Service but continue to be provided by the local authority.

The National Health Service Act 1980 was implemented in April 1982. As a result of this Act, the National Health Service underwent further reorganisation with the elimination of the area level.

Table 13.1 The new structure.

Department of Health and Social Security
↓
Regional Health Authorities
↓
District Health Authorities

Department of Health and Social Security

In 1968, the former Ministries of Social Security and Health were merged to form the Department of Health and Social Security under a Secretary of State for Social Services. The Department of Health and Social Security is responsible for central strategic planning and monitoring. It determines national policy, is responsible for overall budgeting and accounting for health expenditure, determines kind, scale and balance of services to be provided and sets long-term objectives, priorities and standards of care as guidelines for effective regional and area planning. The Secretary of State is answerable to Parliament for the National Health Service.

Regional Health Authorities

There are fourteen Regional Health Authorities covering similar geographical areas to the Local Government Divisions. Each Regional Health Authority has a salaried Chairman appointed by the Secretary of State and members, also appointed by the Secretary of State, who work in a voluntary part-time capacity. The members exercise authority only when meeting as members.

The Regional Health Authority is directly responsible to the Secretary of State and is responsible for general supervision and regional planning. In order to carry out their functions the Regional Health Authority is supported by a team of professionally qualified people who will assist them in planning and monitoring services.

THE REGIONAL TEAM OF OFFICERS

The team consists of: the Regional Medical Officer; the Regional Nursing Officer; the Regional Works Officer; the Regional Treasurer; the Regional Administrator.

These officers will be the 'heads' of their services in the region but will not be the managers of the District Health Authority officers.

The reorganisation that came into effect in April 1982 replaced the 90 Area Health Authorities and the 186 health districts with 200 District Health Authorities.

District Health Authorities

The District Health Authorities serve a population of between 250000–300000 and are responsible for planning, development and management of the health services.

The Authority comprises a chairman, appointed by the Secretary of State, four representatives of the local authority, a consultant, a general medical practitioner, a nurse, a university nominee, a trade union nominee and four Regional appointees. The numbers exercise authority only when meeting as members.

The district

The district is the basic operational unit of the integrated Health Service and an area may comprise up to six districts. A district is defined as a population of 250000–300000 served by the community health services supported by the specialist services of a district general hospital.

THE DISTRICT MANAGEMENT TEAM

The District Management Team comprises a group of officers responsible for planning and coordinating comprehensive health care. Membership: the District Medical Officer; the District or Chief Nursing Officer; the District Finance Officer; the District Administrator.

Two other members one a hospital consultant the other a general practitioner, are representatives of the District Medical Committee. The six members have equal status and decisions are taken by consensus. The members have a joint responsibility for managing the district health services and the officer members of the team also have an individual and collective responsibility to the District Health Authority.

DISTRICT MEDICAL COMMITTEE

Each district has a District Medical Committee to represent all the medical staff and coordinate the medical aspects of health care. Members of the Committee represent particular groupings of doctors. Two members of the Committee are elected as representatives to the District Management Team.

HEALTH CARE PLANNING TEAMS

Health care planning teams are established within districts to determine the health care needs of the community. The teams are composed of general practitioners, consultants, hospital and community nurses and midwives, and health visitors, relevant paramedical staff and representatives of the local authority services, particularly social services. The District Medical Officer coordinates the activities of the teams and provides a link between them and the District Management Team. There are five permanent teams: for the elderly, mentally handicapped, mentally ill, children and maternity cases; other temporary teams may be constituted to look at particular problems.

PRIMARY HEALTH CARE TEAMS

Primary health care teams are composed of general practitioners, health visitors, community nurses and midwives, and are supported by receptionist/ secretarial staff. They constitute a basic health team which has as its objective the provision of health care for families and individuals in the community.

COMMUNITY HEALTH COUNCILS

Community Health Councils have been set up in each health district to monitor the health services on behalf of the community. The Council has the power to secure information and visit hospitals and other institutions. They have access to the officers of the District Health Authority administering the district services. Half of the members of the Council are nominated by the District Council in the district concerned, one-third by local voluntary bodies and the remaining one-sixth by the Regional Health Authority after appropriate consultation. Total membership is between twenty and thirty people. The Community Health Council appoints its own Chairman and publishes an annual report.

The Community Health Council communicates to the District Health Authority the view of the community and their needs and priorities, and the deficiencies of the service.

Joint Consultative Committees

Joint Consultative Committees are the statutory mechanism through which collaboration is achieved between the District Health Authority responsible for the health services within the District and Local Authority responsible for the personal social services. These committees have now been given the job of examining and improving joint planning arrangements.

Family Practitioner Committees

Responsibility for administration of the family practitioner services which involves the work of general practitioners, dentists, pharmacists and opticians resides with the Family Practitioner Committee set up by the Area Health Authority following the 1974 Reorganisation. The Family Practitioner Committees are similar to their predecessors, the Executive Councils, in terms of membership and duties. The Committee consists of thirty members and is responsible for the arrangements for the provision of family practitioner services. Since 1982 one District Health Authority within the boundary of the previous Area Health Authority has monitored the work of these Committees. Further changes are planned.

The unification of the maternity services

Some aspects of the Health Service are of particular relevance to the woman during her pregnancy and after, and these are dealt with in more detail.

Prior to reorganisation of the National Health Service the maternity services were provided by a tripartite structure, hospital specialist services administered by the Regional Hospital Boards, the general practitioner services administered by the Executive Council and the domiciliary midwifery services provided by the Local Health Authority.

Reorganisation brought with it unification of the maternity services under one authority, the Area Health Authority. The community midwifery services were usually run from the District General Hospital, and community midwives practise both in hospital and community. The 1982 reorganisation made few changes in relation to the maternity services which are now organised on a district basis.

Health visiting services

The health visitor is a state registered nurse with midwifery experience who has in addition the statutory Health Visitor's Certificate.

FUNCTIONS

1 The prevention of mental, physical and emotional ill-health and its consequences.

2 Early detection of ill-health and the surveillance of high risk groups.

3 Recognition and identification of need and mobilisation of appropriate resources where necessary.

4 Health education.

5 Provision of care; this will include support during periods of stress and advice and guidance in cases of illness as well as the care and management of children.

Health visitors carry out their duties in people's homes, in doctor's surgeries, health centres and in schools. They work as members of primary health care teams.

Family planning services

Family planning services prior to reorganisation of the National Health Service were provided partly by the Local Health Authority and partly by the Family Planning Association. On 1st April 1974 the Area Health Authority took over the responsibility for the family planning services from the Local Health Authority and subsequently from the Family Planning Association. On 1st April 1982, the District Health Authority assumed responsibility for these services.

The main responsibility for the planning and management of family planning services rests with the District Management Team.

SERVICES AVAILABLE

Since April 1974 the services and supplies have been provided free under the National Health Service.

Services are provided in the following ways.

1 Hospital services: gynaecological wards and clinics; maternity, postnatal wards and clinic.

2 Community services.

3 Domiciliary services.

4 Family practitioner services.

AIMS OF FAMILY PLANNING

To avoid an unwanted pregnancy. Unplanned pregnancy results in stress and unhappiness, it may place stress on an overstretched budget causing others in the family to suffer. Financial and emotional difficulties may lead to the child being taken into care temporarily or permanently.

To improve the physical health of families. Proper spacing and timing of births can contribute to better maternal and child health, and can reduce maternal and perinatal mortality as these increase with maternal age and parity. It can do much to alleviate the emotional stress on overburdened mothers which, in some instances leads to a breakdown in nurturing care.

To reduce the cost to society of abortion and an unwanted child. Numerous studies have shown that family planning is substantially cost saving. It is difficult to assess an overall figure as being the cost to society of unwanted children as opposed to that of wanted children but it is likely to be high. The following figures were given by Dr Owen, the then Secretary of State for Health and Social Security, at a Family Planning Association meeting in March 1976; there are every year 55000 illegitimate births, 45000 conceptions before marriage, and 100000 abortions.

METHODS

There are many factors influencing a woman's decision regarding the method of contraception. They include:

1 Reliability—the success/failure rate of the method.
2 Reason for contraception, i.e. whether she would accept failure of method, therefore a pregnancy.
3 Previous experience.
4 Simplicity of usage.
5 Publicity and propaganda.
6 Influence of husband, partner, friends and relatives.
7 Religious and cultural influences.
8 Age, health and family history.

Birth control methods

Methods of controlling ovulation

ORAL CONTRACEPTIVES

Oral contraceptives contain oestrogen in the form of mestranol or ethinyl-oestradiol and progestogen, or progestogen only.

The progestogen-only pills are taken daily starting from the first day of the menstrual cycle. They act mainly by making cervical mucus impenetrable to spermatozoa, and have a success rate of 96.0–99.2%. They are used for women who are unable to take oestrogens, and during lactation.

Combined pills contain 30–50 μm of oestrogen and varying amounts of progestogen. They are taken daily for three weeks followed by one week without and are started on the fifth day if the normal cycle is more than twenty-six days or on the first day of cycle if the normal cycle is less than twenty-six days. The combined pills act by preventing ovulation, altering the motility of the Fallopian tube, making the cervical mucus impenetrable and preventing normal development of the endometrium. They are virtually 100% reliable if taken according to instructions. The menstrual cycle is regularised by the combined pill and dysmenorrhoea and in some cases premenstrual tension is relieved. The menstrual flow is usually slight.

If a woman has had unprotected sexual intercourse a high dose of an oral contraceptive can usually prevent an unplanned pregnancy. The treatment, which is given under a doctor's supervision, comprises giving a medium dose oestrogen pill such as Eugynon 50 as soon as possible but within three days. The woman is prescribed two tablets and the dose is repeated twelve hours later.

Contraindications

Oral contraceptives are absolutely contraindicated if the woman has a history of thromboembolic disorder, recent or severe liver disorders or a hormone dependent tumour. Relative contraindications include diabetes mellitus, hypertension, renal or heart disease, epilepsy and obesity.

Side-effects of the combined oral contraceptive include headaches, break-through bleeding, obesity, nausea, depression and breast changes.

Special considerations

Ideally, young women should not be prescribed oral contraceptives until they have menstruated for five years or at least have regular periods. Following pregnancy the oral contraceptive may be commenced as soon as the woman wishes to do so. In relation to the menopause the oral contraceptive is stopped at yearly intervals to see if menstruation has ceased.

INJECTABLES

Depo-provera is an injection given at three-monthly intervals and is a good method for poorly motivated women or in areas with a shortage of medical personnel. Progesterone is injected into a muscle and is released slowly into the circulation. Its action is to prevent ovulation and make the cervical mucus impenetrable to spermatozoa. Bleeding may be irregular and fertility delayed by up to six months following cessation of treatment.

PROGESTERONE UTERINE THERAPEUTIC SYSTEM

This system comprises a small flexible T-shaped membrane-enclosed drug reservoir which delivers the progesterone to the lining of the uterus. The hormone is released in a controlled way at a continuous average rate of 65 μg/day. The inserter is an integral part of the system.

This method of contraception is achieved without effecting the hypothalmic-pituitary-ovarian axis for at least a year from a single placement. There is a prompt return to pre-insertion fertility following removal.

Methods of controlling fertilisation

COITUS INTERRUPTUS

The withdrawal of the penis from the vagina before ejaculation. Its reliability is low and is dependent on the control of the male partner and timing. Even so, semen often leaks out before ejaculation. This method places great strain on both partners and often leads to frustration and in some cases psychological disorders.

RHYTHM METHOD OR 'SAFE' PERIOD

This involves avoiding sexual intercourse during the time in the menstrual cycle when conception is likely to occur. The rhythm method is based upon determining the time of ovulation, which is followed by a rise in temperature one or two days later. There are two ways of calculating the 'safe' period, the calendar method and the more reliable temperature method. The calendar method involves recording the first day of the menstrual cycle, i.e. the day bleeding starts, for at least six months, and preferably a year, before using the method. The woman then calculates the 'unsafe' days by determining the shortest and longest cycles and by subtracting eighteen days from the shortest cycle and ten days from the longest. The figure obtained is counted from the first day of the cycle and indicates the first 'unsafe' day.

The temperature method involves the woman recording her temperature first thing every morning and recording it on a special chart. Sexual intercourse is avoided five days before and four days after ovulation. The reliability varies according to the degree of menstrual regularity, and the care taken in applying this method.

The rhythm method is the only method of contraception currently approved by the Roman Catholic Church.

BARRIER METHODS

These include the sheath for men and the diaphragm or cervical cap for women.

The sheath does not require medical supervision and is easily available. The sheath is put on the erect penis leaving the last 1.5 cm of the blind end (or the teat if there is one) empty to receive the seminal fluid. The success rate is increased if the woman uses a spermicide in the form of a contraceptive cream, foam, jelly or pessary.

The vaginal diaphragm is a shallow rubber cap with a coil spring rim which is placed in the vagina to extend from the posterior fornix to behind the pubic bone. It is held in place by muscles and is therefore dependent on good pelvic floor muscles. A spermicidal cream or jelly is applied to each side of the cap which is inserted at any convenient time prior to sexual intercourse, although if longer than three hours a pessary or spermicide should be used in addition. The cap is left in place at least six hours after intercourse.

The size of the cap requires to be rechecked following childbirth or if the woman loses or gains more than 3 kg in weight.

Cervical caps fit over the healthy cervix. The Dumas or Vault cap is placed over the cervix and is held in place by suction. There are five sizes ranging from 50–75 mm in diameter. The cap is dome-shaped and is thicker at the edge. It is used in conjunction with a spermicidal cream or jelly. The Dumas cap is used if the cervix is short.

The vimule fits over the cervix and can only be used if the cervix is long and accessible. There are three sizes ranging from 45–51 mm in diameter. The vimule is used with a spermicidal cream or jelly which is applied only to the outer aspect.

Spermicides are available in the form of jelly, cream, foam, foaming tablets and pessaries. They are not reliable when used on their own but are used to improve the reliability of other methods.

STERILISATION

This is the most effective method of contraception available. It is important that the couple receive counselling so that they are fully aware of the implications of the operation and the alternative methods of contraception available. As a method of contraception it is suitable only for men and women who are married, or have stable unions, and have completed their families or who have serious health grounds for preventing reproduction. Although not a legal requirement, the consent of the partner as well as the prospective patient should be obtained. Tubal ligation is the female method of sterilisation and involves ligating and dividing the Fallopian tubes or in some cases embedding the tubes. The operation may be performed by the abdominal or vaginal route or via a laparoscope usually under a general anaesthetic.

Vasectomy is the male method of sterilisation and involves ligation of the vas deferens usually under a local anaesthetic. This operation is now performed free under the National Health Service.

Because sterilisation cannot be performed with any guarantee of reversibility it is considered to be a permanent method of contraception.

The male genital system

It is appropriate to give a brief description of the male genital system in order for the student to understand vasectomy.

The scrotum. The scrotum is a pouch of dark skin containing the testes and their coverings, the epididymis and the lower end of the spermatic cord. The scrotum is divided into two by a septum, and the division is indicated on the surface by a ridge known as the raphe. The raphe continues forwards along the under surface of the penis, and backwards, to the anus.
The testis. The testis is the male gonad. There are two testes approximately 4 cm long and normally situated one on each side of the scrotum. The testis is surrounded by the visceral layer of the tunica vaginalis, the tunica albuginea. Partitions for the tunica albuginea extend inwards to separate the numerous coiled seminiferous tubules, in which sperms are produced by the process of spermatogenesis (see p. 86).
The epididymis and vas deferens. The spermatozoa are conveyed to the female genital tract in a fluid called seminal fluid, which with the spermatozoa constitutes semen. The seminal fluid is produced in the seminiferous tubules, but fluid from the epididymis, vas deferens, seminal vesicles and prostate are added to it (Fig. 13.1).

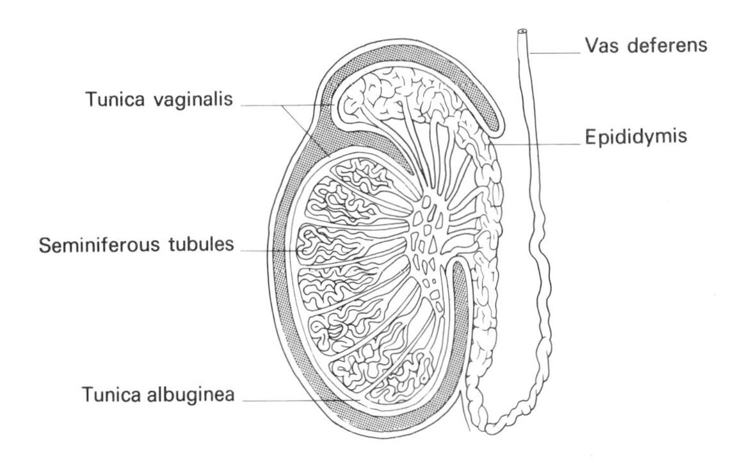

Fig. 13.1 The testis, epididymis and vas deferens.

The epididymis is a highly coiled tube situated in the posterior aspect of the testis. The seminiferous tubules empty their contents by way of small efferent ducts into the epididymis which leads to the vas deferens.

The vas deferens leads off the lower pole of the epididymis and ascends in the spermatic cord. It transverses the inguinal canal, crosses the brim of the pelvis and runs medially towards the posterior aspect of the bladder. Here it hooks over the ureter and then descends towards the posterior aspect of the prostate, where it is joined by the seminal vesicle. The vas deferens is a muscular tube with a narrow lumen and thick wall. In addition to the vas deferens the spermatic cord contains blood vessels passing to and from the

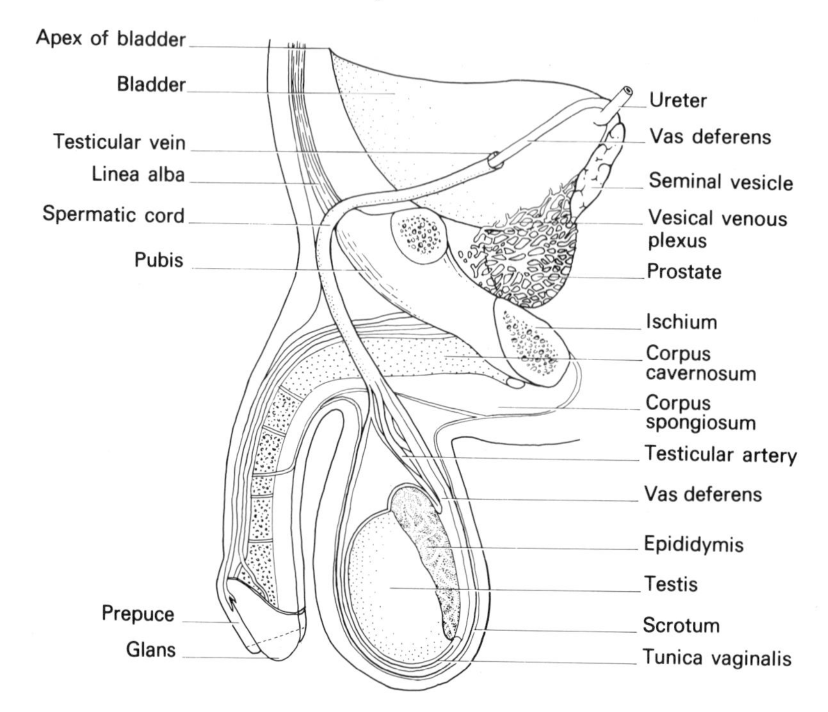

Fig. 13.2 The male genital system.

testis, lymphatic vessels from the testis and muscle which regulates the level of the testis (Fig. 13.2).

The seminal vesicles. Each seminal vesicle is a wide tube which lies coiled behind the prostate and bladder and in front of the rectum. Each vesicle contributes its secretions to semen by way of a short narrow duct that joins the vas deferens to form the ejaculatory duct. This enters the prostate gland (Fig. 13.2).

The prostate gland. The prostate gland consists of glandular tissue embedded in a fibromuscular stroma. It is related anteriorly to the lower part of the symphysis pubis and posteriorly to the seminal vesicles and rectum. It is enclosed in a capsule and surrounded by a rich plexus of veins which receive veins from the penis. The ejaculatory ducts traverse the substance of the gland from its posteriosuperior aspect (Fig. 13.2).

The penis. The penis is a cylindrical organ, slightly extended at its tip to form the glans. The penis is composed of cavernous tissue into which blood vessels can pump blood to make it turgid; this type of tissue is therefore also known as erectile tissue. The penile part of the urethra traverses the entire length of the penis (Fig. 13.2).

Methods of controlling nidation (implantation)

INTRAUTERINE DEVICES

The mode of action of intrauterine devices is unknown but it is thought to alter motility of the Fallopian tube and to result in formation of an unfavourable endometrium by causing an allergic response. There are two kinds of devices available; the Lippe's loop which is made of plastic, and a variety of devices, including Copper 7 and Copper T that are wound with copper which produces a greater allergic response in the endometrium. The devices containing copper are usually replaced every two to three years, but the Lippe's loop is left in place longer.

Intrauterine devices are contraindicated if the woman has fibroids, acute or chronic inflammatory disease, menorrhagia or any unexplained bleeding, a suspicion of carcinoma and suspicion of pregnancy.

Side-effects include heavy periods, cramp-like pain for a day or two following insertion, and perhaps with the next two or three periods, expulsion, uterine perforation, infection and ectopic pregnancy. This method is 97–98% reliable.

An intrauterine device inserted within five days of unprotected sexual intercourse, will usually prevent an unplanned pregnancy.

Other services

In addition to advice regarding methods of contraception and provision of supplies, family planning clinics also provide screening for carcinoma of the cervix and breasts, and undertake pregnancy testing. Some clinics also hold youth advisory sessions and give infertility and psychosexual counselling.

CERVICAL CYTOLOGY

It is a national policy to recommend routine screening for carcinoma of the cervix at five-yearly intervals to all women over the age of thirty-five. Cervical screening is undertaken at yearly intervals at family planning clinics and is usually performed at antenatal booking clinics.

Papanicolau cervical smear provides a means of detecting malignant cells before any cancerous lesion of the cervix is manifest. All epithelia desquamate their surface cells, and malignant epithelia do so more rapidly. An Ayre's wooden spatula is used to scrape off surface cells from the region of the internal os and transfer them to a glass slide where they are 'fixed' by spraying with a fixative solution. The spatula must be rotated 360° keeping the edge in contact with the cervix so that the whole surface is scraped. After being stained, the cells are examined microscopically by a cytologist, who is able to differentiate between normal squamous cells, and abnormal cells. The smear must not be taken from a woman who is menstruating, who is losing lochia, or who has an appreciable vaginal discharge, for red blood cells, pus and debris obscure the squamous cells on the slide and this makes interpretation very difficult.

A national combined request, report and recall form is used with five copies, one each for the woman's general practitioner, the District Health Authority, the sender of the specimen, the laboratory performing the test and the National Health Service Cancer Research Unit.

EXAMINATION OF THE BREASTS

The breasts are routinely examined for abnormal masses at regular intervals at family planning clinics, antenatal booking and postnatal examinations and whenever a cervical smear is taken. The woman is taught self-examination and advised to see her general practitioner if she observes any deviation from normal.

The child health services

UNIFICATION OF THE CHILD HEALTH SERVICES

Responsibility for local authority health services for the pre-school child, for medical and dental inspection and treatment of school children and for services provided by general medical and dental practitioners and the hospital specialist services, was transferred to the Area Health Authorities under the provision of the National Health Service Reorganisation Act 1973 and to the District Health Authorities on 1st April 1982.

COMMUNITY SERVICES FOR THE PRE-SCHOOL CHILD

Child Health Centres

Preventative and advisory services for pre-school children and their parents are based on the Child Health Centres. The community child health services provide regular and systematic supervision of children's physical, mental and emotional health and development progress by doctors, dentists and health visitors. Some family doctors also provide this service for their own child patients and dental care is also provided by general dental practitioners.

Observation or 'At Risk' Register

Since 1963, it has become the practice of health authorities to keep a register of children considered to be 'at risk' of handicapping conditions.

The criteria for admitting children to the observation register vary from area to area but may include the following.

Family history. A family history of deafness or blindness; genetic factors; inborn errors of metabolism, i.e. phenylketonuria.

Prenatal. Infections, i.e. rubella, cytomegalic inclusion disease, syphilis, toxoplasmosis; maternal diseases, i.e. diabetes mellitus, hypertension; obstetric disorders, i.e. threatened abortion, antepartum haemorrhage, pre-eclampsia, polyhydramnios, hyperemesis gravidarum; blood group incompatibilities; other factors including smoking, drugs, X-rays.
Labour. Prolonged or precipitate labour; instrumental delivery; fetal distress; multiple pregnancy; prolonged rupture of membranes.
Neonatal. Pre- or post-term infants; light-for-dates infants; birth asphyxia; respiratory distress syndrome; hypothermia; jaundice; infections; haemorrhagic disease; inborn errors of metabolism; congenital malformation; convulsions; any infant who fails to thrive.

Categories of handicap

Ten categories of handicap are recognised.

1 The blind.
2 The partially sighted.
3 The deaf.
4 The partially deaf.
5 The delicate.
6 The educationally subnormal.
7 The epileptic.
8 The maladjusted.
9 The physically handicapped.
10 Speech defects.

SCHOOL HEALTH AND DENTAL SERVICES

The purpose of medical inspections is to identify as early as possible any deviation from normal, and to ensure that appropriate advice and treatment is obtained. Children are medically inspected as soon as possible during their first year at school or, if they were inspected immediately prior to entering primary school, they are examined again at a later date. Practice for subsequent medical examination varies, in some districts periodic medical examinations are made, in others the school doctor visits the school several times each term and sees children brought to his attention by parents, teachers and school nurses. The school nurse screens all the children's sight and hearing and passes on those whom she thinks need specialist attention to the doctor, who may then refer them to a specialist.

The aim of the school dental service is to provide inspection on school entry, annual reinspection and provision of necessary treatment. Parents are invited and encouraged to attend school medical inspections and the first dental inspection.

Table 13.2 Recommended programme for vaccination and immunisation.

Age	*Type of vaccination or immunisation*
Three months	First injection against diphtheria, whooping cough and tetanus. First dose of oral poliomyelitis vaccine.
Five months	Second injection against diphtheria, whooping cough and tetanus. Second dose of oral poliomyelitis vaccine.
Nine months	Third injection against diphtheria, whooping cough and tetanus. Third dose of oral poliomyelitis vaccine.
Thirteen months	Measles vaccination.
Pre-school	Booster injection against diphtheria and tetanus and oral poliomyelitis vaccine.
Thirteen years	BCG vaccination against tuberculosis and rubella vaccination for girls.

Vaccination and immunisation

From 1st April 1974, Area Health Authorities assumed responsibility for providing and promoting vaccination and immunisation services (Table 13.2). Responsibility for these services was delegated to the community physician. On 1st April 1982, the District Health Authority assumed responsibility for these services.

HEALTH EDUCATION

The purpose of health education is to teach the principles of hygiene and healthy living, and to inform people about the medical and social services provided. Subjects included in health education are: diet, nutrition and weight problems; vaccination and immunisation; smoking; dental care; sexually transmitted diseases; sex education; family planning; antenatal education; home safety; exercise and healthy use of leisure.

THE SOCIAL SERVICES

An introduction

The Department of Health and Social Security was formed in November 1968 when the Ministry of Health and the Ministry of Social Security were merged. The Department, under the Secretary of State, is responsible for the central administration of the social services. Local administration of personal social services is the responsibility of the local authorities.

Under the Local Authority Social Services Act 1970, all personal social services were unified in single local authority departments with their own committee of elected representatives and the appointment of a director of social services.

The present social services cover five main activities namely: services mainly for the elderly (48.2%); services for children (34.1%); services directly for the physically handicapped (7.0%); services for the mentally handicapped (8.4%); services for the mentally ill (2.3%). The percentages indicate the proportion of spending in 1975–76 in the United Kingdom.

The Local Government Act 1972, which came into effect on 1st April 1974, reorganised local government and changed the geographical area, name and status of local authorities. The present local authorities are County Councils, District Councils, Parish Councils, Metropolitan County Councils and Metropolitan District Councils.

The National Health Service Reorganisation Act 1973, which was also implemented on 1st April 1974, brought the health services into line with the local government structure with Area Health Authorities having boundaries corresponding with those of local government County and Metropolitan District boundaries. Joint Consultative Committees were set up to provide liaison between the Area Health Authority responsible for the health services within the area and the local authority responsible for the personal social services. The 1982 reorganisation retained the link between the local authorities and the new district health authorities.

Services for children

Services for children and their families are second only to the services provided for the elderly and accounted for 34.1% of spending in 1975–76. Families with problems make the greatest demand on these services.

Problem families

Factors causing problems within a family are very varied and in some cases insoluble, in spite of all the services available. One or more of the following may be the cause of problems within a family.

1 Housing. Homelessness; overcrowding; substandard accommodation.

2 One-parent families. Unmarried/unsupported mother; lone fathers; separated, temporary or permanent; divorced; widowed; desertion; prison sentence. One-parent families are a large and increasing group in our society. It is estimated that there are 100000 fathers and 500000 mothers in Britain bringing up children alone. The problems and needs of families with only one parent are complex and manifold and include financial hardship, difficulty in finding suitable accommodation and employment, and social and emotional isolation.

3 Financial problems. Unemployed; low income; large family; poor budgeting.

4 Handicap of parent or child. Physically ill or handicapped; mentally ill or handicapped.

5 Immigrant families. Language/communication difficulties; housing—overcrowding, substandard; financial—low income, unemployed.

6 Marital problems. Including wife abuse.

7 Addiction. Drugs, alcohol, gambling.

8 Delinquency.

9 Child abuse. This is a problem causing increasing concern and one for which everyone who comes into contact with children and their families must be constantly alert.

CLASSIFICATION OF CHILD ABUSE

Active. The child is harmed by physical intervention on the part of the parent.

Passive. Harm arises from a process of neglect.

The diagnosis is based on a correlation between the physical signs obtained on injury, the alleged history and the results of investigation into the social background of the family.

Alerting signs include delay in attending hospital following injury; statements such as 'the child bruises easily', 'fell out of someone's arms when being carried downstairs', 'alright when put to bed'; repeated attendance at casualty departments; numerous previous fractures seen on X-ray; child's behaviour especially towards parents; failure to thrive.

Injuries are often unusual and inconsistent with age of the child and include bruises caused by manual pressure. Finger-tip bruises are round or oval and 0.5–2.0 cm in diameter. The child may have a black eye. Burns caused by cigarettes or scalding with boiling water. Bites, fractures, mouth injuries, tender and swollen joints and poisoning.

It is recognised that some children are more susceptible to abuse than others and include low birth weight babies—immature or light-for-dates; unwanted or abnormal children; age—the majority of children are under one year of age, a high proportion are under six months; babies who cry a lot and do not feed or sleep well.

In the same way that some children are more susceptible to abuse, some parents are also more likely to abuse their children. Over 80% of child victims of homicide are killed by their parents. Factors to be considered include:

1 Personality.
   - a Mild: character disorder, emotional immaturity.
   - b Moderate: personality disorder.
   - c Severe: psychopathic.

2 Age. Young, immature couples.

3 Social class. Predominantly of lower social class (see p. 409).

4 General health.
5 Intelligence. Borderline or subnormal intelligence.
6 Criminal record.
7 Marital problems.
8 Battered as a child. The cycle of deprivation.
9 Environmental stress.

The management of these families is usually combined with a care order and includes symptomatic relief, social relearning and teaching appropriate child-rearing skills. When response to treatment appears unlikely, removal of the child from parental care is considered.

It has been estimated that there are fifteen cases of child abuse per day of which twelve require admission to hospital, two die from their injuries and three sustain irreparable brain damage.

Day care for children

CHILD-MINDING

A child-minder is someone, other than a relative, who cares for a child under five years of age for more than two hours per day for payment. The law requires that child-minders must be registered with the Social Services Department of their local authority. Before registration is granted, a social worker checks that the house is safe and makes sure that the applicant is a suitable person. The authority also requires references. The charges vary and are agreed between the child-minder and the parent of the child.

DAY NURSERIES

Day nurseries are provided by the Social Services Department of the local authority to meet the special needs on social or health grounds of families with children under five years of age. Priority is given to one-parent families where the parent has no option but to work to support the family, children with a physical or mental handicap and children whose home conditions are unsatisfactory. Day nurseries are staffed by nursery nurses. Some Social Services Departments also place children in private day nurseries or with child-minders.

PLAYGROUPS

Pre-school playgroups provide a social and educational environment for normal children. They are provided mostly by voluntary associations for children between two and a half and five years of age who attend on average two to five weekly sessions of two and a half hours a day. Mothers actively participate in organising and running playgroups.

Education

NURSERY SCHOOLS

Nursery schools may be separate units independent of schools or part of a primary school. They provide free education for children under five years of age.

Children in care

Prior to January 1971 responsibility for the child care services rested with the Home Secretary. After that date responsibility was transferred to the Social Services Department. The Home Secretary is, however, still responsible for the functions of the courts, the police and the probation and after-care service in relation to children and the law in these matters, and for adoption.

The Local Authority Social Services Act 1970 requires that each local authority should appoint a Social Services Committee and a Director of Social Services who will be responsible for the local authority's personal social services including child care.

The Director will have a duty to look after the interests of children in the following categories.

a Children received into the care of the local authority because they have no parents or guardians, or because their parents or guardians are unable to look after them properly or have abandoned them.

b Children and young persons who appear before a court in either care or criminal proceedings.

c Children placed by a court in the care of the local authority in connection with matrimonial proceedings.

d Children who have been placed in foster homes or who have been placed privately for adoption.

PROVISION OF ACCOMMODATION

Reception centres are short-stay centres where children are assessed for the next move. The next stage may be a home under charge of parent or guardian, a children's home or a home for the very young, a residential nursery or fostering (see p. 431).

PLACE OF SAFETY ORDER

This is an interim care order lasting for twenty-eight days and awarded by a Juvenile or Magistrates Court.

SUPERVISION ORDER

This order, which may last for one to three years, does not have the same legal power as a care order.

CARE ORDER

This is made if a child is committed to care and lasts until the child is eighteen years old or for a minimum of three years. This order can be revoked by the parents or a social worker through the courts.

Fostering

Foster is an old English word for food and is used as an adjective to indicate a relationship in which nursing or bringing up, i.e. provision of food, replaces a blood relationship.

A foster child is a child or young person who is in the care of a local authority or voluntary organisation and who is boarded out with foster parents.

Foster parents are a husband and wife or a woman, with whom a foster child is boarded out. They are registered with the Social Services Department of the local authority. References are required and a check made with the police and health department before registration is granted. The age of the foster parents depends on the ability and personality of the person involved, and the number of children they are permitted to foster on the size of the house.

Foster parents receive an allowance according to the age of the child. The money is to cover general maintenance and pocket money and is paid for from the rates. Extra money is paid to help with holidays or a difficult child.

In the case of fostering, parental rights are retained by the parents if the fostering is voluntary, or transferred to the social worker in the case of a court order or a Social Work Committee if the child has been abandoned and all efforts to trace the child's parents have failed.

Fostering may be short or long-term depending on the reason for the child being in care. The reasons include: mother or father in hospital and no other relative to care for the child; death of parent or parents; abandoned child; child beyond control, at parents request; child appearing before a court in need of care and attention or beyond parental control; prior to adoption.

Some of the difficulties encountered by foster parents and children were overcome by the provisions of the Children Act 1975.

Section 26 offers new safeguards for children who have been in care for longer than six months. Parents may then be required to give twenty-eight days notice of their intention to remove a child. This is intended to protect the child against an abrupt move, and to give everyone time to prepare for the child's return home.

Section 57 sets out new grounds for local authority assumption of parental rights and duties. Where the child has been in the care of the local authority, or partly in the care of a voluntary organisation for three years or more, the local authority may then pass a resolution assuming parental rights and duties on that ground alone. Parents will be given a new right of appeal to a court against such resolutions.

Section 29 deals with restriction on removal of a child pending adoption. People who have looked after a child for five years will be able to start adoption procedures in the knowledge that the child cannot be removed from them before a court hearing without leave of the court. Unlike previous arrangements, this applies whether or not the parents agree to the adoption.

Sections 64 and 65 cover separate representation for children in some court proceedings. Where children or young persons are the subject of unopposed proceedings for the variation or discharge of care or supervision orders, the court may order that their parents shall not represent them or act on their behalf, and may appoint a guardian *ad litem* to safeguard the interests of the child or young person.

In 1983–84 further sections of the Children Act 1975 were introduced and new legislation and regulations affecting children in care and adoption have become effective.

The Child Care Act 1980 states that notice is to be given to a parent when it is proposed to terminate or refuse access to a child in care. The parent may then apply to the juvenile court for an access order. The Act also includes amendments of the law relating to contributions in respect of chidren in care.

Under the Act local authorities are required to serve notice in every case on the person whose rights and duties have been assumed, whether or not they have consented to the action. A guardian *ad litem* may be appointed if court proceedings result because a parent objects.

The Magistrate Courts (Adoption) Rules 1984 includes new rules for adoption proceedings relating to the new roles and duties of Reporting Officers and Guardians *ad litem*, and specific procedure for making applications for freeing and adoption orders, including the documentation which will be required.

Courts will have a new power to appoint a guardian *ad litem* to safeguard the interests of the child in a wide range of proceedings, e.g. care proceedings, applications for variation or discharge of a supervision or care order, parental rights resolution proceedings and access proceedings.

There will be changes in the role of the guardian *ad litem* in adoption proceedings and a new role of Reporting Officer will be introduced.

Parental agreement to adoption will no longer be submitted to the court with the application. The application will indicate whether the parents are willing to agree, but it will be for the Reporting Officer to visit parents who are in agreement and witness their agreement after the application has been placed. Where either or both parents are not in agreement, a guardian *ad litem* will be appointed to investigate the situation.

Sections 14, 15, 16 and 23 of the Children Act 1975, provide for an adoption agency to make an early application to a court to free a child for adoption, either where parents are agreeing to the adoption and it is in their and the child's interest to deal with the matter at an earlier stage than the adoption hearing, or where both parents are opposed to an adoption plan, and there appear to be grounds for asking for the court to dispense with the parent(s) agreement and free the child for adoption.

Section 20 of the Act requires panels for Guardians *ad litem* and Reporting Officers to be established which will be administered by local authorities.

Section 22 deals with the responsibility of the agency placing a child for adoption to provide a report to the court on the background to the placement. In cases where the parent(s) has given consent there may be no other report, since a guardian *ad litem* may well not be appointed. Section 18 requires the local authority to provide a similar report in non-agency cases.

In the case of a baby being placed for adoption, the mother's consent is only valid after the infant is six weeks old. The consent may be unconditional or subject to conditions with respect to religion.

Section 18 requires that only applicants wishing to adopt a child not placed by an adoption agency need notify their local authority of their intention. It is this notice which makes the child a 'protected child' and gives the local authority responsibility for supervising the child's wellbeing while the adoption is pending. For all adoption agency placements, it will be the placing agency's responsibility to monitor the child's wellbeing and carry out welfare supervision.

Section 9 of the Act requires that in non-agency placements, except where the applicant is a parent, step-parent or close relative, the child must be at least twelve months old and must have lived with the applicants (or one of them) throughout the preceding twelve months before an adoption order can be made. The only exception is where the placement is in response to a High Court Order.

In agency placements the requirement remains the same, that the infant has been continuously in the care and possession of the applicant for at least three consecutive months immediately preceding the date of the adoption order and not counting any time before the infant was six weeks old.

Section 19 provides for an Interim Order to be made giving legal custody of the child to the applicants for up to two years, where the placement was not made by an adoption agency.

Section 25 of the Act deals with prospective adopters not domiciled in the United Kingdom. The provisional adoption orders are replaced by orders authorising the adopters to take the child from the country for adoption in their country of domicile.

The Adoption Agencies Regulations 1983 include extensive changes to the way in which adoption agencies must operate, including detailed requirements on the information to be collected about the child, natural parents and prospective parents, and on the way which decisions about adoption must be made.

The Regulations make specific requirements about medical aspects associated with adoption. Adoption agencies have a statutory duty to nominate at least one registered medical practitioner to be the agency's medical adviser, who must be suitably qualified and carry out his functions personally. The medical adviser must have knowledge in paediatrics and general medicine or access to specialist advice. Some local authorities use specialists in those fields; other agencies may nominate a general practitioner with special interests in paediatrics or a specialist in community health. If more than one doctor is involved, good liaison is necessary and one of the advisers should be appointed as co-ordinator. Agencies which care for emotionally disturbed children should have access to a child psychiatrist.

The new Regulations require that the medical adviser (or one of them) must be a member of the Adoption Panel. The Panels have a maximum membership of ten; other people, for example, a psychiatrist or specialist medical practitioner may be invited to attend a particular meeting. Some agencies have joint adoption and fostering panels.

Medical information is obtained about the child. The neonatal report should include the results of any screening tests and the agency must arrange and obtain written reports on 'such other screening procedures or tests on the child and, so far as is reasonably practicable, his parents, as are recommended by the adoption agency's medical adviser'.

Medical information is also required about the natural parents, including, where possible, the father of an illegitimate child and the prospective parents.

The prospective parents will be responsible for obtaining the medical information and lodging it with the court. The court will then forward it to the local authority, which will request its medical adviser to comment and contribute to the Report to the Court.

Adoption

Adoption is a legal procedure by which an adopter is granted an adoption order by a court of law which creates a legal relationship between himself and the adopted person. The person adopting a child takes the place of and assumes the duties and rights of the child's parents or legal guardian. Persons who may be adopted are unmarried and under eighteen years of age.

APPLICATION FOR ADOPTION

Application for an adoption order may be made by two spouses jointly; the father or mother of a child alone or with his or her spouse; an individual acting alone who may or may not be related to the infant.

An applicant or one of the applicants must be over twenty-five years of age the other twenty-one, unless the parent when no age is specified or a relative by blood or affinity when twenty-one years of age is specified. A sole applicant who is a male may not adopt a female without special permission of the court. The applicant must be resident in the United Kingdom or if not ordinarily resident in the United Kingdom must make the application to a High or County Court and notify the local authority in whose area he is living at the time of the application.

METHODS OF PLACING A CHILD FOR ADOPTION

1 By an adoption agency which may be a Social Services Committee or a Local Authority or a registered adoption society.

2 Directly by parent or legal guardian of a child or mother in the case of an ilegitimate child.

Third party adoption was made illegal in February 1983.

An adoption order can only be made in the High Court, the County Court, Magistrate Court or the Juvenile Court. The welfare of the child is the chief consideration of the Court and every care is taken to ensure that the adoption is in the best interest of the child.

THE PUTATIVE FATHER AND ADOPTION

When an affiliation order has been made against the putative father or he has agreed to pay maintenance, the Adoption Rules require that he be given notice of proceedings to adopt the child. The consent of the father of an illegitimate child is not required, but he may in the cases indicated above, appear before the court and state his reasons for objecting to the order.

AFFILIATION ORDER

An application for an affiliation order is made to the Magistrates Court in the area where she normally resides, by a single woman, including a widow or divorced woman or a woman separated and living apart from her husband. The order is made against the putative father for the payment of an appropriate weekly amount and must be made within three years of the child's birth. It continues if the mother marries or adopts her own child but ceases if the child is adopted by persons other than the mother.

ADOPTION CERTIFICATE

The adopted child's new name is entered on the Adopted Children Register which is kept by the Registrar General. A certified copy of the entry, an adoption certificate, replaces the birth certificate. A shortened form of the certificate can be obtained, which is indistinguishable from the short birth certificate.

At the age of eighteen, adopted people are now allowed to obtain a copy of their original birth certificate from the Registrar General by completing an application form obtainable from the General Register Office, Titchfield, Fareham, Hampshire.

A counselling scheme has been introduced to provide assistance and safeguards. An interview is arranged with a counsellor who is a trained social worker, either in London or at a local authority social services department. The counsellor will have information from the adopted person's birth record and can give advice on how to obtain a copy of the actual birth certificate and about other possible sources of information such as the adoption agency that placed them. Efforts to trace birth parents should only be made after careful consideration about the implication of making further enquiries about their background, what this might mean to their adoptive parents, to their natural parents and also to themselves.

Legal adoption was first introduced in 1926 and legislation is now primarily governed by the Adoption Act 1958 and the rules and regulations relevant to the Act. The law regarding the right of adopted adults to obtain a copy of the original birth certificate and also the name of the adoption agency which placed them has been changed by the Children Act 1975.

Useful addresses

The Association of British Adoption and Fostering Agencies, 4 Southampton Row, London WC1.
The Adopted Children's Register, Titchfield, Fareham, Hampshire.
Parent to Parent Information on Adoption Services, 26 Belsize Grove, London NW3. (An informal self-help organisation which works through local groups.)

The handicapped

Approximately 5% of children are born with some degree of mental handicap and about 50% of these have Down's syndrome (see p. 390). Mental illness is rare in childhood but schizophrenia and autism may be present.

Down's syndrome (see p. 390)

Autism

Approximately 2 in 10000 of the child population suffer from the typical syndrome described by Kanner in 1943, and a similar number have characteristics sufficiently marked for them to be included as autistic. Autism can be described as a disorder of effective contact characterised by an inability to develop relationships with people, a delay in speech acquisition, non-communicative use of speech, repetitive manneristic behaviour with distress at change, a good rote memory, and a normal physical appearance.

Diagnosis is made on three special characteristics.

1 A profound and general failure to develop social relationships with a tendency to self-isolation, avoidance of direct eye to eye gaze, and limited attachment to and differentiation of significant adults.

2 Retardation of language development, with impairment of comprehension, echoing of what is heard and reversals of pronouns (calling himself you, and not I).

3 Ritualistic and compulsive phenomena, repetitive play with unusual objects in unusual ways.

Other characteristics not exclusive to autism include: stereotyped repetitive movements of the fingers, hands or the whole body; flicking, spinning or twirling; short attention span; hyperactive behaviour; self injury; feeding difficulties; delayed bladder or bowel control.

Intellectual abilities range from the severely subnormal to the normal, skills often being uneven with better non-verbal skills.

Autism arises in the first year of life and the early onset with the absence of symptoms such as hallucinations or delusional thinking distinguishes it from psychosis of later onset. The family tend to be in a higher social class in contrast to most child psychiatric disorders.

Current research indicates that infantile autism may be the behavioural expression of a wide variety of biological, developmental and psychosocial influences. Psychoanalytic work has indicated that autistic children seem to keep painful, primitive emotional feelings in control by their intense compulsive, obsessional behaviour, maintaining control of a threatening environment as they experience it and feel it. In conjunction with language difficulties such an attitude may distress and discourage parents whose 'appropriate' approaches are ignored. Parents may respond with anger and rejection or with helplessness and withdrawal.

Early intervention is needed to help parents communicate with and maintain contact with their child. Treatment is based on the child's home or a day centre with several techniques to help the parents foster development in all directions. Inpatient management of mother and child may be helpful both diagnostically and to cope with symptoms such as severe feeding difficulties, supporting the mother in facing the autistic child's controls and distancing techniques, and helping her to come close to him.

School-age children appear to benefit most educationally from a structured approach emphasising skills, but there should be small numbers of children with one to one contact of child and teacher if possible. One of the more important prognostic factors seems to be the basic intellectual ability of the child and the schooling he has received. In later adolescence social withdrawal often lessens but language remains impaired.

Useful addresses

Organisations offering advice and support to one-parent families:
Cruse (for the widowed), 126 Sheen Road, Richmond, Surrey.
Gingerbread (self-help groups of one-parent families), Head Office, 35 Wellington Street, London WC2.
National Council for the Divorced and Separated, 13 High Street, Little Shelford, Cambridge.
National Council for One-Parent Families, 255 Kentish Town Road, London NW5.

An organisation offering help to parents with handicapped children is The Joseph Rowntree Memorial Trust, Beverely House, Skipton, Yorkshire. The Trust was set up in 1973 to help the parents of severely congenitally handicapped children under sixteen years of age.

Social security

The Ministry of Social Security and the Ministry of Health were merged in November 1968 to form the Department of Health and Social Security. Local administration of the Social Security Services is the responsibility of the Department's regional and local offices. The services comprise National Insurance Benefits, War Pensions and War Pensioner Welfare, Family Income Supplements, Child Benefits, Attendance Allowances and Industrial Injuries Benefits. The Supplementary Benefits Commission is responsible for the award of supplementary allowances to people under pension age and supplementary pensions for those over pension age, for determining the right to and the amount of family income supplement and for determining the means of a person applying for legal aid.

The following are benefits and allowances of particular interest to the midwife.

Maternity benefits

There are a number of monetary benefits provided for expectant and new mothers, and it is important that the midwife is conversant with these so that she can advise the woman about her entitlements. However, because expectant mothers and their families do not conform to one pattern, there may be considerable variations and the Babies and Benefits Form FB8 gives information about leaflets that cover a variety of circumstances.

Maternity Allowance

This is a weekly allowance that is intended to encourage women to give up work. The allowance is in addition to the Maternity Grant and is payable on the woman's National Insurance contributions. It is usually paid for eighteen weeks; eleven weeks before the expected date of confinement, the week of confinement and the following six weeks. If the pregnancy is prolonged the woman can apply for extra allowance using form BM9. This is given with the first payment of the allowance or can be obtained from a Social Security office. If the woman has not paid enough contributions to claim the full allowance she may be entitled to claim a proportion of it. It cannot be claimed for any period in which the woman is employed, and if the woman is in receipt of maternity pay the allowance is deducted from it, whether or not the woman is entitled to claim the allowance (see p. 409).

The allowance should be claimed not earlier than fourteen weeks nor later than eleven weeks before the week in which the confinement is expected, using form BM4 signed by a midwife or doctor. The current weekly rate for the Maternity Allowance is £27.95 but in certain circumstances the amount may be increased, e.g. if the woman has dependants living with her. If the baby dies, the Maternity Allowance is paid provided the pregnancy has lasted at least twenty-eight weeks.

The woman is provided with a book of orders which she can cash at a Post Office.

Maternity Grant

The Maternity Grant is a non-contributory benefit of £25.00 paid by Giro cheque which can be cashed at a Post Office. It can be claimed from the fourteenth week before the expected week of confinement and up to the end of a period of three months beginning with the date of confinement using form BM4 signed by a midwife or docotor. In the case of multiple births, a grant may be paid for each additional baby who lives for twelve hours or more. The grant is paid if the baby is stillborn.

The Maternity Grant is not deducted from maternity pay nor from a weekly Supplementary Benefit.

Maternity Pay

Paid maternity leave was introduced with the implementation of the Employment Act 1975 (see p. 409). It is paid by the employer at a rate of 90% of the basic pay minus the flat rate maternity allowance. A woman has the right to six weeks' maternity pay if she satisfies certain conditions (see p. 408).

Full details of these benefits are given in a leaflet NI 17A.

Family benefits

CHILD BENEFIT

This benefit replaced the family allowance and the child interim benefit in April 1977. The child benefit is non-contributory, a tax-free cash payment made to anyone, regardless of income, who is responsible for a child under sixteen years of age or under nineteen if still in non-advanced, fulltime education. The weekly rate of the child benefit is £6.85 and is paid by a book of orders cashed at a Post Office.

ONE PARENT BENEFIT

The one parent benefit is paid in addition to the child benefit for lone parents. The benefit is £4.25 a week for the first or only child.

CHILD'S SPECIAL ALLOWANCE

The child's special allowance is a weekly cash payment made to a woman whose marriage has been dissolved or annulled if, at the time of death of her former husband, he was or should have been helping to support one or more of her children. The amount is £7.65 a week for each child.

FAMILY INCOME SUPPLEMENT

This is payable to families whose gross weekly income is less than amounts prescribed by Parliament. The prescribed amount is £85.50 for a family with one child, plus £9.50 for each additional child. Anyone, including a single person, with at least one dependant child can claim, if he or she is in full-time employment, i.e. thirty or more hours a week, or twenty-four hours or more for a single parent. All children who are normally living with the claimant can be included if they are under sixteen or under nineteen and still at school. The amount of the supplement is one-half of the difference between a family's normal gross income and the appropriate prescribed amount. People awarded family income supplement are also entitled to free prescriptions, dental treatment and glasses under the National Health Service, free milk and vitamins for expectant mothers and children under school age, free school meals for children at school and refund of fares for members of the family attending hospital for treatment. The Family Income Supplement is tax-free and is paid by a book of orders which are issued yearly and cashed at a Post Office.

ATTENDANCE ALLOWANCE

This is a tax-free allowance for adults and children over the age of two who are severely disabled either physically or mentally and have required a lot of care for at least six months. The medical requirements are that the person must be so severely disabled physically or mentally that he requires, from another person, frequent attention throughout the day in connection with his bodily functions; or continual supervision throughout the day in order to avoid substantial danger to himself or others; prolonged or repeated attention during the night in connection with his bodily functions; or continual supervision throughout the night in order to avoid substantial danger to himself or others. There are two rates of allowance, the higher rate of £28.60 per week is payable if one of the day requirements and one of the night requirements are satisfied for a period of at least six months. The lower rate of £19.10 per week is payable if one of the four medical requirements are satisfied for a period of at least six months. Claim forms and explanatory leaflets are obtainable from local Social Security offices.

SUPPLEMENTARY BENEFIT

The purpose of supplementary benefit is to provide income on a non-contributory basis for people who are not in full-time work and whose income (if any), whether from benefits or from other sources, is not enough to meet their requirements.

FREE MILK AND VITAMINS

Expectant and nursing mothers and children under school age in families on Family Income Supplement or supplementary benefit get free milk and vitamins automatically, and may get them if on a low income.

Some local education authorities provide free milk to all pupils up to eleven years of age, others for those up to seven. Some provide free milk only to pupils in special schools or where there is a medical need.

Children aged from five up to sixteen years of age who are handicapped or disabled and who do not go to school can get seven pints of milk a week free.

Playgroup organisers and approved childminders can receive one-third of a pint of milk each day the child attends for children up to the age of five who have been in their care for one month.

FREE PRESCRIPTIONS

Expectant mothers and women who have had a baby within the last twelve months, children under sixteen years of age and families in receipt of Family Income Supplement or supplementary benefit are entitled to free prescriptions.

FREE DENTAL TREATMENT

Expectant mothers and women who have had a baby within the last twelve months, children under sixteen, young people under nineteen and still in fulltime education and families in receipt of Family Income Supplement, supplementary benefit or of low income are entitled to receive free dental treatment including dentures.

Young people under eighteen who are not in fulltime education can get free dental treatment but not dentures.

FREE GLASSES

Children under sixteen, young people under nineteen and still in fulltime education and families in receipt of Family Income Supplement, supplementary benefit or of low income can get free glasses.

VOLUNTARY ORGANISATIONS

Many of the existing health services have their origins in the work of voluntary organisations. The term 'voluntary organisation' refers to non-profit-making organisations which are not created by statute. The majority of organisations in the health and social services are registered under the Charities Act 1960. The voluntary organisations supplement the services provided by the health and social services and their contribution is in many cases considerable. Their income is derived from donations, fund-raising activities, legacies and government grants, and in the case of some larger charities from their capital assets.

Voluntary organisations (of interest to midwives)

The Association for Postnatal Illness, 7 Gowan Avenue, London SW6.
Cruse The National Organisation for the Widowed and their Children, 126 Sheen Road, Richmond, Surrey TW9 1UR.
Foresight—The association for the promotion of pre-conceptial care, Woodhurst, Hydestile, Godalming, Surrey GU8 4AY.
Family Services Units, 207 Old Marylebone Road, London NW1.
The Family Planning Association, 27–35 Mortimer Street, London W1.
The Foundation for the Study of Sudden Infant Death (or deaths), 5th Floor, 4 Grosvenor Place, London SW1.
Gingerbread, Head Office—9 Poland Street, London W1 (self-help groups of one-parent families).
The Health Education Council, 78 New Oxford Street, London WC1.
The National Adoption Society, Hoopers Cottage, Kimberly Road, London NW6.
The National Association of Citizen's Advice Bureaux.
The National Association for Maternal and Child Welfare, Tavistock House North, Tavistock Square, London WC1.

The National Association for Mental Health (MIND), 22 Harley Street, London W1.
National Childbirth Trust, 9 Queensborough Terrace, London W2 3TB.
The National Council for One-Parent Families, 255 Kentish Town Road, London NW5.
The National Society for Phenylketonuria and Allied Disorders, 26 Towngate Grove, Mirfield, West Yorkshire.
The National Society for the Prevention of Cruelty to Children, 1–3 Riding House Street, London W1.
Parent to Parent. Information on Adoption Services, 26 Belsize Grove, London NW3. (An informal self-help organisation which works through local groups.)
Royal Society for Mentally Handicapped Children and Adults, 123 Golden Lane, London EC1.
The Spastics Society, 12 Park Crescent, London W1.
The Stillbirth and Perinatal Death Association, 15A Christchurch Hill, London NW8 1JY.

ACTS OF PARLIAMENT

Abortion Act 1967.
Adoption Acts 1958 and 1960.
Children (or Children and Young Persons) Acts 1908–1975.
Education (Handicapped Children) Act 1970.
Family Allowances Acts 1944–1959.
Health Services and Public Health Act 1968.
Local Authority Social Service Act 1970.
Local Government Act 1972.
Mental Health Act 1959.
Midwives Act 1902–1951.
Misuse of Drugs Act 1971.
Misuse of Drugs Regulation 1973.
National Assistance Act 1948.
National Health Service Act 1946.
National Health Service (Family Planning) Act 1967.
National Health Service (Family Planning Amendment) Act 1972.
National Health Service Reorganisation Act 1973.
National Insurance Acts 1946 and 1953.
Notification of Births 1907 and 1915 (later included in the Public Health Act and amended by National Health Services Act 1946).
Nurseries and Child-minders Regulations Act 1958.
Public Health Acts 1848–1961.
Registration of Births and Deaths Acts 1874 and 1936.
Social Services Act 1970.

VITAL STATISTICS

Statistics are numerical facts collected systematically. Facts about the population which concern their health and the incidence of disease are collected together for the purpose of comparison and research, and with the object of improving health and eliminating disease. The facts are expressed in figures which are given in rates per thousand of the population or a particular group concerned.

The vital statistics that are of interest and importance to the midwife are those relating to birth, and to deaths associated with childbearing.

Birth rate

The birth rate, i.e. live birth rate, is the number of registered live births per 1000 of population (Table 13.3), i.e.

$$\text{Birth rate} = \frac{\text{Number of registered live births} \times 1000}{\text{Population}}$$

A live birth is defined as follows: an infant born at any stage of pregnancy who breathes or shows other signs of life after complete expulsion from its mother is born alive.

Table 13.3 Births: England and Wales

Year	*Total births*	*Live births*	*Live birth rate*	*Illegitimate live births as percentage of all live births*
1977	574664	569259	11.6	9.7
1978	601573	596461	12.1	10.2
1979	643153	638028	13.0	10.9
1980	661007	656234	13.3	11.8
1981	638659	634456	12.9	12.8
1982	629870	625931	12.6	14.4

The 574664 births in England and Wales in 1977 was the lowest since records began. This fall was followed by an increase in each of the following three years. This upward trend was reversed in 1981, since then there has been a gradual reduction.

During the same period it will be noted that the percentage of illegitimate live births has increased from 9.7 to 14.4%.

Notification of birth

The Public Health Act 1936 requires that all births must be notified in writing: to the District Medical Officer; by any person in attendance upon the mother at the time of, or within six hours of the birth; within thirty-six hours of birth.

The purpose of the notification is to provide a means of alerting those responsible for the subsequent care of the mother and child and also to provide the basis of various health records used by the District Health Authority to ensure periodical recall for screening, vaccination and immunisation. Information from notifications can also be used for statistical and epidemiological purposes.

The following information is included in the notification.

1 Surname.
2 Mother's full name, date of birth and, if known, National Health Service number.
3 Mother's usual address, and if different, the address to which she will proceed immediately after discharge from hospital.
4 Date, time and place of birth.
5 Live or stillbirth.
6 Single or multiple birth.
7 Period of gestation.
8 Mother's previous pregnancies.
  a Live births.
  b Stillbirths.
  c Miscarriages.
9 Sex of baby.
10 Birth weight.
11 Nature of any congenital abnormality observed at birth.
12 Name and address of mother's general practitioner.

Registration of birth

The Registration of Births and Deaths Registration Act 1953 requires all births to be registered with the Registrar of Births and Deaths for the district in which the birth occurs; by the parent or any person in attendance at the birth; within forty-two days of birth.

District Health Authorities arrange for particulars of Registration of Births to be checked against the notifications to ensure that all births registered have been notified. If notification has been omitted, the District Health Authority should investigate and remind the person who attend at the birth of the statutory obligation to notify.

The District Medical Officers send Registrars particulars of notifications of births so that the information supplied to the Registrar can be checked to ensure the registration of all births. The following information is passed on to the Registrar:

1 Date, time and place of birth.
2 Live or stillbirth.
3 Full name of mother.
4 Mother's postal address.
5 Sex of baby.
6 Birth weight. This is to enable the Office of Population Census and Surveys to produce national and local statistics on the incidence of low birth weight, and on the relationship between birth weight and infant mortality.

Certification of birth

A certificate of birth is issued at the time of registration by the Registrar. A short certificate which gives the full name and sex of child and the date and place of birth is issued free. A full certificate which includes details of parentage is issued on payment of a small fee. An illegitimate child is registered by the mother. The father's name can only be entered on the birth certificate if he accompanies her and gives his consent or on production of an order made under the Affiliation Proceedings Act 1957, without his consent being required.

Stillbirth rate

An infant who has issued forth from its mother after the twenty-eighth week of pregnancy and has not at any time after being completely expelled from its mother breathed or shown any sign of life is a stillborn infant.

$$\text{Stillbirth rate} = \frac{\text{Number of registered stillbirths} \times 1000}{\text{Registered total (live and still) births}}$$

Table 13.4 Stillbirths: England and Wales

Year	*Stillbirths*	*Stillbirth rate*
1977	5405	9.4
1978	5112	8.5
1979	5125	8.0
1980	4773	7.2
1981	4203	6.6
1982	3939	6.3

There has been a decrease in the number of stillbirths and in the stillbirth rate during the period under review. The largest numerical fall was in 1981 when there were 570 fewer babies stillborn. In percentage terms the largest fall (0.9) was between 1977 and 1978, with a marginally smaller decrease (0.8) between 1979 and 1980.

Stillbirths continue to constitute the larger percentage of perinatal deaths (see below), and with the exception of 1978 when it was 52.4% it has remained approximately 55%.

Causes

1 Intrauterine anoxia.
2 Congenital abnormalities.

Predisposing causes

1 Pre-eclampsia and eclampsia.
2 Antepartum haemorrhage.
3 Multiple pregnancy.

Notification of stillbirth

The notification of a stillbirth is as for a live birth (see p. 445).

Midwife's responsibility. The midwife is required by the United Kingdom Central Council to send to her Local Supervising Authority a notification that a stillbirth has occurred in her practice. A statutory form is supplied for this purpose. The midwife undertakes the care of the woman for a minimum of ten days following the birth and offers support and assistance to the family as a whole.

Certification of stillbirth

A certificate of stillbirth is signed either by a registered medical practitioner or by a certified midwife who was present at birth or examined the body. If there is doubt that the infant was stillborn the Coroners' Office is informed. The Coroner may order an enquiry or inquest and is responsible for completing the certificate.

Registration of stillbirth

Stillbirths have been registered in England and Wales since 1927 when the rate was approximately forty per 1000 births. The stillbirth is registered with the local Registrar, usually within a few days. The Registrar issues a certificate of burial/cremation, without which the body may not be buried, unless on a Coroner's order. This is taken to the undertaker and cremation or interment in a burial ground is arranged.

No death grant is payable in the case of a stillborn infant but the hospital or District Health Authority in the case of a home confinement are required by the Department of Health and Social Security to meet the cost of the burial.

Stillbirths are included in perinatal deaths which are discussed below.

Perinatal mortality rate

The perinatal mortality rate is the number of stillbirths and deaths in the first week of life per 1000 registered total births, i.e.

$$\text{Perinatal mortality rate} = \frac{\text{Number of stillbirths and deaths under one week} \times 1000}{\text{Registered total births}}$$

Stillbirths form the larger proportion of perinatal deaths (see above). The deaths occurring in the first week of life are referred to as early neonatal deaths which are also included in the neonatal mortality rate.

Table 13.5 Perinatal mortality: England and Wales

Year	*Perinatal deaths*	*Perinatal mortality rate*
1977	9757	17.0
1978	9353	15.5
1979	9432	14.7
1980	8807	13.3
1981	7557	11.8
1982	7087	11.3

There was a sharp fall in perinatal deaths in England and Wales from 8815 in 1980 to 7557 in 1981 with a further fall in 1982. The fall in the perinatal mortality rate from 13.3 per 1000 registered total births in 1980 to 11.8 per 1000 in 1981 was the largest percentage fall in this rate since perinatal mortality statistics first became available in 1928. However, although the fall in the perinatal mortality rate was general, there are still considerable regional variations with the rate ranging between 7 and 17 per 1000 registered total deaths.

Causes

1 Congenital malformations.
2 Fetal anoxia and asphyxia neonatorum.
3 Immaturity.
4 Birth trauma.

The three principal causes of perinatal mortality account for between 70 and 80% of all perinatal deaths and affect the infant mortality figures more than anything else that happens in the first year of life.

Predisposing causes

1 Hypertension, pre-eclampsia and eclampsia.
2 Threatened abortion and antepartum haemorrhage.
3 Multiple pregnancy.
4 Breech presentation and delivery.
5 Maternal age, parity and social class.
6 Intrauterine infections, i.e. rubella.
7 Rhesus haemolytic disease.
8 Maternal disease, i.e. diabetes mellitus.
9 Teratogenic drugs.

Perinatal Surveys undertaken in 1958 and 1970 have contributed to knowledge of perinatal deaths and identified measures which should be taken to reduce perinatal mortality, namely:
1 Improved standard of antenatal care.
   a Early booking.
   b Selection of place for antenatal care and confinement.
   c Frequent and thorough supervision leading to early detection and treatment of disorders such as pre-eclampsia.
   d Follow-up of 'defaulters'.
   e Identification of high risk groups and more frequent and specialised supervision.
   f Advice regarding diet, smoking, alcohol and drugs.
2 The recognition of intrapartum hypoxia and active resuscitation of an asphyxiated infant.
3 Special care of low birth weight babies.
4 Prevention of Rhesus haemolytic disease.

Neonatal mortality rate

The neonatal mortality rate is the number of deaths within four weeks of birth per 1000 registered live births, i.e.

$$\text{Neonatal mortality rate} = \frac{\text{Number of deaths within four weeks} \times 1000}{\text{Number of registered live births}}$$

Deaths in the first week of life, early neonatal deaths, are also included in the perinatal mortality rate. The majority of neonatal deaths occur on the first day of life and are equivalent to those in the next fifteen years; deaths in the first month of life are equivalent to those in the next thirty years.

Table 13.6 Neonatal mortality: England and Wales

Year	*under 4 weeks*	*Neonatal deaths under 1 week*		*under 24 hours*		*Neonatal mortality rate*
1977	5278	4352	7.6	2381	4.2	9.3
1978	5185	4241	7.1	2226	3.7	8.7
1979	5253	4307	6.8	2354	3.7	8.2
1980	5018	4034	6.1	2206	3.4	7.6
1981	4224	3354	5.3	1871	2.9	6.7
1982	3925	3148	5.0	1768	2.8	6.3

The causes and predisposing causes of, and the reasons for the reduction in neonatal mortality are closely related to perinatal deaths. In addition improvement in paediatric surgery and improved techniques for sterilisation of feeding equipment have contributed to the falling rate.

Infant mortality rate

The infant mortality rate is the number of deaths of infants under one year per 1000 registered live births, i.e.

$$\text{Infant mortality rate} = \frac{\text{Number of deaths of infants under one year} \times 1000}{\text{Number of registered live births in the year}}$$

Table 13.7 Infant mortality: England and Wales

Year	*Infant deaths*	*Infant mortality rate*
1977	7841	13.8
1978	7454	13.2
1979	8161	12.8
1980	7883	12.0
1981	7019	11.1
1982	6775	10.8

The infant mortality rate for England and Wales fell in 1981 and the decrease was in percentage terms the largest fall for a single year since 1975/6. However, although this fall was reflected in more than two thirds of all areas, there was considerable national variations.

There was a marked increase in the number of infant deaths in 1979 (707), and it was not until 1981 when there was an even greater decrease (864) that the number of infant deaths fell below that of 1978.

Deaths within four weeks of birth, neonatal deaths, are included in infant mortality and in 1982 accounted for 45.6% of the total. Therefore the causes and predisposing causes and the reasons for the reduction in infant mortality are closely related to neonatal deaths.

Other causes of infant deaths include:

1 Infections—gastroenteritis and respiratory tract infections such as pneumonia and bronchitis.

2 Accidental suffocation.

3 Accidents in the home.

Measures which have reduced infant mortality from 140 per 1000 live births in 1900 include:

1 Vaccination and immunisation.

2 Improved social conditions, i.e. housing and sanitation.

3 Improved techniques for sterilisation of feeding equipment.

4 Improvement in artificial milk preparations.

5 A pure milk supply.

Today we are concerned not simply with survival but with the quality of health in those who survive, and the following facts show that there is no room for complacency:

1 Of all infants, 2% have substantial malformation evident at birth or in pre-school years.

a 5% suffer from mental handicap.

b 3% suffer from retarded growth.

c 0.3% suffer from blindness, deafness and cerebral palsy (1500 babies a year).

2 One-third of all children born with mental subnormality have Down's syndrome.

3 One in 400 are paralysed with spina bifida.

The most promising strategy for conquering these disorders is to try and prevent them occurring in the first place by prenatal diagnosis and selective abortion (see p. 473).

Statistics relating to childbearing are influenced by many factors but in particular by the marital status, age, parity and social class of the mother.

The tables overleaf show how these factors affected the statistics in 1980.

The breakdown of the 1980 statistics as they relate to the marital status, age, parity and social class of the mother reveal the following:

1 In percentage terms, the baby of an unmarried mother is at greater risk in all categories but in particular in relation to perinatal and infant deaths.

2 The optimum age to have a baby is between twenty-five and thirty-four years with a highest percentage of stillbirths occurring in women over

Table 13.8 Vital statistics by marital status of mother 1980

		Total	*Legitimate*	*Illegitimate*
Stillbirths	Number	4773	4007	696
	*Rate	7.2	7.0	8.9
Perinatal	Number	8796	7480	1316
deaths	*Rate	13.3	12.8	16.9
Neonatal	Number	4987	4233	754
deaths	**Rate	7.6	7.3	9.7
Infant	Number	7790	6499	1291
deaths	**Rate	11.9	11.2	16.7
Live births		656234	578862	77372
Total births		661007	582939	78068

* Per 1000 Total births.
** Per 1000 Live births.

Table 13.9 Vital statistics by age of mother 1980

Age		Under 16	16–19	20–24	25–29	30–34	35+
Stillbirths	Number	8	500	1387	1460	953	463
	*Rate	6.2	8.3	6.8	6.5	7.3	11.3
Perinatal	Number	24	991	2698	2700	1655	728
deaths	*Rate	18.6	16.5	13.3	12.0	12.6	17.7
Neonatal	Number	18	600	1625	1546	874	324
deaths	**Rate	14.1	10.1	8.1	6.9	6.7	8.0
Infant	Number	24	1042	2612	2361	1283	468
deaths	**Rate	18.7	17.5	13.0	10.6	9.9	11.5

* Per 1000 Total births.
** Per 1000 Live births.

Table 13.10 Vital statistics by parity of mother 1980

Parity		0	1	2	3	4+
Stillbirths	Number	1856	1130	627	267	197
	*Rate	7.7	5.4	7.1	9.3	12.4
Perinatal	Number	3384	2168	1155	455	318
deaths	*Rate	14.1	10.4	13.1	15.8	20.0
Neonatal	Number	1889	1313	642	233	156
deaths	**Rate	7.9	6.3	7.3	8.2	9.9
Infant	Number	2564	2241	1064	377	253
deaths	**Rate	10.7	10.8	12.2	13.2	16.1

* Per 1000 Total births.
** Per 1000 Live births.

Table 13.11 Vital statistics by social class of mother

Social Class		I	II	III	IV	V
Stillbirths	Number	204	745	1963	708	313
	*Rate	5.0	6.0	7.1	8.0	9.5
Perinatal	Number	398	1377	3521	1324	560
deaths	*Rate	9.7	11.1	12.8	15.0	17.0
Neonatal	Number	232	787	1933	761	319
deaths	**Rate	5.7	6.4	7.1	8.7	9.8
Infant	Number	364	1171	2893	1185	523
deaths	**Rate	3.9	9.5	10.6	13.5	16.0

* Per 1000 Total births.
** Per 1000 Live births.

thirty-five years of age and perinatal, neonatal and infant deaths occurring where the mother is under sixteen years of age.

3 The second born child is at least risk in all categories except infant deaths where the first born child is marginally less at risk. The differences are most marked in relation to perinatal deaths.

Children who are fifth or more in birth order are at greatest risk in all categories but in particular in relation to perinatal deaths.

4 The lower the social class the greater the risk in all categories but especially in relation to infant mortality where the difference between social class I and social class V is 12.1. The smallest difference in percentage terms (4.1) is seen in relation to neonatal death.

Maternal mortality rate

The maternal mortality rate is the number of maternal deaths associated with pregnancy and child bearing per 1000 registered total births, i.e.:

$$\text{Maternal mortality rate} = \frac{\text{Number of maternal deaths associated with pregnancy and child bearing} \times 1000}{\text{Number of registered total births}}$$

Causes

The causes of death directly ascribed to pregnancy and childbirth for England and Wales in 1976–78 are given in Table 13.13. There were a total of 227 in that period and the details are discussed in the *Report on Confidential Enquiries into Maternal Deaths in England and Wales 1976–78* (HMSO, London).

A maternal death is defined as 'the death of a woman while pregnant or

Table 13.12 Maternal mortality rates: England and Wales

Year	*Number of maternal deaths associated with pregnancy and childbearing per 1000 registered total births*
1977	0.12
1978	0.10
1979	0.10
1980	0.10
1981	0.10
1982	0.10
1983	0.10

Table 13.13 Major causes of maternal deaths: England and Wales 1976–78

Cause of death	*Number of deaths*
Pulmonary embolism	45
Hypertensive diseases of pregnancy	29
Haemorrhage	26
Puerperal sepsis	24
Ectopic pregnancy	21
Abortion	19
Ruptured uterus	14
Amniotic fluid embolism	11
All other causes	38
Total	227

within forty-two days of termination of pregnancy irrespective of duration and the site of the pregnancy, from any cause related to or aggravated by the pregnancy or its management but not from accidental or incidental causes'.

An international system of classification is now used to sub-divide maternal deaths into direct as those resulting from obstetric complications of pregnancy, labour and the puerperium; and indirect as those resulting from previous existing disease, or disease that developed during pregnancy that was not due to obstetric causes. A third sub-division classifies deaths from other causes which 'fortuitously' occur in pregnancy or the puerperium, and are excluded from the maternal mortality rate. The 1976–78 Report made enquiries into 427 deaths: 227 (53%) direct deaths; 97 (23%) indirect deaths; and 103 (24%) fortuitous deaths.

The major causes of maternal death are included under the appropriate section as are deaths due to complications of anaesthesia, diabetes mellitus, cardiac disease, epilepsy, Caesarean section and suicide.

Enquiries into maternal deaths

The causes and circumstances surrounding each maternal death in England and Wales have been studied since 1928 and a triennial report produced since 1952–54.

A report on each maternal death is sent to a regional assessor by the obstetrician concerned, and information is also received from the coroner. The report is commented on by central advisors and the information is then put on to a punch card and analysed by a computer. Death certificates pertaining to obstetrics are sent to the Department of Health and Social Security from St Katherine's House every three months. If no report has been received, the regional assessor is informed and investigates the lack of information.

Seventy-six of the deaths associated with pregnancy were classified as indirect maternal deaths and one hundred and three as fortuitous deaths. In addition, there were twenty-one deaths from cardiac disease (see p. 226) that were also classified as indirect maternal deaths.

Table 13.14 Deaths from miscellaneous causes 1976–78

Cause of death	*Number*
Sudden death of unknown cause in puerperium	6
Sudden death of unknown cause in pregnancy	1
Liver disorders in pregnancy	7
Air embolism	1
Malignant neoplasm of placenta—choriocarcinoma	1
Excessive vomiting in late pregnancy	1
Cerebral anoxia following obstetric surgery—cerebral sinus thrombosis	1
Other complication of delivery—inhalation of gastric contents	1
Venous complication of pregnancy and the puerperium—	1
retroperitoneal haematoma	1
Total	20

Notification, certification and registration of maternal death

Notification of a maternal death is sent by the obstetrician to the Area Medical officer. The midwife must notify her local supervising authority, by means of a statutory form, if a maternal death occurs in her practice.

The certificate of death is completed by the doctor and the death registered with the local Registrar within five days.

The decline in the numbers of maternal deaths from four per 1000 in 1900 has been contributed to by the following measures:

Table 13.15 Associated causes of maternal deaths 1976–78

Cause of death	*Number*
Adrenal disorders	2
Arterial aneurysms	5
Alcoholic disorders	1
Autoimmune diseases—systemic sclerosis	1
Blood diseases	
Sickle cell disease	4
Acute leukaemia	4
Thrombocytopenic purpura	1
Thrombotic thrombocytopenic purpura	1
Cerebral infarction	3
Diabetes mellitus	3
Encephalitis	2
Epilepsy	3
Diseases of gastrointestinal tract	
Diaphragmatic hernia	2
Spontaneous rupture of stomach	1
Gastric ulceration	1
Gastroenteritis	1
Intestinal obstruction	1
Peritonitis	1
Intussusception	1
Volvulus	1
Diseases of colon:	
Crohn's disease	2
Ulcerative colitis	2
Hepatic failure	2
Intracranial haemorrhage	24
Kyphoscoliosis	1
Meningitis	1
Neoplastic diseases	33
Pituitary infarction	1
Respiratory diseases	
Asthma	4
Bronchiectasis	1
Pneumonia	12
Interstitial pulmonary emphysema	1
Renal diseases	
Pyelonephritis	2
Renal failure	2
Septicaemia	2
Sudden death of unknown cause after the puerperium	4
Sudden unnatural deaths	
Suicide	18
Open verdict or misadventure verdict	14
Accidental deaths	6
Road traffic accidents	6
Manslaughter	2
Total	179

1902 Training of midwives.
1915 Introduction of antenatal care.
1932 Introduction of ergometrine.
1935 Sulphonamides introduced.
1942 Penicillin introduced.
1948 National Health Service: provision of complete antenatal care for all pregnant women; emergency obstetric unit; blood transfusion service.

Other factors include: improved antenatal care; active management of the third stage of labour; increase in number of maternity beds; early ambulation; improved social conditions; improved surgical, anaesthetic and laboratory techniques—classification of bacteria and testing sensitivities; improved X-ray facilities.

Further reading

Barber D. (ed.) (1975) One Parent Families, Davis-Poynyer, London.

Butler N.R. & Alberman E.D. (eds) (1969) *Perinatal Problems. The Second Report of the 1958 British Perinatal Mortality Survey*. E & S Livingstone Ltd, Edinburgh.

Chamberlain R., Chamberlain G., Howlett B. & Claireaux A. (1975) *British Births 1970, Volume 1: The First Week of Life*. Heinemann Medical Books Ltd, London.

Ferri E. (1976) *Growing Up in a One-Parent Family*. National Foundation for Educational Research Publishing Company Ltd, Windsor.

Ferri E. & Robinson H. (1976). *Coping Alone*. National Foundation for Educational Research Publishing Company Ltd, Windsor.

Report on Confidential Enquiries into Maternal Deaths in England and Wales 1976–78. HMSO, London.

Jepson M.E. (1983). *Community Child Health*. Hodder and Stoughton.

Keywood O. (1982). *Personal and Community Health*. Blackwell Scientific Publications. Oxford.

Chapter 14
Psychological Aspects in Relation to Childbearing

PSYCHOLOGICAL ASPECTS OF PREGNANCY, LABOUR AND THE POSTNATAL PERIOD

Emotional and behavioural adaptation to pregnancy and parenthood is very complex and individual, and is influenced by the woman's previous experiences and relationships, and is dependent upon her psychological maturity.

Childbearing is a time of profound change not only physically, but also psychologically and emotionally. It is probably the most important experience in a woman's life and challenges her ability for psychological adaptation.

Pregnancy, especially the first, is often associated with a feeling of detachment and introspection, and the woman becomes preoccupied with her pregnancy and her reactions to it. She may experience a feeling of depression and, although this may be related to the complex hormonal and chemical changes, she needs help in understanding these feelings. It is difficult for her to understand these feelings, particularly if this is a planned pregnancy and she is longing for a baby.

There are many causes of psychological stress in pregnancy, including anxiety, which is an integral part of the normal process of adapting to change. The effect of this on the woman will be determined by many factors, including her attitudes and beliefs about childbearing and her social circumstances.

Factors which may cause anxiety and adversely affect the woman's adaption to pregnancy include financial worries. The loss of income when the woman gives up work may cause problems regarding financial commitments. The maternity allowance or maternity pay may help to overcome this problem. Most women are worried about whether the baby will be normal and this is an anxiety they have difficulty in sharing, even with their husband. Women who have had a previous termination of pregnancy may experience a delayed grief reaction or feelings of guilt. They may fear retribution in the form of harm to this baby. Some women may become anxious about their appearance and fear that they will no longer be attractive to their husband.

The woman should be given every opportunity to discuss her anxieties and fears, and the midwife should develop the way of talking to a woman and asking questions that conveys not only a willingness to listen, but also an understanding of her anxieties. The woman looks to the midwife for reassurance and clarification of the problems and appropriate information and advice.

All women have individual expectations and fears concerning childbirth and motherhood, and our care should be planned to help her to meet these expectations and overcome her fears and anxieties. Responses to care will vary from one woman to another, and it is the recognition of the individual needs of the woman that is so important in the provision of care if we are to meet the needs of all women. Some women prefer to let the professionals caring for them to make the decisions and may not want to know why a particular course of action is to be taken. Other women are satisfied with the decisions being made for them, but want an explanation of what is happening, whilst some women expect and even demand to be consulted and for their views to be taken into account.

Many women look forward to labour with fear and trepidation. If this is their first baby, then it is the fear of the unknown, and teaching in preparation for labour may be helpful in explaining the process of labour and the care provided. The pain associated with labour is the cause of most anxiety; the woman may be concerned that she will be unable to cope and will, as she feels, make a fool of herself. It is therefore important that the preparation for labour includes not only adequate information about the methods of pain relief, but also instruction on relaxation, so that the woman can learn to relax and have control over the contractions.

The mental attitude with which a woman approaches labour has an effect on her tolerance of the discomfort or pain that she experiences, and it is also now accepted that a woman's pain threshold is significantly lowered by loneliness and lack of emotional support in labour. Therefore it is important to encourage her to have someone with her during her labour to ensure she is not left on her own. Many husbands now remain with their wives during labour, and it is important to involve them in the preparation classes so that they can be a useful participant in the birth of their baby.

Some women express strong preferences about the conduct of their labour. These preferences may be extremely important to individual pregnant women if the experience of childbirth is to be satisfactory and fulfilling. An individual care plan gives the opportunity to discuss a woman's wishes, and where possible these should be met. The midwife and obstetrician should determine the framework of a safe standard of care while leaving women and their husbands free enough to make their own decisions.

The emphasis placed on natural childbirth can place pressure on some women who cannot or do not want to comply to these ideals, and those women who are unable to meet this often idealised view of childbirth often feel they have failed and have a sense of guilt.

The birth of a first baby is the greatest and most significant change in life style experience. The mother is caught up in unending demands on her time and energy. Women who have adjusted well to their pregnancy and to becoming a mother, and who are in good health and well-rested, are able to cope with this change, but a woman who has not adjusted may resent these demands, may feel neglected now that the attention has been diverted from her to the baby.

If childbirth has not been an emotionally fulfilling experience, then it can have far-reaching effects on the mother's ability to relate to her baby. Studies have indicated that mothers who experience feelings of indifference, detachment or dislike for their babies in the first few days have often had labours that were in some way unsatisfactory. Most frequently the women had had intervention in labour and assessed labour as being painful.

The mother needs help and support in coping with the new routine, but it is important to develop the mother's confidence and self-esteem and to provide advice and support without undermining the mother's confidence in her own responses. The midwife's approach needs to be spontaneous, flexible and non-threatening as well as practical.

The emphasis placed on breast feeding can place an unfair burden on a mother who does not want to or cannot breast feed her baby. Mothers who choose to bottle feed their babies often suffer from discrimination, however unintentional; for example, they may not receive advice about breast care during pregnancy, although general care applies regardless of the intended method of feeding.

It has become accepted practice to encourage the mother who wishes to breast feed her baby to do so soon after delivering to facilitate a good mother–baby relationship. This response is no less important for the mother and baby when bottle feeding is planned, but how many mothers are given the opportunity to bottle feed their baby following delivery?

Again, breast care in the early postnatal period is directed very much towards the mother who is breast feeding, as is supervision at feeding time, and the mother who is bottle feeding may receive less attention and advice. This subtle form of discrimination may undermine the mother's confidence in her choice at a time when every effort should be made to develop self-confidence.

Depression in the postnatal period is often mixed with anxiety and concern, sometimes about herself, but more often about her baby or other children. The relaxing of visiting rules to allow children to visit their mothers in hospital and the early transfer home of mother and baby to the care of the community midwife have done much to overcome this problem.

Bereavement

A stillbirth or neonatal death is not only a tragedy for the parents and their family, but for those that are involved in the care, who also share in the sense of loss. Distress of parents raises feelings of anxiety in those involved and if the parents' reaction is one of anger and hostility directed against the hospital, medical staff or midwives, our instinctive reaction is to become defensive. It takes courage and strength of character to submit oneself to the parents' intense grief, and react in an appropriate way. But the impact of the care and support they receive can affect the way they come to terms with or fail to come to terms with their loss. If proper mourning has not occurred, there may be problems during a subsequent pregnancy or after the birth of the next baby.

Bereavement is not an illness, but a process that must be allowed to run its course, and this takes time. However, a bereaved person may experience physical symptoms such as sleep disturbances, loss of appetite and a prolonged feeling of depression, and those involved in the care must be alert to when the normal mourning reaction is becoming abnormal.

Grief as a concept conjures up a dignified picture of sadness, but the reality may be very different. Each person will grieve in his or her own way, and reactions may occur at different times and be of different intensities, but there are some common patterns in the way most people react.

There are several stages in the grieving process:

The most immediate reaction is one of shock. The person denies reality by distancing themself from what is happening. This stage usually does not last for very long. The bereaved person is numb and experiencing everything in slow motion as though it is happening to someone else. Shock is a coping mechanism, sedating the person and giving them time to come to terms with what has happened at their own pace and in their own way. Later they will be able to recall in detail what occurred.

The midwife may find herself coping with this distressing situation at the birth of a stillborn baby. The sense of loss in giving birth to a dead baby makes the delivery very distressing for the parents and for the midwife and doctor. The parents may be overwhelmed at the delivery and the mother may be under the influence of drugs. It is therefore important to remember that at this time it is difficult for them to understand what people are saying to them and for them to make decisions. They should be invited to see and hold their dead baby, but there should be no pressure either way but the opportunity left open. Women who have a stillborn baby experience a sense of unreality and often have more difficulty in coming to terms with their loss than mothers of a neonatal death. Seeing and holding the baby and giving the baby a name helps to create a reality.

The midwife may feel reluctant to let the parents see a deformed baby, believing the sight of the baby would be distressing, but fantasies about the appearance of the baby are probably more frightening than the reality. We often underestimate the parents' ability to cope and, if handled sensitively, it can be a reassuring not frightening experience. Even a grossly abnormal baby will have some normal features and if these are revealed first and the baby gradually uncovered, even an anencephalic baby can appear unfrightening to the parents. It may be appropriate to give the parents time alone with their baby.

A later reaction may be one of anger. The anger may be directed against someone close or against those involved in the care. It is partly the loss of experience in the future that makes stillbirth and neonatal death such a tragic and deeply frustrating experience and sometimes this frustration is expressed as anger. It is important to encourage the bereaved parents to express their feelings and not to be shocked or upset by what they say.

Guilt and self-accusation may also occur. Guilt may be associated with fantasies that their thoughts or actions have caused the baby's death, for example, the mother may not have wanted the baby or may have had a previous pregnancy terminated. Shame may be associated with a sense of having failed as a woman and a mother, and an important part of the care is to help the woman regain self-confidence and a sense of worth.

Non-rational thoughts and actions can be part of the normal mourning process. The woman may have an urge to search for and find her lost baby and may be found wandering in the nursery or ward; she may hear a baby crying and think it is her baby. She becomes preoccupied with thoughts of her baby. At this time the woman may be showing psychological aspects of anxiety and be unable to eat or sleep. If she has not seen or held her baby, now might be an appropriate time for her to do so, or if she has done so she may need to repeat the experience. It is important at this time that she has something to 'find'. A photograph of the baby may also be of help.

Some bereaved parents want to discuss repeatedly the details surrounding the death, but others prefer to be alone with their grief and some may be withdrawn and unresponsive. It is important to encourage the parents to talk, but not to force the issue. Listening is an important activity which does not need a reply. It is better to say nothing than to say something that adds to the parents' distress. Some well-meaning attempts to comfort can have the opposite effect, for example, referring to existing children or a future baby may be seen as an attempt to deny the existence of this baby. The parents may need reassurance about a future pregnancy, but it must not be used as a means of reducing the impact of this loss.

A side-ward should be made available for the mother, but she should not be put in a single room for the benefit of others, but because it is her choice. She must not feel isolated or alone—she needs privacy without isolation. Also sending a grieving mother home within a few days may not be the right decision; she may prefer to be at home with her family or she may want to remain in hospital. It should be left to the woman and her husband to decide. Whether in hospital or at home there is a need for continuity of both midwifery and medical staff. A visit from the hospital chaplain or someone of the parents' own choice may be a source of comfort and reassurance.

In coping with the parents' distress some other aspects of care may be overlooked, for example, the problem of lactation. The production of milk is a very upsetting experience for the mother and it may help to reduce her distress if she is prepared for this occurrence and lactation is inhibited as soon as possible with the minimum of discomfort.

It is natural that as midwives our first concern is for the mother, but the father also needs help and support; it was his child too. He needs the opportunity to talk and help with the distressing formalities of registration and burial. He may be tired and shocked and not able to take in the facts. Facilities should be made available for him to stay with his wife; not only is he the best person to provide her with much needed love and physical contact, but the alternative may be for him to return to an empty house and be alone in his grief.

The parents may need help in coping with other children who may find the situation incomprehensible and frightening. It is important that they are not forgotten and the community midwife may be able to help the parents to explain to the children what has happened. The mother may not want to see her other children and she will need help in coping with and overcoming this reaction.

If the parents gave permission for a post-mortem examination, the results should be given to them as soon as possible, as the wait increases anxiety and delays recovery. This may also be an appropriate time to discuss a future pregnancy and for advice to be given on contraception, as it is important for the parents to come to terms with their loss before considering a future pregnancy.

Bereaved parents have to make enormous readjustments to life. They have anticipated and planned for their baby throughout pregnancy, and because the outcome is not as they anticipated they have to organise their feelings differently. Death is an emotionally painful experience to come to terms with and one of the problems for parents of a stillborn baby is that they have no memories, and memories facilitate mourning. They should be encouraged to take an active part in the formalities such as registration and burial, as these activities create memories which assist the recovery process.

A funeral is a ritual that gives the parents something tangible to remember. The way to overcome some of the difficulties to normal mourning that occur as the result of a stillbirth is to make the most of what is tangible and can be remembered. If parents are helped to grieve it may help to avoid some of the psychological difficulties which follow stillbirth.

Staff also have to come to terms with their own feelings and hence cope with the process of bereavement and mourning. It is perhaps more difficult in midwifery, as we are used to coping with life and the joyous occasion of birth, not death and sadness.

Counselling

Counselling is an enabling relationship; it provides the means in which one person is in a position to help another. How that situation is developed will depend on many factors, some relating to the counsellor, others to the person needing/seeking help. For example, the relationship of a midwife to a woman during pregnancy and labour and the mother and baby during the postnatal period, will be influenced not only by her professional training and experience, but also by her personal experience. The relationship of a woman to a midwife will be dependent on her previous experience and her expectations regarding the present pregnancy.

Too often counselling is interpreted as giving advice, but it is or should be much more than that. The disadvantage of just giving advice is that it can make the advised dependent on the advisor. This is not necessarily a problem in the first instance but it can become one if the situation does not develop. Therefore the counsellor should be progressing towards a relationship where she is helping the person to understand her own difficulties, and to identify the choices that are available and take responsibility for the decisions that are made. In this way the counsellor is developing the self-confidence of that person so she can have more control over her own life and face problems in the future with less anxiety and tension.

This is particularly relevant in the midwife–mother relationship. It is very easy for the midwife to take over from the mother and sometimes, however unintentional, undermine the mother's confidence in her ability to care for her baby. The role of the midwife is to encourage the mother's natural reaction to her baby so that she develops confidence. If the midwife helps the mother to decide the right course of action when she is not sure what to do or if she has responded in an inappropriate way, the mother will eventually develop the ability to solve her own problems but, what is more important, she will learn to trust her own reactions and to become a more confident and contented wife and mother. The value of including the father as much as possible is that he can provide the support and understanding that his wife needs when professional help is less readily available.

It must be borne in mind that communication in counselling as in all interpersonal relationships may be verbal or non-verbal. What the person is not telling you or is unable to put into words may be as important if not more important than what is being said. Also the midwife's attitude is an important form of non-verbal communication; an attitude that is offhand or too moralistic will create barriers and lead to ineffective communication.

Attitudes are affected by personal experiences some of which can be helpful and others that may come between the counsellor and the person seeking help and create a situation that is counter-productive. Counselling relies on a good interpersonal relationship between the counsellor and the person seeking help. You cannot help someone unless you can relate to them and, just as important, they can respond to you. It is important to recognise one's limitations and to know when to ask someone else to take over. The art of successful counselling is to know when to be involved and when to become uninvolved.

What must never be overlooked is that whilst it is essential for a midwife to develop counselling skills and increase her efficiency in counselling, it does not make her a counsellor. Counselling is an integral part of the midwife's practice and as such interacts with her other skills, but there are limits and it is important for her to be aware of her limitations and recognise when the skills of a trained counsellor are needed.

Counselling skills are important to the midwife because she comes into close contact with a woman at one if not the most important time of her life; a time when her heightened awareness makes her particularly vulnerable. This is a very privileged and responsible position and if handled skilfully can be a very rewarding experience for mother and midwife. The midwife must establish a helping relationship with the mother, she must listen to what she has to say, encourage her to examine her feelings, and respond in an appropriate way. This will require the midwife to adjust personal attitudes and develop a flexible approach to care. This will enable the woman to express her feelings—her expectations, anxieties and fears, and to come to terms with them and through this experience gain personal development. This will also help the woman and her husband to face the responsibilities of parenthood with greater confidence.

Chapter 15
An Introduction to Genetics

GENETICS

A consequence of the successful control of diseases due to exogenous factors is the increasing relative importance of genetically determined diseases and congenital malformations among the main causes of death and disease. This is particularly relevant in relation to deaths in the first year of life, for example, in 1900 the infant mortality rate was 154 per 1000 registered live births in England and Wales, and one in every thirty deaths was due to congenital malformation. By 1982 the infant mortality rate had fallen to 10.8 and one in every four deaths was due to congenital malformation.

In recent years there has been an increasing interest in clinical genetics and a growing demand for genetic counselling and, linked with this, a developing interest in prenatal diagnosis as a means of reducing the number of babies born with severe abnormalities. In addition, the recent advances made in the fields of cytogenetics, biochemistry and haematology have increased the knowledge and understanding of the hereditary aspects of many diseases.

Genetics may seem very academic and not relevant to the day to day practise of midwifery, however, if we consider that congenital malformation is the cause of 25% of all stillbirths and 20% of deaths in the first week of life, it becomes obvious that some knowledge of the causes behind these statistics is required. In addition, the midwife will have early contact with parents of babies born malformed, and an understanding of the aetiology will assist the midwife in providing care and support.

Fetal development is the result of the interaction between genetic inheritance and the intrauterine environment, and in many cases of congenital abnormality the exact cause may not be apparent whereas in others a specific causative factor(s) can be identified. The diagnosis is further complicated by the knowledge that some conditions may be caused by either a genetic or an environmental factor; for example, a mentally defective child may be the result of genetic action or intrauterine hypoxia and in addition to the known teratogens there are others as yet unknown which further complicates an exact diagnosis of the causative factor(s).

Environmental factors

1 Hypoxia, anoxia (see p. 325).
2 Infection. The rubella virus is known to cause serious abnormality including mental retardation, deafness and cataracts (see p. 372). Other infecting organisms which can cause fetal damage are the cytomegalovirus and the protozoan responsible for toxoplasmosis (see pp. 373, 374).
3 Drugs. Some drugs given to women in early pregnancy have been shown to be the cause of abnormality, e.g. thalidomide, and are no longer prescribed. Steroids are known to cause changes in the genitalia of female fetuses, and the anticonvulsant, epanutin, may be a cause of cleft lip.
4 Alcohol. Excessive intake of alcohol may result in mental retardation.

Genetic factors

An inherited factor is responsible for the abnormality or causing the teratogenic effect. The transmission of the condition may be from the mother or father or a combination of both parents (see below).

A gene comprises a group of chemicals situated on chromosomes which determine the characteristics. The name chromosome derives from their ability to take up basic stains—chromos (colours)—some (body). Chromosomes are the main source of chemical information which determines that a cell becomes like the parent cell and endows the animal or plant, with all the characteristics of its species. They are fine coiled thread-like structures in the nucleus of a cell and consist of protein and a substance known as deoxyribonucleic acid (DNA). The deoxyribonucleic acid molecule is double stranded and the two strands are twisted to form a spiral known as the double helix. Each strand is composed of hundreds of smaller chemical units called nucleotides consisting of a sugar, a phosphate, and a base. Another nucleic acid, ribonucleic acid is also present in the nucleus in small quantities but the majority is in the cytoplasm of the cell.

There are a definite number (diploid number) of chromosomes in each cell of any species of plant or animal, for example, man has forty-six chromosomes but a mouse only forty.

The genetic code

Information (coded instruction) is stored in chemical form in the nucleus of the cell and is contained within the chromosomes in the form of genes.

CELL DIVISION

The single stranded chromosomes condense and at a certain stage in the division the chromosomes split into two, remaining attached at a junction point referred to as a centomere. It is at this stage that further development is halted when a karyotype is prepared and a karyotype is, therefore, a preparation of chromosomes as they appear during the activity involved in nuclear division. The two parallel strands of each divided chromosome are known as chromatids.

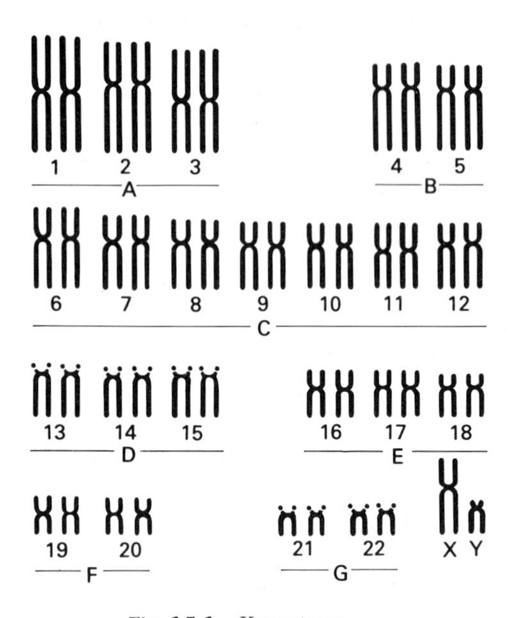

Fig. 15.1 Karyotype.

Somatic cells contain a total of 46 chromosomes; 23 matching pairs composed of chromosomes from each parent known as autosomes which are similar in males and females, and a pair of sex chromosomes which are different; the female comprises XX and the male XY.

Somatic cells divide by a process of mitosis, the chromosomes divide longitudinally one passing to each resultant cell. Therefore each new cell has the same complement of chromosomes exactly reproduced as the parent cell.

The gametes—the ova and spermatazoa—undergo a series of mitotic divisions resulting, in the case of the male gametes, in a vast increase in numbers. The final divisions, which give rise to the mature gametes are not miotic. Instead of producing cells with 46 chromosomes, the ovum and spermatozoa have only 23 chromosomes so at fertilisation the resulting zygote contains the diploid number of 46 chromosomes. The division which gives rise to a reduction in the chromosomes is known as meiosis. During the formation of the ovum (oogenesis) the cytoplasm is not divided equally; after the first meiotic division one nuclei receives more of the cytoplasm, and the other nuclei is separated off to form the first polar body which eventually degenerates. The next meiotic division produces a second polar body and a mature ovum.

Genetic counselling

Many factors have led to more couples receiving genetic counselling. The 574 664 births in England and Wales in 1977 was the lowest since records began. The average number of children in a family was less than two, therefore expectations of parents are that they should have normal healthy children able to enjoy an active life. Planning of pregnancy has also resulted in miscarriage becoming a more significant event. Changing patterns of disease have placed more emphasis on the preventative aspects of care, and social changes such as the liberalisation of the laws on abortion and improved methods of contraception, and the recent advances in prenatal diagnosis have enabled couples to prevent pregnancy if there is a high risk of an abnormal baby, or to decide to proceed with a pregnancy with the option of prenatal testing and, if necessary, termination of pregnancy.

Those seeking or referred for genetic counselling include:

1 Parents who have had an abnormal child and wish to know the risk of recurrence in a subsequent child or where studies on aborted material have identified an abnormal conceptus.

2 Premarital/preconception counselling where there is a specific problem, e.g. where there is a known family history of an abnormal child or inherited disease.

Genetic counselling consists essentially in indicating the nature and degree of the risk of transmitting inherited or partially inherited conditions, with the aim of preventing the birth of a handicapped child.

The formulation of genetic prognosis requires an accurate clinical diagnosis and adequate information about the family history. The estimation of risk may be very simple or extremely difficult according to the mode of inheritance. In some cases an exact diagnosis, as in phenylketonuria or cystic fibrosis, is all that is required for the risk to be identified. Difficulties occur in conditions which are partially genetic in which aetiology is not fully understood. In some cases the risk estimates have to be empirical, i.e. based on published data.

As in all forms of counselling a sympathetic understanding attitude is essential. But also, because of the complex nature of the subject, it is important to make sure the couple understand the risks. The use of clear diagrams showing the method of inheritance will assist the couple in understanding the significance of information they are receiving.

Mode of inheritance

Some diseases are transmitted from generation to generation but others are only recognised when more than one child is born to unaffected parents. A child inherits from its parents characteristics common to all humans but in addition other characteristics peculiar only to his parents.

Human characteristics are determined by the genes, and are paired in the same way as the chromosomes so that a child inherits one of a pair from each parent. The genes are referred to as alleles and if they transmit the same information the individual is homozygous for those genes, but if they have a different action the individual is heterozygous. An example of this is the Rhesus factor. The Rhesus system comprises several different antigens the main ones being classified as C, D, E, c, d, e. The presence of the D antigen confers Rhesus positive status on an individual; if it is absent the person is Rhesus negative. If a child inherits the D antigen from both its parents he is Rhesus positive homozygous (DD), if he inherits the D antigen from one parent but not the other he is Rhesus positive heterozygous (Dd). A child who does not inherit the Rhesus factor from either parent is Rhesus negative (dd). An individual's genetic makeup is referred to as his genotype and the interaction between that and the environment his phenotype.

If an individual inherits an abnormal gene from one of his parents and a normal gene from the other the outcome will vary. If the inheritance results in a disease or abnormality despite the presence of one normal allele, the effect of the abnormal gene is dominant and the resultant disease or abnormality dominantly inherited. However, if the gene does not produce any disease or abnormality the effect is recessive. But if the individual inherits a similar defective gene from both parents, the combined effect may produce a disease which is said to be recessively inherited.

Most genes are located on the autosomes and a disease or abnormality resulting from genes located on these chromosomes is referred to as an autosomal disease, i.e. autosomal dominant or recessive condition. The term sex-linked is used when the abnormal gene is located on the sex chromosomes, but, because there are no known Y-linked conditions, the term X-linked is also used.

Variation in mode of inheritance

MUTATION

Mutation is a change which takes place spontaneously in a chromosome or gene and may produce an alteration in the characteristic under its control.

Chromosome mutation

a Polyploidy. There is duplication (double or treble) of the entire set of chromosomes in the gametes (ovum or spermatazoon) or zygote.
b Translocation. A chromosome breaks and the fragment joins another (non-homologous) chromosome.
c Centric fusion. Two chromosomes with terminal centromeres join and function as one chromosome.
d Aneuploidy. One or more chromosome is duplicated or missing, e.g. Down's syndrome. Trisomy 21 (see p. 390).

Gene mutation

This occurs when a section of the deoxyribonucleic acid molecule in a chromosome is not copied exactly in cell division, e.g. phenylketonuria, and sickle cell anaemia. Phenylketonuria is an autosomal recessive disease where there is an inability to convert phenylalanine to tyrosine (see p. 379).

The haemoglobin molecule consists of a sequence of eight amino acids. In sickle cell anaemia (disease) one of the DNA bases has not yet correctly paired prior to meiotic division which formed the gamete and the property of the haemoglobin is altered (see 219).

The incidence of inherited diseases

Dominant. If uncomplicated this type of inheritance raises few problems: there is a one in two chance that any child of an affected person will be similarly affected.

Examples of dominant conditions

1 Achondroplasia.
2 Huntingdon's Chorea.
3 Osteogenesis Imperfecta.

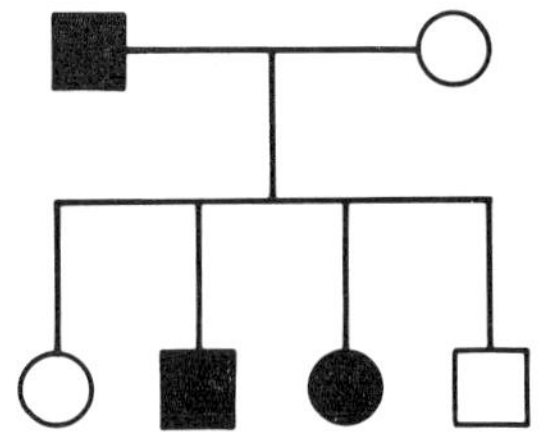

Fig. 15.2 Autosomal dominant inheritance.

Recessive. Where a couple are known to be carriers because they have already had an affected child, the risk is one in four that any future child will be similarly affected. Apart from cousin marriages the risk to the children of affected people or to children of their normal sibs is very small.

Examples of recessive conditions
1 Cystic fibrosis (see p. 381).
2 Phenylketonuria (see p. 379).
3 Sickle cell disease (see p. 219).

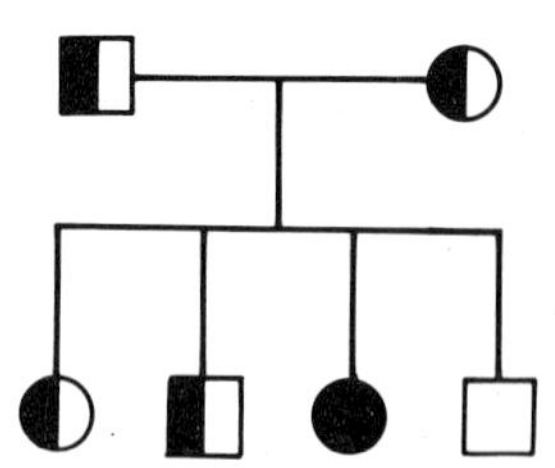

Fig. 15.3 Autosomal recessive inheritance.

Sex-linked. In practice these conditions are X-linked as there are no known Y-linked conditions. If a woman is heterozygous for an X-linked gene, i.e. she carries the abnormal gene on one of her two X chromosomes, there is a one in two chance that her son will be affected or that her daughter will be a carrier. The advances in the detection of heterozygous carriers has improved the reliability of genetic counselling, especially in X-linked conditions.
Examples of X-linked conditions
1 Haemophilia.
2 Duchenne muscular dystrophy.
3 Christmas disease (factor IX deficiency).
4 Glucose-6-phosphate dehydrogenase deficiency (see p. 365).

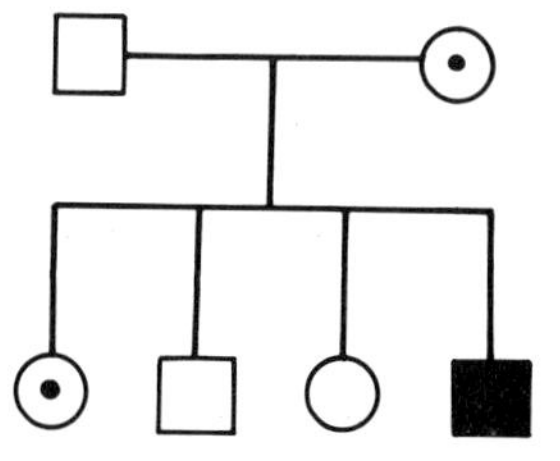

Fig. 15.4 Sex linked inheritance.

Examples of conditions which may have more than one type of genetic determination are:
1 Congenital deafness. Most types are recessive, but X-linked and dominant types occur.
2 Muscular dystrophy. The severe Duchenne type is X-linked, the milder limb-girdle form recessive and the facio-scapula-humeral form dominant.
3 Gargoylism. The Hunter type is X-linked, the Hurler type is recessive.
4 Retinitis pigmentosa. Dominant, recessive and X-linked forms occur.

Examples of common conditions with partial and complex inheritance and approximate empirical recurrence risks.

1 Infantile pyloric stenosis. There is a 1 in 20 risk for brothers or sons and a 1 in 40 risk for sisters or daughters of affected males. There is a 1 in 5 risk for brothers or sons and a 1 in 10 risk for sisters or daughters of affected females.

2 Spina bifida cystica; anencephaly. The risk for siblings of affected persons is 1 in 20.

3 Cleft lip with or without Cleft palate. There is a 1 in 30 risk for siblings or sons and daughters of affected persons.

4 Congenital dislocation of the hip. There is a 1 in 40 risk for brothers and sons, and a 1 in 10 risk for sisters and daughters of affected females. There is a somewhat higher risk for relatives of affected males.

5 Talipes equinovarus. There is a 1 in 50 risk for siblings of affected persons.

6 Down's syndrome. In regular trisomy 21 there is about a 1 in 100 risk for siblings of affected persons independent of maternal age. The risk may be higher if a translocation is present.

7 Congenital malformation of the heart. There is about a 1 in 30 risk, in all types of heart malformation taken together, for siblings of affected persons.

With multifactorially determined conditions the recurrence risk is raised if there is already more than one affected person in the family; for example, if parents have already had two children with spina bifida cystica, or anencephaly, the recurrence risk rises to about 1 in 8; where a parent affected with cleft lip with or without cleft palate has already had one affected child, the risk for further children rises to about 1 in 10.

Prenatal screening and diagnosis

Many congenital and inherited abnormalities can now be diagnosed antenatally by analysis of maternal blood or amniotic fluid obtained by amniocentesis or by ultrasonography, techniques that are now widely available. In addition, new techniques such as fetoscopy are being used in some centres to diagnose other disorders.

Congenital malformation is the major cause of perinatal mortality and in human terms causes untold grief and also feelings of guilt that are difficult to overcome. The relative importance of congenital malformations as a cause of death and disease, has led to advances in prenatal screening and diagnosis as a means of preventing the birth of an abnormal child.

The major causes of congenital abnormality include many conditions which can now be diagnosed in utero by the various techniques and tests that are currently available, and others where work is being undertaken to extend the scope of prenatal screening and diagnosis.

Major causes of congenital abnormality:

1 Neural tube defects—spina bifida, meningomyelocele, anencephaly and some cases of hydrocephaly.
2 Congenital heart disease.
3 Severe mental retardation.
4 Down's syndrome.
5 Cleft lip and palate.
6 Talipes.
7 Cerebral palsy.
8 Blindness.
9 Deafness.
10 Abnormalities of limbs.
11 Others including renal tract abnormalities.

Methods of prenatal screening

MATERNAL BLOOD SAMPLING

Testing the maternal serum for alpha-fetoprotein is a screening test for open neural type defects. In some units this has been introduced as a routine test but in others it is used selectively. The most accurate results are obtained between sixteen and eighteen weeks gestation. Alpha-fetoprotein levels above the 95th centile, which is twice the median value, are suspicious but not conclusive of a neural tube defect, as high levels are also associated with a multiple pregnancy. But it is an indication to perform further investigations such as ultrasonic examination and amniocentesis.

ULTRASONIC EXAMINATION

Visualisation of the fetus by ultrasonography is performed routinely in many units. In addition to assessing the period of gestation by measuring the crown-rump length and later the bi-parietal diameter (see p. 317), the examination may also reveal abnormalities of head and limbs and even cardiovascular and renal defects. The presence of open neural tube defects such as spina bifida and anencephaly may confirm a diagnosis suspected when raised maternal serum alpha-fetoprotein levels were found.

AMNIOTIC FLUID ANALYSIS

Amniotic fluid is obtained by the technique of amniocentesis which involves introducing a needle transabdominally into the uterine cavity. Amniocentesis is performed after the fourteenth week of pregnancy and following an ultrasonic scan to localise the placenta and the position of the fetus. The woman empties her bladder and is made comfortable in the supine position. Using an aseptic technique, the skin is infiltrated with a local anaesthetic and a spinal needle with stylet is inserted into the amniotic cavity. The stylet is withdrawn and clear fluid should be seen. A syringe is connected to the needle and 20 ml of amniotic fluid is withdrawn.

Amniocentesis is not without risk and should not therefore be performed unless there is a good indication. The risks include abortion, fetal death and later in pregnancy, antepartum haemorrhage. In a Rhesus negative woman with a Rhesus positive fetus there is a risk of Rhesus isoimmunisation and 5 μg of anti D immunoglobulin should be given as a precaution.

Cytology

The amniotic fluid contains fetal cells and following culture a karyotype can be prepared (see p. 468) and changes in the number of chromosomes or the presence of chromosomal abnormalities detected. In this way abnormalities such as Down's syndrome can be diagnosed.

In addition, the sex of the fetus can be determined and sex-linked disorders detected (see p. 472).

Recent advances in cell culture techniques have made it possible to diagnose metabolic disorders such as phenylketonuria (see p. 379) and Tay-Sachs Disease where there is a deficiency of the enzyme hexosaminidase-A resulting in mental retardation.

Biochemical studies

Biochemical studies of the amniotic fluid have been used for many years to estimate liquor bilirubin levels in the management of Rhesus incompatibility (see p. 368) and to assess fetal maturity in late pregnancy by estimating the lecithin-sphingomyelin ratio as a means of determining fetal lung maturity (see p. 318).

In recent years biochemical studies have included measurement of alpha-fetoprotein levels as a means of detecting open neural tube defects. Levels of liquor alpha-fetoprotein above 20 μg/ml indicate the presence of such a defect.

FETOSCOPY

This technique enables visualisation of the fetus through a fine endoscope with a fibre optic telescope placed transabdominally into the amniotic cavity. As with amniocentesis, this is an aseptic technique performed under local anaesthetic. The woman is sedated to minimise maternal and fetal activity, and the procedure is carried out under ultrasonic guidance to avoid injury to the fetus or placenta.

The procedure, which requires great skill and expertise, can be used to detect any gross structural abnormality. In addition, the umbilical cord can be visualised and a specimen of fetal blood obtained by a needle passed via the endoscope and inserted into an umbilical vessel either at the umbilicus or insertion of the cord into the placenta.

The fetal blood sample can be used to detect haemoglobinopathies such as thalassaemia and sickle cell disease—autosomal recessive disorders. The test involves an analysis of the haemoglobin chains that the fetal red blood cells are synthesising.

Assays for Factors VIII C and IX C can also be performed to detect haemophilia, and blood typing to determine if the fetus is at risk of Rhesus haemolytic disease.

Diagnosis of chromosomal abnormality and metabolic disorders can be made as well as the X-linked condition Duchenne muscular dystrophy.

Biopsy of fetal skin and liver has also been performed using this technique.

Another technique that has been used more recently involves obtaining embryonic tissue from the non-placental part of the trophoblast for genetic analysis to detect blood disorders. An endoscope is introduced into the vagina and a biopsy taken from the trophoblast. This procedure is carried out at about eight weeks gestation before the villi disappear.

Increasing experience with amniocentesis and the introduction of ultrasound has made prenatal screening and diagnosis possible and safer, and the recent advances in cytogenetics and fetoscopy has further increased the scope of this field of fetal medicine.

However, one of the problems associated with prenatal screening for congenital abnormality and disease is that many of the tests available cannot be performed until pregnancy is several weeks advanced; for example maternal serum alpha-fetoprotein levels are most accurate between sixteen and eighteen weeks gestation and amniocentesis is performed after fourteen weeks gestation. The analysis may take several weeks as in the case of tissue culture for chromosomal analysis which takes up to three weeks. This delay means that the pregnancy is advanced beyond the optimal time for termination if this is indicated. Also because of the risks associated with amniocentesis, it should not be performed unless the couple agree to the pregnancy being terminated if the results of the studies confirm a fetal abnormality.

Appendix: Terminology

Alleles. Alternative forms of a gene which may occupy the same site on homologous chromosomes.

Autosomes. Chromosomes other than sex chromosomes.

Chromatids. The two parallel strands of the divided chromosome.

Chromosome. One of a number of structures contained in the cell nucleus and bearing the genes.

Centomere. The junction point between the two parts of the divided chromosome.

Cytogenetics. The study of chromosomes and their abnormalitics.

Dominant trait. One which is determined by the presence of a gene in heterozygous form.

Gene. A group of chemicals situated on chromosomes which determine characteristics.
Genetics. The study of the method of inheritance of the characteristics.
Heterozygous. Having a different allele at the gene locus.
Homozygous. Having the same allele at the gene locus.
Karyotype. A preparation of chromosomes numbered and grouped according to size.
Meiosis. Reduction of the number of chromosomes in a germ cell by means of two consecutive nuclear divisions during maturation.
Mitosis. Cell division during which the chromosomes split longitudinally and are distributed in equal numbers to resultant cells.
Recessive trait. One which is determined by the presence of a gene in heterozygous form.
Sex chromosomes. A pair of chromosomes responsible for sex determination.
Sex-linked trait. One determined by the presence of a gene on the sex chromosome.
Teratogen. Agent which causes abnormality of formation and growth of fetal organs.
Translocation. A chromosome breaks and the fragment joins another chromosome.

Chapter 16
Medico-Legal Aspects in Relation to Childbearing

Congenital Disabilities (Civil Liability) Act 1976

An Act to make provision as to civil liability in the case of children born disabled in consequence of some person's fault; and to extend the Nuclear Installations Act 1965, so that children so born in consequence of a breach of duty under the Act may claim compensation (22nd July 1976).

This introduction to the Act identifies the reason why a midwife needs to have some knowledge of its contents. The special role of the midwife as a practitioner in her own right means that she makes, and takes responsibility for, her own decisions and if as a consqeuence a baby is born disabled, the midwife could be liable under the provisions of this Act. This would be in addition to any liability relating to professional conduct as identified in the Handbook Incorporating the Rules and the Notices Concerning a Midwife's Code of Practice, and other policies and procedures laid down by the employing authority.

The importance of accurate and detailed records is not only a professional responsibility invested in the midwife but also a sensible precaution to protect herself in the event of litigation. The need for attention to detail both in the provision of care and the maintenance of records cannot be over-emphasised, and a midwife's records should be able to withstand the scrutiny of another professional acting for the plaintiff in a case of litigation.

1 Civil liability to a child born disabled.

1 If a child is born disabled as the result of such an occurrence before its birth as is mentioned in subsection (2) below, and a person (other than the child's own mother) is under this section answerable to the child in respect of the occurrence, the child's disabilities are to be regarded as damage resulting from the wrongful act of that person and actionable accordingly at the suit of the child.

A child that is born disabled can, under this Act, sue either through its parents or guardian, or later on its own behalf for up to twenty-one years. This reinforces the advice contained in the Handbook regarding the preservation of records, namely that 'A midwife must not destroy or arrange for the destruction of official records made whilst she is in professional attendance on a case and required to be kept by these rules; if she finds it impossible or inconvenient to preserve them she must transfer them to the local supervising authority or her employing authority, and details of the transfer must be duly recorded'. You will note that it is important for the midwife to have a record of the transfer of the responsibility for the safe keeping of her records.

2 An occurrence to which this section applies is one which:

a affected either parent of the child in his or her ability to have a normal, healthy child; or

b affected the mother during her pregnancy, or affected her or the child in the course of its birth, so that the child is born with disabilities which would not otherwise have been present.

The first of these two subsections refers to an occurrence at the time of conception of the child and therefore it is unlikely to involve the midwife. However, the nature of the midwife's work means the second subsection is relevant particularly in relation to care in labour, where failure to provide proper care could result in the birth of a disabled child and therefore a breach of duty by the midwife.

3 Subject to the following subsections, a person (here referred to as 'the defendant') is answerable to the child if he was liable in tort to the parent or would, if sued in due time, have been so; and it is no answer that there could not have been such liability because the parent suffered no actionable injury, if there was a breach of legal duty which, accompanied by injury, would have given rise to the liability.

Note that the 'defendant' is answerable to the child not to the parent. Tort is derived from the medieval Latin word *tortum* meaning wrong, and 'in tort' refers to a duty imposed by law—not contract—making the offender liable to action for damages in the event of a breach of duty. A duty of care is assumed when the woman is booked; no contract is signed but nonetheless the duty has legal implications.

The 'due time' refers to the time during which the mother could have sued for a breach of duty of care.

This subsection also refers to the fact that although the duty of care is to the mother, the liability to the unborn child still applies even though the woman herself did not suffer any 'actionable injury'.

4 In the case of an occurrence preceding the time of conception, the defendant is not answerable to the child if at that time either or both of the parents knew the risk of their child being born disabled (that is to say, the particular risk created by the occurrence); but should it be the child's father who is the defendant, this subsection does not apply if he knew of the risk and the mother did not.

The point of interest in this subsection is the knowledge or otherwise of the parents or parent regarding the risk of their child being born disabled. The growing demand for genetic counselling (see p. 469) and pre-conception care and advice (see p. 7) brings more prospective parents into contact with professionals, and again emphasises the importance of accurate record keeping.

An example of a 'particular risk created by the occurrence' is vaccination against Rubella. Because the live attenuated vaccine is used, the fetus would be at risk if the woman conceived within three months of receiving the vaccine. Therefore she must be advised against pregnancy and an effective method of contraception prescribed.

Notice that the father is answerable to the child if he knew of the risk of the child being born disabled and the mother did not.

5 The defendant is not answerable to the child for anything he did or omitted to do when responsible in a professional capacity for treating or advising the parent, if he took reasonable care having due regard to then received professional opinion applicable to the particular class of case; but this does not mean that he is answerable only because he departed from received opinion.

The term 'reasonable care' is somewhat ambiguous but in most cases a standard of care is recognised and documented, and midwives are referred to the Handbook and Code of Practice. The time lag between the occurrence and the suit means that professional opinion and therefore practices may have changed. This subsection recognised that fact and protects a professional from being answerable to the child based on practices that were introduced after the time when he was responsible. It does, however, underline the importance of the midwife keeping up to date with current practices.

This subsection also makes the point that it is not only when a professional has departed from received opinion that he is liable.

6 Liability to the child under this section may be treated as having been excluded or limited by contract made with the parent affected, to the same extent and subject to the same restrictions as liability in the parent's own case; and a contract term which could have been set up by the defendant in an action by the parent, so as to exclude or limit his liability to him or her, operates in the defendant's favour to the same, but no greater, extent in an action under this section by the child.

A contract is a mutual agreement enforceable by law, and this subsection explains how a contract entered into by the parent also pertains to the child in the same way as in subsection three. This is important in relation to the current situation where many women express strong preferences about their care which may conflict with professional opinion. Ideally a compromise should be reached that does not put the fetus at risk but this may not be possible. Again, the need for detailed and accurate record keeping cannot be overemphasised.

7 If in the child's action under this section it is shown that the parent affected shared the responsibility for the child being born disabled, the damages are to be reduced to such extent as the court thinks just and equitable having regard to the extent of the parent's responsibility.

As with the above, the problem of a 'woman's' wishes with regard to her care conflicting with professional opinion is relevant. How far professionals can go in carrying out procedures in the interest of the unborn child and against the wishes of the expectant mother is currently under debate. This could have an influence in the Court's decision because a right (justice) recognised by the court of equity supersedes common and statute law when they conflict.

2 A woman driving a motor vehicle when she knows (or ought reasonably to know) herself to be pregnant is to be regarded as being under the same duty to take care for the safety of her unborn child as the law imposes on her with respect for the safety of other people; and if in consequence of her breach of that duty her child is born with disabilities which would not otherwise have been present, those disabilities are to be regarded as damage resulting from her wrongful act and actionable accordingly at the suit of the child.

This subsection makes the woman liable if as a result of carelessness during pregnancy her child is born disabled. It raises the question of who would bring the prosecution on behalf of the child against its mother? The 'child' may do so when he is old enough to know his rights.

3 Civil liability to a child born disabled due to radiation.

1 Section 1 of this Act does not affect the operations of the Nuclear Installations Act 1965 as to liability for, and compensation in respect of, injury or damage caused by occurrences involving nuclear matter or the emission of ionising radiations.

2 For the avoidance of doubt anything which:

a affects a man in his ability to have a normal healthy child; or

b affects a woman in that ability, or so affects her when she is pregnant that her child is born with disabilities which would not otherwise have been present, is an injury for the purposes of that Act.

This subsection clarifies the term injury under the Nuclear Installations Act 1965, and it is worth noting that it is not the ability of the man or woman to have a child, but their ability to have a normal healthy child that is at issue.

3 If a child is born disabled as a result of an injury to either of its parents caused in breach of a duty imposed by any of sections 7 to 11 of that Act (nuclear site licensees and others to secure that nuclear incidents do not cause injury to persons, etc.) the child's disabilities are to be regarded under the subsequent provisions of that Act (compensation and other matters) as injuries caused on the same occasion, and by the same breach of duty, as was the injury to the parent.

4 As respects compensation to the child, section 13 (6) of that Act (contributory fault of person injured by radiation) is to be applied as if the reference there to fault were to the fault of the parent.

These two subsections confirm the liability and the right of the child to compensation as a result of a breach of duty to its parents under the Nuclear Installations Act 1965 and on the same basis as its parents.

5 Compensation is not payable in the child's case if the injury to the parent preceded the time of the child's conception and at the time either or both of the parents knew the risk of their child being born disabled (that is to say, the particular risk created by the injury).

There is a link between this exclusion clause and 1 (4) above. The onus is on either or both the parents to be aware of the risk to a child of an 'injury' that occurred subsequent to conception. Professionals may be involved if advice is sought by the parents prior to a pregnancy.

4 Interpretation and other supplementary provisions

The following sections and subsections seek to clarify the meaning of some of the words used in the Congenital Disabilities (Civil Liability) Act 1976, and makes additional statements relevant to it.

1 Reference in this Act to a child being born disabled or with disabilities are to its being born with any deformity, disease or abnormality, including predisposition (whether or not susceptible of immediate prognosis) to physical or mental defect in the future.

Disabled (disability) refers to a physical incapacity caused by injury or disease; a deformity is a malformation; and abnormality means deviating from type. A 'predisposition to physical and mental defect in the future' means that the disability does not have to be diagnosed at birth.

2 In this Act:

- **a** 'born' means born alive (the moment of a child's birth being when it first has a life separate from its mother), and 'birth' has a corresponding meaning; and
- **b** 'motor vehicle' means a mechanically propelled vehicle intended or adapted for use on roads.

Although the wording is not the same, sub-section 2 (a) has the same meaning as the definition of a live birth as included in the Code of Practice, i.e. 'A baby born at any stage of pregnancy who breathes or shows other signs of life after complete expulsion from its mother is born alive'.

3 Liability to a child under Section 1 or 2 of this Act is to be regarded:

- **a** as respects all its incidents and any matters arising or to arise out of it; and
- **b** subject to any contrary context or intention, for the purpose of construing references in enactments and documents to personal or bodily injuries and cognate matters,

as liability for personal injuries sustained by the child immediately after its birth.

This subsection refers to that part of the Act concerned with persons other than the child's own mother (Section 1) and the mother herself (Section 2), but does not refer to liability due to radiation (Section 3).

4 No damages shall be recoverable under either of these sections in respect of any loss of expectation of life, nor shall any such loss be taken into account in the compensation payable in respect of the child under the Nuclear Installations Act 1965 as extended by section 3, unless (in either case) the child lives for at least forty-eight hours.

This subsection raises again the importance of accurate record keeping, in this case with regard to the exact time of birth and death; the parents right to compensation could depend on this attention to detail.

5 This Act applies in respect of births after (but not before) its passing, and in respect of any such birth it replaces any law in force before its passing, whereby a person could be liable to a child in respect of disabilities with which it might be born; but in section 1 (3) of this Act the expression 'liable in tort' does not include any reference to liability by virtue of this Act, or to liability by virtue of any such law.

The liability under this Act applies only to babies born after the 22nd July 1976, and supersedes any previous Act in respect of these babies.

6 References to the Nuclear Installations Act 1965 are to that Act as amended; and for the purposes of section 28 of that Act (power by Order in Council to extend the

Act to territories outside the United Kingdom) section 3 of this Act is to be treated as if it were a provision of that Act.

This subsection reaffirms that the statements made in section 3 subsections 1 to 5 of the Congenital Disabilities (Civil Liability) Act 1976 and section 28 of the amended Nuclear Installations Act 1965 are interchangeable.

5 This Act binds the Crown.

The 'Crown' refers to the Government and Legislature.

6 1 This Act may be cited as the Congenital Disabilities (Civil Liability) Act 1976.

The correct title of the Act is reiterated.

2 This Act extends to Northern Ireland but not to Scotland.

Note that the Act does not extend to Scotland which has its own separate legal system.

The Congenital Disabilities (Civil Liability) Act 1976 reinforces the importance of midwives maintaining a high standard of care in line with current accepted practises, maintaining accurate and detailed records of the care provided and ensuring that the records are not destroyed. This is not only the professional duty of all midwives but a sensible precaution against possible future litigation.

SECTION V

THE MIDWIFERY PROFESSION

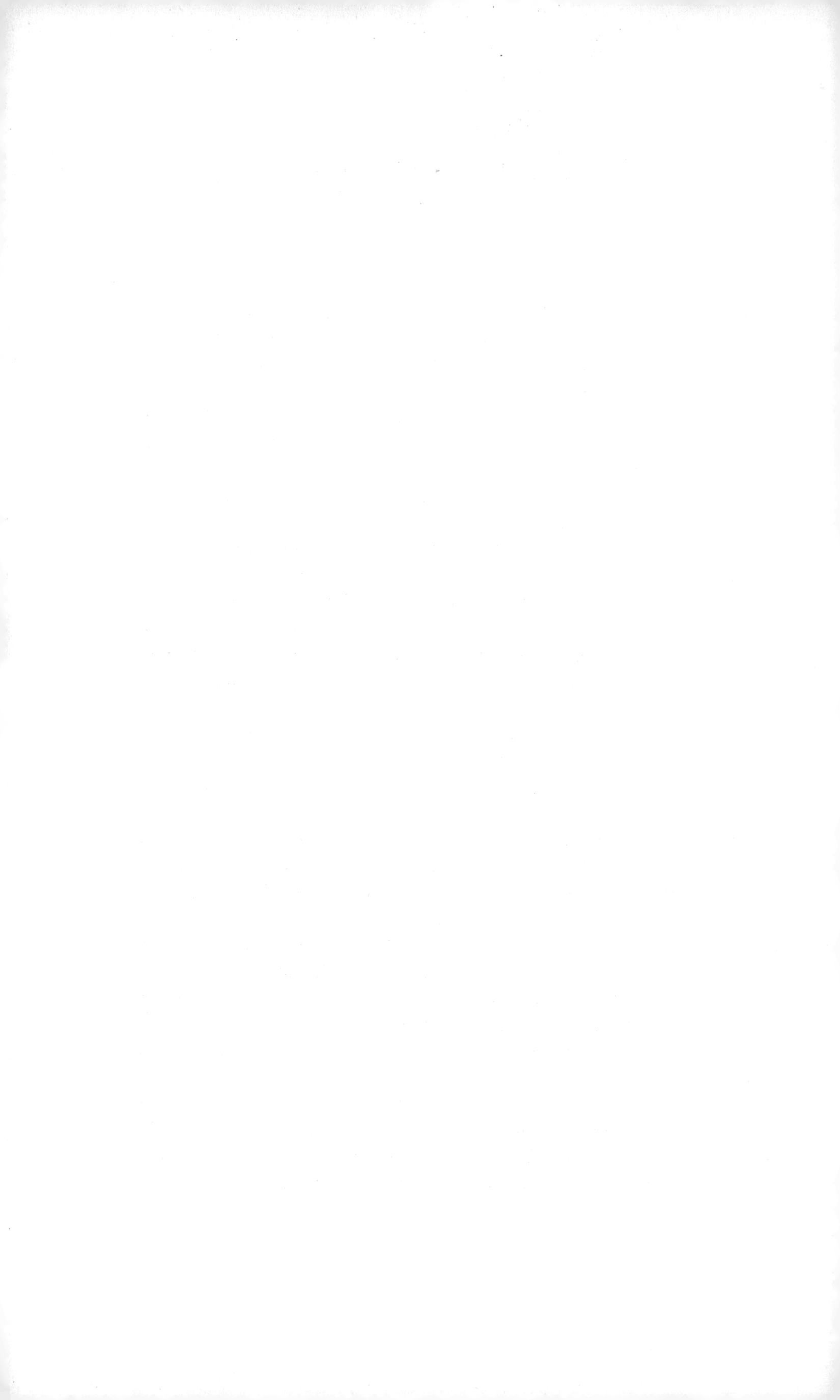

Chapter 17
The History of Midwifery

The changes in the practice of midwifery are a reflection of the changes that have taken place in the maternity services and midwives have progressed from the unqualified birth attendants of previous centuries to the highly trained professional of the 1980s.

From the seventeenth century doctors became involved in what had previously been the all-female world of childbirth and the woman-midwives were relegated to practise among the poor. Although a small number were trained in the lying in hospitals that were established in the mid-eighteenth century, the majority were uneducated, ignorant women. The Obstetrical Society of London set up a Board of Examiners in 1872, introduced a voluntary examination for midwives and issued a certificate of proficiency. About one-third of the 22 308 women admitted to the first Roll of Midwives in 1905 held the certificate of the London Obstetrical Society; just over two thousand held hospital certificates but the majority were bona fide midwives who held no certificates but had practiced for at least one year and were of good character.

The Midwives Institute was founded in 1881 with the aim of raising the efficiency and improving the status of midwives and to petition Parliament for their recognition. The Institute changed its name to the College of Midwives in 1941 and was granted the Royal prefix in 1947.

Many attempts were made to regularise midwives in the late nineteenth century. A Committee of the Royal College of Physicians was appointed to consider a Bill that had been rejected by Parliament in 1891. The Committee recommended the need for legislation to educate, examine and register midwives and that a Parliamentary Select Committee be asked for. A Committee was appointed in 1892, and in its report stated that 'evidence has shown that there is at present serious and unnecessary loss of life and health and permanent injury to both mother and child in the treatment of childbirth, and that some legislative provision for improvement and regulation is desirable'.

Many Bills were introduced and rejected between 1895 and 1900, but in 1902 a Bill was introduced which received the Royal Assent on 31st July 1902. The Midwives Act 1902 was designed to protect women and babies of the poor, and its objective was to secure the better training of midwives and to regulate their practice. The body created to administer the Act was the Central Midwives Board.

The Midwives Act 1902 sanctioned the setting up of the Central Midwives Board (CMB), prescribed its constitution and laid down its duties and powers. The CMB was authorised to frame rules:

1 Regulating its own proceedings.

2 Regulating the issue of certificates and the conditions of admission to the roll of midwives.

3 Regulating the course of training and the conduct of examinations and the remuneration of examiners.

4 Regulating the admission to the roll of women already in practice as midwives at the passing of this Act.

5 Regulating, supervising and restricting within due limits the practice of midwives.

6 Deciding the conditions under which midwives may be suspended from practice.

7 Defining particulars required to be given in any notice under Section 10 of this Act.

Amendments were made to the Midwives Act 1902 in 1918, 1926, 1934, 1936 and 1950. The Midwives Act 1951, consolidated all previous Acts.

The Central Midwives Board

The Board (1983) consisted of seventeen members of whom seven (of whom two were certified midwives and one was a fully registered medical practitioner engaged in general practice) were appointed by the Secretary of State after consultation with such bodies and persons as appeared to him to be concerned.

Four were fully registered medical practitioners appointed, as to one each, by the Royal College of Physicians of London, the Royal College of Surgeons of England, the Royal College of Obstetricians and Gynaecologists and the Society of Community Medicine.

Four were certified midwives appointed by the Royal College of Midwives.

Two (not being midwives) were appointed, as to one each, by the County Council's Association and the Faculty of Community Medicine.

The function of the CMB was to protect the public by providing well trained midwives who were required to carry out a code of practice as laid down by the Board.

The rules of the CMB together with the Midwives' Code of Practices were incorporated in a Handbook. The rules were divided into nine Parts and seven Schedules.

Part I. Preliminary including interpretation of terminology used in the Rules and a revocation of previous Midwives Rules.

Part II. Rules Regulating the Proceedings of the Board.

Part III. Rules Regulating Training, Examinations and Admission to the Roll.

Part IV. Regulating, Supervising and Restricting Within Due Limits The Practice of Midwives.
Part V. Refresher Courses.
Part VI. Advanced Diploma in Midwifery.
Part VII. Midwife Teachers Diploma.
Part VIII. Uniform and Badge.
Part IX. Transitional Provision.

Schedule I. Certificate of Enrolment as a Midwife.
Schedule II. Subjects to be included in the Course of Training.
Schedule III. Length of Training for Persons with a Nursing Qualification.
Schedule IV. Notice of Intention to Practise.
Schedule V. Advanced Diploma in Midwifery.
Schedule VI. Midwife Teachers Diploma Course.
Schedule VII. Uniform for State Certified Midwives.

Notices concerning a midwife's code of practice

The Notices indicated a standard of practice to be observed by all midwives, and covered eighteen areas of the midwife's practice and responsibility. The last Notices to be prepared by the Board were adopted with only minimal changes by the new statutory body, and will be discussed later (see p. 498).

The Nurses, Midwives and Health Visitors Act 1979

The Nurses, Midwives and Health Visitors Act, 1979, sanctioned the setting up of the United Kingdom Central Council and the four National Boards for Nursing, Midwifery and Health Visiting, and on 1st July 1983 they replaced the nine existing statutory bodies which had been responsible for basic and postbasic education and training, and professional conduct of nurses, midwives and health visitors in the United Kingdom including the Central Midwives Board.

The United Kingdom Central Council

The United Kingdom Central Council for Nurses, Midwives and Health Visitors is responsible for maintaining a single professional register of all nurses, midwives and health visitors in the United Kingdom, developing standards of education and training, establishing and improving standards of professional conduct and protecting the public from unsafe practitioners.

The membership of the UKCC comprises seven members from each of the National Boards.

The National Boards for Nursing, Midwifery and Health Visiting

There are four National Boards, one each for England, Northern Ireland, Scotland and Wales. The original members of the Boards were appointed by the Secretary of State after consultation with the professions.

In March 1983, professional elections were held and nurses, midwives and health visitors who had opted on to the electoral role had the opportunity to vote for candidates from their profession to represent them on one of the National Boards.

The membership of the National Boards is as follows:

English National Board: thirty elected members and fifteen members appointed by ministers.

Northern Ireland National Board: twenty-four elected members and eleven members appointed by ministers.

Scottish National Board: twenty-four elected members and fifteen members appointed by ministers.

Welsh National Board: twenty-four elected members and eleven members appointed by ministers.

The elected members are in the ratio of four nurses to one midwife and one health visitor.

Each National Board appoints seven members to serve on the United Kingdom Central Council for five years.

After the elections the United Kingdom Central Council and the National Boards took over the responsibilities of the nine existing statutory bodies bringing for the first time education, training and regulation of nurses, midwives and health visitors in the United Kingdom into one co-ordinated system. Elections are to be held every five years.

Standing Midwifery Committee

The Nurses, Midwives and Health Visitors (Midwifery and Finance Committees of the National Boards) Order 1982 (1569) was laid before Parliament in November 1982 and came into operation in December 1982. It made provision for the Standing Midwifery Committee to:

> consist of not less than nine and not more than fourteen persons appointed by the Board of whom a majority shall be persons who work or have worked in the professional field of midwifery.
>
> Each National Board may appoint as members of its Midwifery Committee persons who are not members of the Board: provided that at all times each Committee shall include at least four persons who are also members of the Board which appointed them.
>
> The members of the Midwifery Committee shall include at least two registered medical practitioners appointed after consultation with bodies representative of

those parts of the medical profession from which the appointment is to be made. Each National Board shall, after consultation with its Midwifery Committee appoint one of the members of that Committee who is also a member of that Board to be Chairman of that Committee.

Functions of the Standing Midwifery Committee to the Board

1 The execution of all matters concerning midwifery practice.
2 Within the agreed policy extant at the time, the execution of matters concerned with the approval of training institutions, examinations and initiation courses.

The Professional Officer (Midwifery) is the serving officer to the Midwifery Committee.

The English National Board Midwifery Committee

The Committee comprises fourteen members; ten Board members and four co-opted non-Board members. The ten Board members are made up of five midwives, an obstetrician, a general medical practitioner, a health visitor, a registered nurse tutor and a registered sick children's nurse. The four non-Board members are midwives.

Local supervision of midwives

Local Supervising Authorities were set up under the Midwives Act 1902 to exercise general supervision over all midwives practising in their areas in accordance with the rules of the Central Midwives Board. On 1st April 1974 in accordance with Schedule 4 of the National Health Service Reorganisation Act 1973, the statutory responsibility of local supervising authorities under the Midwives Act 1951 was transferred from Local Health Authorities to Regional Health Authorities. The Nurses, Midwives and Health Visitors Act 1979 provides for all the continuance of the system of local supervision in accordance with the United Kingdom Central Council's Rules (see p. 495). The scope of these responsibilities extends not only to midwives employed in the National Health Service but also to those employed by voluntary and religious organisations, other Government Departments, i.e. Ministry of Defence and the Home Office, private nursing homes, employment agencies and midwives in private practice.

The duty of every local supervising authority is as follows:
1 To receive, see and act on notifications of intention to practise from all midwives within the geographical area.
2 To receive, see and act on all other notifications of intention to practise from midwives in domiciliary, institutional, public and private practice.

3 To ensure that all midwives in the area of the local supervising authority who have notified their intention to practise shall comply with the rules of attendance at a Statutory Postgraduate Course. Special attention should be paid to the organisation of refresher courses for midwives returning to practice after six years.
4 To prepare a report for the National Board on midwives who have been charged with misconduct under the Council's Disciplinary Rules.
5 To ensure that the Health Authorities arrange for the supervision of midwives referred from the Council for a probationary period.
6 Appropriate professional support for midwives in dealing with the medical practitioner in accordance with notice Number 1 of the Midwives' Code of Practice would be provided in the first instance by the Health Authority but if necessary ultimate responsibility must be with the Regional Health Authority.
7 Duties under Statute (as amended), other than the Nurses, Midwives and Health Visitors Act 1979 and Regulations, e.g. Misuse of Drugs Regulations 1973 and the Misuse of Drugs (Amendment) Regulations 1974, Notification of Births Act 1907, Population Statistics Act 1960 (cause of stillbirths), Births and Deaths Registration Act 1936.
8 Other responsibilities under Section 10 (1) of the Nurses, Midwives and Health Visitor Act 1979 not covered.

Rule 63 of the United Kingdom Central Council sets out the statutory duty of the local supervising authority regarding suspension of a midwife from practice.

1 It shall be the duty of the local supervising authority to suspend a midwife from practice when necessary for the purpose of preventing the spread of infection, whether or not she has contravened any of the rules laid down by the Council.
2 The local supervising authority may suspend from practice until the case has been decided:

a a midwife against whom it has taken proceedings before a Court of Justice;
b a midwife against whom it has reported a case for investigation to a Board;
c a midwife who has been referred to the Professional Conduct Committee of the Council;
d a midwife who has been referred to the Health Committee of the Council.

3 A local supervising authority, in discharging any duty imposed on it by section 16 (1) (b) of the Act, or in exercising the power given in sub-paragraph 2 of this rule to suspend a midwife from practice, shall:

a notify the midwife concerned in writing of any decision to suspend her; and
b in the case of a suspension authorised by paragraph 2 of this rule, forthwith report any such suspension and the grounds thereof to a Board and/or the Council, as may be appropriate.

The National Health Service Reorganisation Act 1973 placed responsibility for the supervision of midwives on the Regional Health Authority (RHA) but although the ultimate responsibility remains with the RHA there are many of the functions of supervision that were carried out through the Area Health Authorities until 1st April 1983, when these bodies were taken over by the District Health Authorities.

It is the responsibility of the Regional Health Authority or, in Wales, the District Health Authority, as the supervising authority to ensure that each Health District has local Supervisors of Midwives to carry out the duties of supervision of midwives.

Supervisor of Midwives

Prior to reorganisation of the Health Service, the Medical Officer of Health for the Local Health Authority was designated supervisor of midwives. Many of the tasks were delegated to a senior midwife working in the community who was known as the non-medical supervisor of midwives. After 1st April 1974, the role of supervisor of midwives was invested with a senior midwife working in the health district.

Qualifications of Supervisors of Midwives

1 A person to be appointed under section 16 of the Act by a local supervising authority to exercise supervision of midwives shall:

- **a** be a registered midwife; and
- **b** have had three years' experience as a practising midwife, not less than one year of which shall have been in the two years immediately preceding the appointment; and
- **c** except in the case of a person who has given a written undertaking to attend an induction course within six months of appointment, shall have completed such a course not more than three years prior to the appointment.

'The supervising authority is responsible through the local Supervisor of Midwives for providing/organising training facilities for all midwives to acquire and maintain a satisfactory level of competence. For this purpose the Supervisor of Midwives should be familiar with the post-basic training requirements of all midwives practising under her jurisdiction and should satisfy herself of the competence of the individual midwife to ensure she is not proposing to undertake procedures for which she has not been properly trained. In undertaking these statutory responsibilities the Supervisor will need to work with those midwives responsible for specific areas of midwifery practice within her supervisory boundaries.'

The system of supervision should provide the midwife with the appropriate professional support which she may require in the general conduct of her practice. In any case of difficulty or doubt the midwife should consult with her supervisor; for example, if a woman requests a home confinement and the midwife considers the accommodation and facilities to be unsuitable, she should notify her Supervisor of Midwives; if a midwife is asked for confidential information by the police, she should immediately report such a request to her supervisor.

The Supervisor of Midwives authorises the Drug Supply Order which enables the midwife to obtain a supply of pethidine for use in her practice.

The Supervisor of Midwives is responsible for the day to day supervision of midwives and receives the Notices of Intention to Practise on behalf of the local supervising authority.

Chapter 18
The Practice of Midwifery

Handbook of Midwives Rules

The United Kingdom Central Council for Nursing, Midwifery and Health Visiting issues a Handbook of Midwives Rules which comprises Part V of the Nurses, Midwives and Health Visitors Rules Approval Order 1983, Statutory Instrument 1983 No. 873.

The Midwives Rules are divided into four sections:

Section A Rules regulating Kind and Standard of Training and Examination;

Section B Diplomas in Midwifery;

Section C Rules Regulating, Supervising and Restricting Within Due Limits the Practice of Midwifery;

Section D Refresher Courses.

The following is a summary of Section C of the Rules as they relate to midwives practising in England and Wales:

Section C Rules Regulating, Supervising and Restricting Within Due Limits the Practice of Midwives.

53 Form of notice of intention to practise

1a Every registered midwife shall, before holding herself out as a practising midwife or commencing to practise as a midwife in any area, give notice of her intention to do so to the local supervising authority, and shall give a like notice in the month of January in every year thereafter during which she continues to practise in that area.

b Such notice shall be given to the local supervising authority of the area within which the midwife carries out her practice, and the like notice shall be given to every other local supervising authority within whose area she at any time practises or acts as a midwife, within forty-eight hours at the latest after she commenced so to practise or act.

c Every notice shall contain such particulars as may be required by the Council using the form prescribed in Schedule 11 which shall include date of attendance at an appropriate refresher course.

d The local supervising authority shall supply the Board during the month of February each year, the names and addresses of all midwives who during the period of twelve months ending with the 31st January in that year, have notified the authority of their intention to practise within that area.

54 Restriction of treatment

A practising midwife shall not, except in an emergency, give any treatment which she has not been trained to give either before or after registration as a midwife, or which is outside her sphere of practice.

55 Restriction of the use of drugs

1. A practising midwife shall not on her own responsibility administer any drug, including an analgesic, unless in the course of her training, whether before or after registration as a midwife, she has been thoroughly instructed in its use and is familiar with its dosage and methods of administration or application.

2a A practising midwife shall not, except on the instructions and in the presence of a registered medical practitioner, administer an inhalational analgesic to a patient unless:

(i) she is satisfied from an examination of the patient by a registered medical practitioner during pregnancy that there is no contraindication to the administration of the analgesic;

(ii) she has, either before or after registration as a midwife, received, at a training school approved by a Board for the purpose, instruction in the essential of obstetric analgesia.

b A practising midwife shall not administer an inhalational analgesic by the use of any type of apparatus unless:

(i) that type of apparatus is for the time being approved by the Council on the recommendation of a Board as suitable for use by midwives; and

(ii) where the Council on the recommendation of a Board so directs in relation to certain types of apparatus, the type of apparatus has been inspected and approved by or on behalf of the Council (within such period before the date of administration as the Council may determine), as fit for use by midwives and a certificate to that effect, signed on behalf of the Council is in the possession of the body or person by whom the apparatus is held.

c The type of apparatus approved by the Central Midwives Board prior to the 1st July 1983 shall be deemed to have been approved by the Council and any certificate shall be treated as having been signed by the Council unless the Council gives notice to the contrary.

56 Restriction on administration of anaesthetics

Unless special exemption is given by the Council to enable a particular hospital to investigate new methods, a practising midwife must not administer any anaesthetic otherwise than on the instruction and in the presence of a registered medical practitioner.

57 Duty to record administration of drugs

A practising midwife who administers or applies in any way any drug other than an aperient must make a proper record of the name and dose of the drug and the date, time and method of its administration or application.

58 Duty to carry out instructions of registered medical practitioner

In any case where a registered medical practitioner responsible for providing maternity services to a patient is exercising personal supervision and direction the following provisions shall apply:

a where the medical practitioner is personally present, a practising midwife must carry out the instructions of the medical practitioner in relation to the care and treatment of the patient;

b where the medical practitioner is not present, a practising midwife must exercise her professional skill and judgment in accordance with these rules, and in doing so she must comply with the wishes of the medical practitioner save insofar as in so complying she would break any of these rules or act outside her sphere of practice.

59 Duty to keep records

1 A midwife must record her personal observations and details of the care of her patient during pregnancy, labour and the postnatal period, using for the purpose the form approved by the Council from time to time.

2 In a hospital, nursing home or similar institution where a register or record is kept which incorporates the requirements prescribed in the approved form, it shall be the duty of the midwife in attendance on a patient to see that the appropriate records are completed.

3 A midwife must not destroy or arrange for the destruction of official records made whilst she is in professional attendance on a case and required to be kept by these rules; if she finds it impossible or inconvenient to preserve them she must transfer them to the local supervising authority or to her employing authority, and details of the transfer must be duly recorded.

60 Emergency medical treatment

1 In the event of an emergency a practising midwife shall call in to her assistance a registered medical practitioner, and shall forthwith report the matter to the local supervising authority stating the nature of the emergency and the name of the practitioner called in.

2 A practising midwife who in compliance with paragraph 1 of this rule has called in a registered medical practitioner to assist her in an emergency shall:

a note the facts in her records

b obtain the instructions or learn the wishes of the practitioner to enable her to comply with rule 58 and note such instructions or wishes in her records.

61 Duty to allow inspection

A practising midwife shall give to her supervisor of midwives every reasonable facility to inspect her methods of practice, her appliances, her personal register of cases and other records and such part of her residence as may be used for professional purposes.

62 Duty to be medically examined

A practising midwife shall, if the local supervising authority deem it necessary for preventing the spread of infection, allow herself to be medically examined.

Section D Refresher Courses

85 Duty to attend courses

1 Subject to paragraph 2 of this rule and to rule 88 every registered midwife who gives notice of intention of practise under rule 53 shall within the period of twelve months beginning with the date of such a notice, attend a course of instruction approved by a Board for the purpose of this rule.

2 Paragraph 1 of this rule shall not apply to a registered midwife:

a to whom rule 86 applied, or

b who has within the period of five years immediately preceding the date of giving notice of intention to practise attended a course or passed an examination prescribed by a Board.

86 Courses for midwives who have not practised for six years or more

Subject to the provision of rule 88, every midwife who gives notice of her intention to practise under rule 53 and who has not practised as a midwife at any time during the period of six years immediately preceding the date of giving such notice, although on the part of the register for midwives throughout such period, shall, within a period of three months beginning with that date, attend a course of practical and theoretical instruction approved by a Board for the purpose of this rule; and she shall not practise as a midwife without the consent of the local supervising authority before she has satisfactorily completed such a course.

The Handbook of Midwives Rules contains schedules. The Schedules relating to England and Wales are:

Schedule I	Rule 28 Subjects to be included in the course of training
Schedule II	Rules 53, 66 and 80 Notice of Intention to Practise
Schedule III	Rule 44 Advance Diploma in Midwifery Course in Preparation for the above Diploma
Schedule IV	Midwife Teacher's Diploma Course Requirements for Approval of Courses of Teacher Training leading to the award of the Midwife Teacher's Diploma
Schedule V	Rule 47 Uniform for Midwives

United Kingdom Central Council for Nurses, Midwifery and Health Visiting Notices concerning a Midwives' Code of Practice for Midwives practising in England and Wales 1983.

The Notices are not Rules and are not included in a statutory Instrument. They are complementary to the United Kingdom Central Council Midwives Rules for England and Wales and indicate a standard of practice to be observed by midwives. Failure to maintain that standard may render a midwife liable to a charge of negligence or misconduct.

Notices Concerning a Midwives' Code of Practice

1 Midwife/Doctor Relationship

The Notice recognises the variations in and therefore the impracticability of defining the professional relationship of practising midwives with registered medical practitioners, but indicates principles which midwives should follow in their relationships with doctors.

The midwife is required to carry out the instructions of the doctor when he is present and his wishes if he is not present unless, in the latter, they would conflict with any of the Council's Rules, in which case she must exercise her skill and professional judgement in accordance with the Rules. The Notice reminds the midwife of the support of the local Supervisor of Midwives and the over-riding importance of the welfare of the mother and baby.

2 Limits of Practice

The original midwifery legislation was designed to protect mothers and babies of the poor, and all subsequent legislation has continued this high ideal; therefore, the statutory body required to administer the Act, previously the Central Midwives Board and now the United Kingdom Central Council, determines the limits within which the midwife is allowed to practise and places the responsibility on the midwife to be aware of the limits and for maintaining her competence to work within those limits.

3 Prevention of Infection
'A midwife must recognise the dangers of infection. Sterilised surgical gloves must be worn during the delivery and when making vaginal examinations.'
4 Drugs which may be Carried and Used by Midwives
This Notice lists drugs and preparations which should ordinarily be carried by a midwife. They are antiseptics, aperients, sedatives and analgesics, a local anaesthetic, an oxytoxic preparation and approved agents for neonatal and maternal resuscitation. The actual drugs and preparations the midwife carries is determined by the employing authority.
5 Supply of Prescription Only Drugs to Midwives
'Certain drugs which are normally only available on a prescription issued by a medical practitioner may be supplied to midwives for use in their practice under Part III of the Medicines Act 1968. These drugs are listed in Schedule IV Part III of the Medicines (Prescriptions Only) Order 1980, and any subsequent amendments.'
6 Use of Controlled Drugs
'The use of controlled drugs by midwives is covered by the Misuse of Drugs Regulations 1973, and the Misuse of Drugs (Amendment) Regulations 1974.'

This Notice distinguishes between midwives working in hospital and midwives working in domiciliary practice. In hospital all controlled drugs must be checked by a second responsible person (preferably a trained nurse or a student), who must also witness the administration. Neonatal drugs must be checked by two professionally qualified persons. 'The senior midwife on duty is responsible for the contents of the drug cupboard, and these must be checked each time she assumes responsibility.'

The Misuse of Drugs Regulations provide for the suppply of pethidine to midwives in domiciliary practice. If the woman is cared for or transferred to a hospital those drugs must not be used.
7 Destruction of Controlled Drugs
'The Misuse of Drugs Regulations lay down a procedure by which midwives may surrender stocks of unwanted drugs to an appropriate medical officer, but not to a Supervisor of Midwives, and also a procedure for the destruction of pethidine no longer required. This may be done by a midwife herself, but only in the presence of an 'authorised person', who may be one of the following: a police officer; an inspector of the Home Office Drugs Branch; an inspector of the Pharmaceutical Society of Great Britain; the senior administrative officer employed in the administration of a National Health Service hospital; a regional pharmaceutical officer in England or a pharmaceutical advisor in Wales; and medical officers of the Welsh Office Regional Medical Service.'
8 Arranging a Substitute
'A midwife must not arrange for any other person than a midwife or registered medical practitioner to act as her substitute.'

9–12 Duties of a Midwife During the Antenatal Period, Labour, the Postnatal Period and to the Baby

These Notices indicate a standard of practice for midwives when providing care during the antenatal period, labour, the postnatal period and to the baby, and include the requirement that in the event of any illness or abnormality becoming apparent the midwife has a duty to seek medical aid. The role of the midwife in health education is emphasised, including promotion of breast feeding.

13 Duties to Regard Information as Confidential

This Notice deals with the confidential nature of any information derived from professional attendance on a woman and offers the following guidelines:

a 'A midwife should not supply information to the police or anyone else simply in response to a police request for information, even though the matter being investigated appears to be a serious one;

b She should immediately report such a request to her Supervisor of Midwives;

c She must make a note in her records of the request, nature of the request and the fact of her report to her Supervisor;

d She should not allow herself to be drawn into conversation with the policeman, however pressing his request for information may be.'

14 Advertising

This Notice gives guidance about advertisement of a midwife's service which is not prohibited by the Rules, but must not seek 'to promote professional advantage by indicating a standard of practice superior to that of other members of the profession'. Failure to adhere to this Notice could leave the midwife open to a charge of misconduct.

15 Calling in of Medical Aid

This Notice explains that 'illness' and 'abnormality' includes past illness and abnormality. It also draws attention to the importance of the strictest observance of the provision of the Rules relating to the calling in of medical aid and refers the midwife to the arrangements for maternity medical services in the National Health Service. In the first instance the midwife should contact the medical practitioner who has accepted responsibility to the maternity medical services of the woman; if he or his deputy is not available or if the woman has no doctor who has accepted responsibility for her maternity care, the midwife should call a doctor whose name is on the list of medical practitioners having obstetric experience. If the medical aid is required after the fourteenth day, but before the twenty-eighth day of the postnatal period, the doctor providing general medical care or, if he is not available, any other registered medical practitioner should be called.

16 Record Keeping

'In accordance with the Rules the midwife is required to keep detailed records of all cases she attends.

It is important that these records should be made at the time of attendance, that they should be as clear and as detailed as possible, since in the event of any query subsequently arising in a particular case, they may be required as proof that the midwife has carried out her duties correctly.'

17 Preservation of Records

'The Congenital Disabilities (Civil Liability) Act 1976 provides that a child may be entitled to recover damages where he has suffered as a result of a breach in a duty of care owed to the mother or the father, unless that breach of duty of care occurred before the child was conceived and either or both parents knew of the occurrence (see p. 478). It follows, therefore, that the preservation of records relating to birth may require special consideration and no midwife should take responsibility for the destruction of such records. The duty of the midwife is set out in the Rules (see p. 495).

18 Notification of Change of Name and/or Address

'A midwife is required to notify, in writing, the United Kingdom Central Council and her Local Supervising Authority of any change of name and/or address which may occur.'

19 Duties Imposed on a Midwife by Rules

This Notice refers to the midwife's duty regarding notice of intention to practise (see p. 495).

20 Duties Imposed on Midwives by Statute

'Under the Births and Deaths Registration Acts and the Public Health Acts, a midwife must in certain cases notify the Registrar of Births and Deaths and the appropriate medical officer (see p. 445).

This Notice also includes, for the purpose of the registration of births and deaths, the definition of a live birth (see p. 444) and a stillbirth (see p. 446).

Chapter 19
The Midwife

The World Health Organisation's definition of a midwife is as follows:

A Midwife is a person who, having been regularly admitted to a midwifery educational programme, duly recognised in the country in which it is located, has successfully completed the prescribed course of studies in midwifery and has acquired the requisite qualification to be registered and/or legally licensed to practise midwifery.

Sphere of Practice

She must be able to give the necessary supervision, care and advice to women during pregnancy, labour and the postpartum period, to conduct deliveries on her own responsibility and to care for the newborn and the infant. This care includes preventative measures, the detection of abnormal conditions in mother and child, the procurement of medical assistance and the execution of emergency measures in the absence of medical help. She has an important task in health counselling and education, not only for patients but also within the family and community. The work should involve antenatal education and preparation for parenthood and extend to certain areas of gynaecology, family planning and child care. She may practise in hospitals, clinics, health units, domiciliary conditions or in any other service.

Article 4 of the European Economic Community Midwives Directives (1) states:

Member States shall ensure that midwives are at least entitled to take up and pursue the following activities:

1 to provide sound family planning information and advice;

2 to diagnose pregnancies and monitor normal pregnancies; to carry out the examinations necessary for the monitoring of the development of normal pregnancies;

3 to prescribe or advise on the examinations necessary for the earliest possible diagnosis of pregnancies at risk;

4 to provide a programme of parenthood preparation and a complete preparation for childbirth including advice on hygiene and nutrition;

5 to care for and assist the mother during labour and to monitor the condition of the fetus in utero by the appropriate clinical and technical means;

6 to conduct spontaneous deliveries including where required an episiotomy and in urgent cases a breech delivery;

7 to recognise the warning signs of abnormality in the mother or infant which necessitates referral to a doctor and to assist the latter where appropriate; to take the necessary emergency measures in the doctor's absence, in particular the manual removal of the placenta, possibly followed by manual examination of the uterus;

8 to examine and care for the newborn infant; to take all initiatives which are necessary in case of need and to carry out where necessary immediate resuscitation;
9 to care for and monitor the progress of the mother in the postnatal period and to give all necessary advice to the mother on infant care to enable her to ensure the optimum progress of the newborn infant;
10 to carry out the treatment prescribed by a doctor;
11 to maintain all necessary records.

The term midwife is universal, but the training status and legal responsibility vary widely. In the United Kingdom the midwife is recognised as a practitioner in her own right entitled to practice within a limited sphere. She is trained and qualified to give comprehensive care and advice during pregnancy, labour and the postnatal period, and to care for the newborn baby.

Antenatal care

Care during the antenatal period involves monitoring the physical and emotional well being of the expectant mother and the growth and well being of the fetus by regular clinical examinations that will detect any deviations from normal. The midwife may work in general practitioners' surgeries, health centres or in hospital antenatal clinics, and make visits to expectant mothers in their homes to make examinations and discuss arrangements for home confinement or early transfer home after the birth of the baby. In addition the midwife prepares couples for labour and parenthood, and advises about the social services and benefits available to the woman and her family.

Management of labour

The midwife is trained to use her skills and judgment to provide physical care and psychological support for women during normal labour and immediate care of the newborn, and to recognise deviations from normal that require referral to a doctor. She is the senior person present at over 70% of deliveries. The midwife is authorised to use specific drugs for the relief of pain in labour and to control haemorrhage.

Postnatal care

The midwife's duties during the postnatal period include care of the mother and baby up to twenty-eight days following delivery, and the initiation of an infant feeding regime. While the midwife should encourage mothers to breast feed their babies she is responsible for teaching alternative methods of feeding and providing support to the mother in achieving a satisfactory feeding routine. She should discuss the various methods of contraception and family planning services available.

The midwife must at all times be able to recognise abnormal or potentially abnormal conditions which necessitate referral to a doctor. She is also trained to carry out emergency measures until the arrival of a doctor.

Factors that have influenced the practice of the midwife in the maternity services in recent years include:

1 The reorganisation of the National Health Service in 1974 involving the integration of the maternity services under the direction of the new Health Authorities resulting in the midwifery services being centred on the place where the confinement occurs and being organised from the hospital.

2 Shared antenatal care in many cases was interpreted as care provided by the obstetric medical team in hospital and the general practitioner relegating many midwives working in hospital and in the community to the role of maternity nurse.

3 The progressive fall in the birth rate between 1964 and 1977.

4 A hospital confinement rate of over 98%. The decline in domiciliary confinements led to a reduction in midwives employed by local authorities before the integration of the maternity services. Following reorganisation, many midwives based in the community have attended women in labour in hospital for whom they have given antenatal care and will continue care during the postnatal period.

5 The role of the midwife in the management of labour changed with the introduction of mechanical aids to induce or accelerate labour and monitor the fetus and the midwife was required to develop expertise in using technical aids as well as retaining her traditional skills. In this environment the midwife worked more closely with obstetricians who became more actively involved, although the immediate care of the woman remained largely the concern of the midwife. Not surprisingly, many midwives found difficulties in adopting and adjusting to the changes and suffered a crisis of identity that has taken some time to resolve. A more rational approach to intervening in the progress of labour has resulted in midwives once more beginning to re-establish their role although there is still some progress to be made.

6 The upsurge of consumer groups critical of the dehumanising effects of the hospital-based maternity services and the interventionist approach to labour has led midwives to evaluate their practice and adopt a more flexible approach to care that takes account of the woman's preference for her personal care and that of her baby.

7 Early transfer of mothers and babies from hospital to home. This has reduced the involvement of the hospital-based midwife in postnatal care beyond the third day and increased the involvement of the community-based midwives.

Index

Abbreviations 3–5
ABO blood group
  incompatibility 365
    and jaundice 363
  investigations 39
Abdominal examination 39, 46–49
  abnormal lie and shoulder presentation 263
  antepartum haemorrhage 182–3
  in breech presentation 253
  in brow presentation 262
  in cephalopelvic disproportion 266
  in face presentation 259–60
  labour, first stage 146, 147, 150–51
  in occipitoposterior position 250
  postnatal 164, 168
  in prolonged labour 270
Abdominal wall abnormalities, neonatal 388–9
Abnormal lie and shoulder presentation 263–4
  cause 263
  diagnosis 263
  management 264
Abortion 171–6
  Act 175
  illegal 176
  induced 175–6
  legal (therapeutic) 175
  obstetric history 36
  septic 176
  spontaneous 171–4
    causes 172
    complete 173
    conceptus abnormality 172
    habitual 174
    incomplete 173
    missed 174
    threatened 172–3
  tubal 178
Abrasions, birth trauma 350
Abscess, breast 298
Acidosis, correction, in asphyxia 346
  in respiratory distress syndrome 362
Acts of Parliament 443
Admission, first stage of labour 144
Adoption 434–6
  Act 436
  affiliation order 43
  application 435
  certificate 435–6
  court proceedings 432–4
  methods of placing 435
  putative father 435
Adrenal glands in pregnancy 29
Air embolism 286
Alcohol 9, 41, 467
Alcopar (bephenium hydroxynaphthoate) in hookworm 218
Alphafetoprotein
  amniotic fluid 475
  maternal serum 40
Alkaline phosphatase, heat stable, placental 324
Amenorrhoea 17, 20, 22
Aminophylline in pulmonary oedema 224
Aminion, anatomy 95
Amnionitis 373
Aminotic fluid 102–5, 311
  amount 102
  biochemistry and cytology 317–8, 475
  circulation 102
  composition 102
  embolism 285–6
  functions 102–3
  oligohydramnios 105
  polyhydramnios 103–5
Amniotomy 238–9
  contraindications 238
  dangers 239

Amniotomy (*cont.*)
management 239
technique 238
Ampicillin in pyelonephritis 202, 203,
Anaemia 215–21
in Asian, women 405
children 406
chronic, following haemorrhage 187
effects on pregnancy 221
folic acid deficiency 218–19
haemoglobinopathies 219–21
haemolytic anaemia 221
heart disease 222
iron deficiency anaemia 216–18
parasitic infestation 218
physiological 215
in pregnancy 216
in pre-term infant 357
sickle cell 219–20
thalassaemia 220–21
twin pregnancy 207
Anaesthesia
hazards 291–4
causes of death 292
hypoxic cardiac arrest 294
intubation difficulty 294
Mendelson's syndrome 292–3
management 293
prevention 292–3
misuse of apparatus 293
Analgesia
epidural, in maternal heart disease 224–5
inhalational, administration by midwife 153, 496
first stage of labour 153
regional, first stage 153–5
caudal 154
epidural 153–5
Analgesics 152–3
Ancoloxin 189
Anencephaly 389
Anoxia causing birth trauma 347
Antenatal care 32–56
aims 32
Antepartum haemorrhage 179–88
Caesarean section 184, 185
classification 179–80
differential diagnosis 182–3
indication for induction of labour 237
labour 185
management 183–5
maternal dangers/complications 186–7
mortality 187
placental localisation 184
signs and symptoms 182–3
in twin pregnancy 207
see also Placenta praevia: Placental abruption
Antibody screening 39, 49
Anticoagulants, intravenous and oral, in phlebothrombosis 300–1
Anticonvulsant drugs in epilepsy 230
Antigen D
absence 364
anti-D immunoglobulin 367–8
Apgar score 344–5
Asphyxia neonatorum 343–6
Apgar Score 344–5
causes 343–4
endotracheal intubation 345–6
in light-for-dates infants 359
management 345–6
mild 344, 362
in pre-term infant 353
resuscitation 345
severe 344, 345–6
types of asphyxia 344
Asthma, during pregnancy 229
mortality 229
Asynclitism
'At risk' fetus 318–20
fetal factors 319–20
maternal factors 318–9
'At risk' infants 346, 397–8
categories 397
family 397
labour 397
neonatal 397–8
prenatal 397
handicap register 398
'At Risk' Register 424–5
criteria for admitting 424
handicap, categories 425
Atrial septal defect 222, 384
Attendance allowance 440–1
Auscultation, during pregnancy 48–9
Autism 436–8
Axis traction forceps 288

Bacillus proteus causing pyelonephritis 203
Backache in pregnancy 25

Bacterial endocarditis 223
Bacteriuria in renal disease 202
  asymptomatic 202
Ballottement, internal and external 21
Bandl's ring 245
Barlow's modification of Ortolanis's test 336, 382
Barrier methods of contraception 419–20
Barrier nursing 375
Bartholin's glands, anatomy 59
Bathing, baby, teaching 53
Battledore placenta 98
BCG vaccination 228
Bephenium hydroxynaphthoate (Alcopar) in hookworm 218
Bereavement 460–4
Bile duct, atresia or absence causing jaundice 365
Bilirubin, conjugation 364
  serum levels 363, 368
Birth
  certification 446
  control, methods 417–23
  notification 445
  rate 444
  registration 445–6
  trauma 346–50
    extracranial 346–7
    eyes, injury 350
    cerebral irritation, signs 348
    intracranial 347–9
    muscular injury 350
    nerve injury 349
    skeletal injury 349
    skin injury 350
Bladder
  anatomy and physiology 139–41
    blood supply 141
    ligaments 141
    lymphatic drainage 141
    micturition, physiology 141–2
    structure 140–1
  care during fast stage 146
    in prolonged labour 269
  postnatal 162, 164
Blastocyst 15
  anatomy 87
  implantation 88
Bleeding in early pregnancy 171–9
  abortion 171–6
  carcinoma 179
  causes 172
  cervical erosion 179
  decidual 171
  ectopic pregnancy 178–9
  hydatidiform mole 176–7
  implantation 171
  polyp, cervical 179
Blood
  changes at birth 332
  coagulation, and antepartum haemorrhage 186
  groups and haemolytic disease of the newborn 364
    see also ABO blood group: Rhesus factor
  investigations, in pregnancy 39–40, 49
  mole 174
  normal values in pregnancy 28–9
  pressure in eclampsia 196–7
    estimation 39, 45
    in pre-eclampsia 191, 195
    in pregnancy 28
    in puerperium 163
  transfusion in iron deficiency anaemia 218
  volume in pregnancy 27
Booking arrangements for confinement 43
  home assessment 44–5
Bowel, care
  during first stage 146
  in puerperium 164
Brachial neuralgia in pregnancy 26
Brachial plexus injuries 349
Bradycardia, fetal 326
Braxton Hicks contractions 21, 46, 70
Breast
  care during pregnancy 42
    in puerperium 166
  changes, early, in pregnancy 17–18
    second trimester 20
  examination, routine 38
  feeding after birth 162, 337
    advantages 339
    complementary feeds 339
    contraindications 340
  infections 297–8
    abscess 298
    predisposing causes 297–8
    signs and symptoms 298
  milk, composition 133
    flow 131–2
    inhibition 167

Breast (*cont.*)
production 131
withdrawal 132
see also Mammary gland 129–32
Breech presentation 252–9
antenatal management 253
assisted delivery 257–8
delay of aftercoming head 257–8
delay in descent 257
extended arms 257
Burns-Marshall technique 257, 258
dangers 259
diagnosis 253
external cephalic version 253–4
dangers 254
extraction 259
indication for induction 254
Lovsett manoeuvre 257
management of labour 254–5
first stage 254–5
mechanism 255
second stage 255
Mauriceau-Smellie-Veit manoeuvre 257–8
mechanism 255–6
mortality rate 259
positions 253
spontaneous delivery 256–7
Bromocriptine 167
Bronchitis, chronic, during pregnancy 229
Brow presentation 261–3
cause 262
diagnosis 262
management 262–3
Bruising at birth 350
Bupivocaine (Marcain) 354
Burns-Marshall technique 257, 258
Buttocks, sore 395–6

Caesarean section 289–91
in abnormal lie and shoulder presentation 264
in antepartum haemorrhage 185, 186
in breech presentation 253
in brow presentation 263
in face presentation 261
indications 290
maternal mortality 290
risk to fetus 291
types 290
Candicidin (Candeptin) 232
Candidiasis 232
Caput succedaneum 125, 346
Cardiac catheterisation 385
Cardiac disease in pregnancy 221–7
causes 222
contraceptive advice 226
cyanotic heart disease 224
grades of functional capacity 222
management, general 222–6
of labour 224–5
of pregnancy 222–3
of puerperium 255
maternal mortality 227
specific malformations 226
pulmonary oedema 224
social aspects 226
Cardiac output in pregnancy 27
Cardiff Infusion Unit 240
management 253
Cardiff inhaler 153
Cardiovascular
aspects of pregnancy 27–29
system, abnormalities 384–5
changes at birth 332
Care plan, midwifery 38, 144
Carneous mole 179
Central Midwives Board 152, 153, 155, 487–9
constitution 488
Handbook Incorporating Rules 448–9
Central nervous system, abnormalities 389–90
Cephalhaematoma 125, 346
Cephalopelvic disproportion 265–7
abdominal examination 266
cause 265
Caesarean section 267
indications 265
for induction of labour 237
management 267
pelvic assessment 266
prolonged labour 267–73
first stage 268–271
second stage 272–3
third stage 273
trial of labour 266–7
X-ray examination 266
Cerebral irritation, at birth
management 348–9
signs 348
Cervical cap 420
Cervical cytology 423–4

Cervical dystocia 246
Cervix, uterine
  anatomy 64–5
  changes during pregnancy 18, 68
  effacement and dilation 75–6
  reforming 79
Chest in pre-term infant 353
Chignon, caused by vacuum extractor 347
Child, children
  abuse 428–9
  benefit 440
Child Care Act 432
Children Act 431, 432, 433, 436
  health services 424–6
    'at-risk' registers 424–5
    centres 424
    pre-school 424–5
    school 425
    unification 424
    vaccination and immunisation 426
  minding 429
  social services 427–38
    adoption 434–6
    children in care 430–2
    day care 429–30
    education 430
    fostering 431
    handicapped 436–8
  special allowance 440
Chilling, neonatal
  management 393
  prevention 392
  results 393
Chloasma 19
Chlorpromazine (Largactil) 304
Choanal atresia 385–6
Chorion
  epithelioma 177
  frondosum 92, 94
  hydatidiform mole 176–7
  laeve 95, 96
  primitive 91
Chorionic gonadotrophin, human
  excretion levels 321
    and hydatidiform mole 176–7, 321
    multiple pregnancy 321
    normal pregnancy 100
  function 16, 100
Chorionic somatomammotrophin 101
Chromosomal abnormalities 390–2
Chromosomes 467
  mutation 470–1
Circulation, fetal 312–5
Clavicle, fracture at birth 349
Cleft lip and cleft palate 386
Clinitest/stix 380
Clitoris, anatomy 58
Clothing during pregnancy 41
Coagulation disorder, causing haemorrhage 186, 277
Coarctation of the aorta 385
  pregnancy complicating 222
Coccygeus muscle 116
Coccyx, anatomy 107
Coitus
  during pregnancy 42
  interruptus 419
Cold injury, neonatal 392–3
  chilling
    prevention 392
    results 393
  management 393
Colostrum, composition 133
Community Health Councils 414–5
Compound presentation 265
  management 265
Congenital abnormalities, neonatal 381–92
  in pre-term infants 354
Congenital Disabilities (Civil Liability) Act 1976 478–83, 501
Congenital dislocation of the hip 382–3
Conjunctivitis 376
Constipation in pregnancy 25
Continuous positive airway pressure 363
Contraception 417–23
  postnatal 168
Contraceptive(s) 417–23
  advice, and heart disease of pregnancy 226
  history and pregnancy 34
  injectables 418
  methods 417–23
  oral 417–18
    contraindications 418
    effects 16, 418
    pre-conception 8
Contractions, uterine
  abnormal 243–6
    hypertonic 245–6, 268, 270
    hypotonic 244, 268, 270

Contractions (*cont.*)
  Braxton Hick 21, 46, 70
  delay in recommencement in twin pregnancy 209
  and fetal distress 326
  first stage of labour 72–4, 147
  hypertonic, prolonged labour 268, 270
  hypotonic and post partum haemorrhage 274–5
    prolonged labour 268, 270, 272
    and retained placenta 278
  muscles, first stage 72–6
  suppression, in premature labour 242–3
    drugs 242–3
    infusion 242
    intramuscular injection 243
    oral 243
Convulsions
  in eclampsia 195–6
    control 196
  neonatal 396
Cord, umbilical, *see* Umbilical cord
Corpus albicans 86
Corpus luteum 14, 85
Corticosteroids in pregnancy 29
Counselling 464–5
Cow's milk allergy 395
Cramp in pregnancy 26
Cravings in pregnancy 30
Cri du chat syndrome 391
Cyanotic heart disease 224
Cystic fibrosis, clinical features 381
  diagnosis 381
  incidence 381
  treatment 381
Cytology, cervical 423–4
  fetal 318, 475
Cytomegalovirus, neonatal 373, 467
Cytotrophoblast 90, 91

Day care, children 429–32
Day nurseries 429
Deafness, congenital 372
Decidua
  formation 91
  parts 91
  shedding 79
Deep transverse arrest 251
Definitions 5–7
Delivery
  conduct 157–60
  estimated date 35
  preparation 157
  of twins 208–10
  see also Labour
Demand feeding 166, 339
Dental
  care during pregnancy 41
  pre-conception 9
  caries 222
  treatment, free 441–2
Department of Health and Social Security 412
Depo-provera 418
Depressive psychosis 304
Diabetes mellitus 211–5
  chemical 211
  classification 211–2
  clinical 211
  neonatal 394
  in pregnancy 213–4
    effect on diabetic state 212
    effect on fetus 213, 393–4
    effect on infant 215
    effect on placenta 97
    effect on pregnancy 213
    indications for induction of labour 237
    latent 211–2
    management of labour 214
    management of pregnancy 213–4
    management of puerperium 215
    maternal mortality 215
    potential 212
  signs and symptoms 211
Diaphragm as contraceptive 420
Diaphragmatic hernia, neonatal 386
Diarrhoea, neonatal 395
Diazepam (valium) in eclampsia 196
Dibenyline (phenoxybenzamine) 201
Dichloralphenazone (Welldorm) 152
Diet
  during first stage of labour 151
  during pregnancy 41, 51–2
    daily requirements 51
  in prolonged labour 269
  in puerperium 165–6
  in pre-conception care 8
  see also Nutrition
Digits, extra 383
Discus proligesus 84
District Health Authorities 413
District Management Team 414

District Medical Committee 414
Doriden (glutethimide) 152
Down's syndrome 390–1
Drugs
  advice 9, 37
  causing respiratory centre dysfunction 343
    antidotes 345
  during pregnancy 41, 467
Ductus arteriosus 314
Ductus venosus 313
Duodenal atresia 387
Dyspnoea, neonatal 396

EACA (epsilon amino caproic acid) 186
Eclampsia 195–8
  aetiology 195
  convulsions 195–6
  delivery 197–8
  differentiation from epilepsy 230
  indication for induction 237
  management 196–8
  maternal mortality 198
  nursing care 197
  observations 197
  perinatal mortality 198
Ectopic pregnancy 178–9
  secondary abdominal 179
  tubal 178
Edward's syndrome 391
Electrophoresis, blood 40
Embolism, air 286
  amniotic fluid 285–6
  pulmonary 286, 301–2
Emergencies, obstetric 274–86
Emphysema during pregnancy 229
Employment
  Act 1980 407, 408
  following childbirth 407–9
  in pregnancy 407–9
  Protection (Consolidation) Act 1978 407
  rights 408
Endocrine factors in pregnancy 29
Endometrium
  anatomy and physiology 64–5
  changes during pregnancy 69
Endotracheal intubation 345–6
Engorgement, breast 297
Entonox apparatus 153
Enzymes, placental 324–5
Epilepsy in pregnancy 230–1
  differentiation from eclampsia 230
  maternal mortality 231
  status epilepticus 231
  treatment 230–1
Episiotomy 158–9, 286
  face presentation 261
  indications 158
  prolonged labour 272
  technique 159
    perineal infiltration 159
  types of incision 158
Epispadias 388
Epsilon amino caproic acid (EACA) 186
Erb's palsy 349
Ergometrine 160, 173, 276
Erythroblastosis fetalis 97
Escherichia coli causing pyelonephritis 203
Estimated date of delivery 35
Estrovis (quinestrol) 167
Ethinyl-oestradiol 417
Ethnic groups 403–7
Exchange transfusion, *see* Transfusion, exchange
Exercises, postnatal, in puerperium 165
Exomphalos 388
External caphalic version 253–4
  contraindications 253
  dangers 254
  procedure 254
Eyes
  infection, postnatal 376
  injury, birth trauma 350

Face presentation 259–61
  cause 259
  dangers 261
  diagnosis 259–60
  management 261
  mechanisms of labour 260–1
  positions 259
Facial palsy 349
Fainting in pregnancy 26
Fallopian tubes
  anatomy and physiology 80–2
  blood supply 81
  changes in pregnancy 82
  changes in puerperium 82
  ectopic pregnancy 178
  lymphatic drainage 83
  nerve supply 83
  relations 83

Fallot's tetrology 385
Falx cerebri 126
Family
  benefits 440–2
  history 33
  income supplement 440
  planning services 416
  in society 401–7
    extended 401
    nuclear 401
Family Practitioner Committees 415
Fat
  fetal 312
  necrosis, birth trauma 350
Feeding
  artificial (bottle) 340–2
    complementary to breast 339
    hazards 340–1
    preparation and giving 341–2
    requirements 340
    sterilisation of utensils 342
  pre-term infant 356–7
  see also Breast feeding
Ferrivenin 217
Ferrous preparations
  in folic acid deficiency 218
  in iron deficiency anaemia 217
Fertilisation 15, 87
  controlling 419–20
Fertility history and pregnancy 34
Fetus (fetal) 309–30
  abnormality, indication for induction 237
  in antepartum haemorrhage 186
    dangers 187–8
  at risk factors 318–20
  axis pressure 76
  blood sampling 329–30
    complications 329
    Singer test 330
  breathing, ultrasound 321
  circulation 312–5
    temporary structures 315
  development 309–11
  distress 325–30
    aetiology 325–6
    fetal causes 326
    labour, first stage 328–30
      second stage 330
    management 328–30
    maternal causes 325
    placental causes 325
    signs 326–8
    twin pregnancy 209
    umbilical cord causes 326
    uterine causes 326
  growth and maturity 315–6
    assessment 316–18
  head, engagement 47, 48
    first stage of labour 147, 148
  heart, after amniotomy 239
    auscultation 48
    changes 326–7
    first stage of labour 146
    monitoring, ultrasound 321
    in occipitoposterior position 250
    physiology 312–5
    in prolonged labour 270
    second stage 156
    sounds, normal 21
    in twin pregnancy 206
  hormone excretion 322–4
  malpresentations 252–65
    abnormal lie 263–4
    breech 252–9
    brow presentation 261–3
    compound 265
    face presentation 259–61
    shoulder presentation 263–4
  and maternal diabetes mellitus 213
  and maternal pyelonephritis 204
  and maternal renal disease 200
  movements 21, 311, 321
  papyraceus 205
  physiology 311–12
  placental function and well-being 320–25
  position 47
  in pre-eclampsia 193, 194
  presentation 47
  second stage 156
  size 47
  skull 119–27
  vault 120–4
    bones 120
    diameters 121–3
    fontanelles 121
    head circumferences 124
    internal structures 126–7
    moulding 124–5
    regions 121
    scalp 125
    sutures 120–1
  well-being, assessing 320–5
Flagyl (metronidazole) 232
Folate requirements 218

Folic acid
deficiency in pregnancy 218
in epilepsy 230
Follicle stimulating hormone 13, 14
releasing factor 13, 14
Follicles, ovarian 83–5
Folvite 218–9
Fontanelles, fetal skull 121
Forceps delivery 286–8
indications 288
preparations 288
types of forceps 287
Forewaters, formation 76
rupture 238
see also Amniotomy
Fostering 431–2
Fractures, birth trauma 349
Frusemide with morphine sulphate in pulmonary oedema 224
Fundal dominance 73
Fundus
height 46
palpation 46
uteri 64

Galactosaemia 365, 380–1
clinical features 381
diagnostic test 380
management 381
Gastroenteritis 376
Gastrointestinal tract
abnormalities, neonatal 386–8
changes at birth 333
postnatal infections 376–7
in pregnancy 30
Gastroschisis 389
Genes 467
mutation 470, 471
Genetic(s) 466–77
code 467
counselling 469
environmental factors 467
factors 467
inheritance, mode 470
variation 470–1
prenatal screening and diagnosis 473–6
amniotic fluid analysis 474–5
biochemical studies 475
cytology 475
fetoscopy 475–6
maternal blood sampling 474
methods, 474–6
ultrasonic examination 474
terminology 476–7
Genital system, male 420–2
Genital tract, female
anatomy and physiology 57–85
external 57–60
blood supply 60
internal 60–85
see also specific organs
infection 295–6
causative organisms 295–6
complications 296
management 296
maternal mortality 296
signs and symptoms 296
Genitalia in pre-term infant 353
Genitourinary tract, abnormalities 388
Glasses, free 442
Glucocorticoids in pregnancy 29
Glucose-6-phosphate dehydrogenase 221, 365
Glutethimide (Doriden) 152
Glycosuria in pregnancy 30, 212
Gonadotrophic hormones in pregnancy 29
Gonads, female, *see* Ovaries
Gonorrhoea and pregnancy 234–6
complement fixation test 235
danger to infant 235, 376
penicillinase production 235–6
strains 235–6
treatment 235–6
Graafian follicles 13, 14, 84–5
Gravindex test 20
Grief (grieving) 461–2
stages 461–2
Group-B streptococci 233
neonatal 378–9
Growth of fetus 315–7
amniotic fluid studies 317
assessment 316–7
radiology 316
ultrasound 317
weight 316

Haemoglobin
and anaemia of pregnancy 215, 217
concentration at birth 332
conversion from fetal to adult 332
estimation 40, 49
in pregnancy 29

Haemoglobin (*cont.*)
in puerperium 164
variants 219
Haemoglobinopathies in pregnancy 219–21
management 220, 221
Haemolytic anaemia
in infant 364
in pregnancy 221
Haemolytic disease of the newborn 364
see also Rhesus
Haemorrhage
antepartum, *see* Antepartum haemorrhage
labour, third stage, control 78, 160
and obstetric shock 280, 281
postpartum, *see* Postpartum haemorrhage
in pre-term infant 354
Haemorrhagic disease of the newborn
aetiology 371
clinical manifestations 371
prevention 337, 371
treatment 371
Haemorrhoids in pregnancy 25
Handicap register 398
categories 398,425
Handicapped children, services 436–8
Head circumference and appearance, pre-term infant 351–2
Health Care Planning Teams 414
Health education 426
Health visiting services 416
Heart
defects, congenital 402–4, 372, 384–5
disease, *see* Cardiac disease
rate in pregnancy 28
fetal, *see* Fetal heart
Heartburn in pregnancy 24, 30
Hegar's sign 19
Height 38
Hepatic immaturity, in the newborn 364
Herpes genitalis 233
Hexoestrol diproprionate 167
Hiatus hernia 387
High risk groups 43–4
conditions presenting at pregnancy 44
high parity 44
multigravida 44
primigravida 44
Hindwaters, formation 76
rupture 238
Hirschsprung's disease 387
History, background 32–7
contraception 34
family 33
fertility 34
medical 33–4
menstrual 34–5
obstetric 35–7
surgical 34
Home assessment, for confinement 44–5
early transfer 44
Hookworm infestation in pregnancy 218
Hormones
administration, in
induction of labour 239–41
management 241
excretion during pregnancy 321–4
human chorionic gonadotrophin 321
human placental lactogen (somatomammotrophin) 322
oestrogen 322–4
placental enzyme production 324–5
progesterone 324
in pregnancy 29
Human chorionic gonadotrophin, *see* Chorionic gonadotrophin
Human placental lactogen, *see* Placental lactogen
Humerus, fracture at birth 349
Hydatidiform (vesicular) mole 97, 104, 176–7
clinical features 177
diagnosis 177
HCG levels 177, 321
follow-up care 177
management 177
and pre-eclampsia 192
Hydrallazine (Apresoline)
in eclampsia 196
Hydrocephaly, neonatal 389
Hydrocortisone 293
Hydrops fetalis 365
Hydroxyprogesterone caproate (Primolut Depot) 172–3
Hyperemesis gravidarum 188–9
aetiology 188

Hyperemesis gravidarum (*cont.*)
clinical signs 188–9
management 189
Hypernatraemia, neonatal 396–7
Hypertension
during pregnancy 190–1, 198–9
aetiology 199
associated disorders 190–1
essential 199, 229
management 199
and heart disease 223
in pre-eclampsia 191
essential 192
Hypertonic uterine action 245–6
Hypnosis during labour 55
Hypnotics, during first stage of labour 152
Hypocalcaemia
in light-for-dates infants 359
neonatal 396
Hypofibrinogenaemia
and antepartum haemorrhage 186
and postpartum haemorrhage 275
Hypogastric arteries 315
Hypoglycaemia
in light-for-dates infants 359
maternal, effect on fetus 213
neonatal 393, 396
in pre-term infant 353
Hypothrombinaemia
after birth 332, 371
in haemorrhagic disease of the newborn 371
prevention 337
Hypospadias 388
Hypotensive drugs in pre-eclampsia 194
Hypothermia
in light-for-dates infants 359
in pre-term infant 353
Hypothyroidism
diagnostic test 338
Hypotonic uterine action 244
Hypoxia
causing birth trauma 347
extrauterine 343
intrauterine 268, 325–30
aetiology 325–6
labour, first stage 328–30
second stage 330
signs 326–8
see also Asphyxia neonatorum

Icterus gravis neonatorum 365
Identification at birth 334
Imferon 217–8
Immaturity, neonatal 251–7
Immunisation programme 426
Immunoglobulin, Anti-D 367–8
Immunological tests for pregnancy 20
Imperforate anus 388
Implantation, controlling 423
Inborn errors of metabolism 379–81
Incontinence, in puerperium 297
Infant
feeding, teaching 341–2
see also Feeding
light-for-dates 351, 357–9
mortality rate 450–1
pre-term 351–7
Infection
in cardiac disease 222, 223
in diabetes mellitus 213
neonatal 371–9
barrier nursing 375
causative organisms 374
environment 375
equipment 375
Group-B streptococci 378–9
investigations 378
meningitis 378
mothercraft 375
personnel 374–5
prevention 374
sites of infection 376–8
treatment 378
prenatal 371–4
prevention, pre-term infant 355–6
in light-for-dates infant 359
in prolonged labour 269
see also specific headings
Inherited diseases 471–3
dominant 471
incidence 471–3
recessive 471
sex-linked 472
Innominate bones, anatomy 108–9
Insulin 211, 214, 215
Intermittent positive pressure ventilation 363
Intrauterine death
in diabetes mellitus 213
indication for induction of labour 237
Intrauterine devices 423
Intravascular transfusion 368

Intravenous feeding, pre-term infant 357
Investigations in pregnancy 39–40
Iron deficiency anaemia 216–8
  causes 216
  daily requirement of iron 216
  diagnosis 217
  haemoglobin 218
  iron levels 217
  management 217–8
  signs and symptoms 216
  types of iron 217–8
Iron supplements, pre-term infant 357
Irritation, cerebral, *see* Cerebral irritation
Ischiococcygeus muscle 116
Ischium 106
Isthmus, uterine 64

Jacquemier's sign 18, 62
Jaundice
  in hyperemesis gravidarum 189
  neonatal 363–70
    ABO incompatibility 365
    causes 364–5
      rare 365
    conjugation of bilirubin 364
    degrees 363
    haemolytic disease of the newborn 364–5
  hepatic immaturity 364
    infection causing 365
    kernicterus 370
    management 367–9
    'physiological' 364
    phototherapy 370
    Rhesus incompatibility 365–9
  in pre-term infant 353–4
Jectofer 217
Joint Consultative Committees 415

Karyotype 468, 475
Kernicterus 370
Kidney
  anatomy and physiology 134–8
  blood supply 138
  effects of pregnancy 143
  effects of puerperium 143
  fetal 311
  functions 138
  lymphatic drainage 138
  nephron, structure 136
  nerve supply 138
  relations 135
  structure 135–6
  supports 135
  urine formation 136–7
Kjelland's forceps 287
Kleihauer test 183, 367
Klumpke's palsy 349
Konakion (phytomendadione) 353, 390

Labia majora, anatomy 57
Labia minora, anatomy 57–8
Labour
  abnormal 237–94
    lie and shoulder presentation 263–4
  accelerated 268
  active management 268
  and antepartum haemorrhage 184–6
    maternal care 185
  changes in uterus 70–9
  and heart disease in pregnancy 224–5
  induction 237–41
    amniotomy 238–9
    hormone administration 239–41
    indications 237–8
    methods 238–41
  management 144–62
    first stage 144–55
      abdominal examination 146, 147, 150–1
      acceleration phase
        multigravida 72
        primigravida 71
      admission 144
      analgesics 152–5
      assessment of progress 147–51
      diet 151
      drugs 152–5
      history 145
      hypnotics 152
      latent phase
        multigravida 72
        primigravida 71
      observations and recordings 145–6
      position 151–2
      tranquillisers 155
      vaginal examination 147–50, 151
    second stage 155–9
      analgesia 157

Labour (*cont.*)
episiotomy 158–9
general care 156
instructions 156
observations and recordings 156
position 156
delivery 157
preparation 157
conduct 157–9
third stage 159–61
drugs 160
placenta and membranes, delivery methods 160–1
inspection 162
postnatal care, immediate 161–2
mechanism 127–8
onset, causes 70–1
physiology, first stage 72–6
second stage 76–77
third stage 77–8
precipitate 245
premature 241–3
causes 241–2
definition 241
drugs 242–3
induced 242
management, labour 243
pregnancy 242
spontaneous 242
preparation for 52, 54–5
hypnosis 55
Leboyer method 55
natural childbirth 54
psychophysical 54
psychoprophylaxis 54–5
prolonged, active management 267–73
definition 267
fetal distress and danger 268, 271
first stage 268
causes of delay 268
monitoring progress 270
observations and recordings 269–70
specific management 270
management, active (accelerated labour) 268
maternal distress 268
maternal mortality 271, 273,
nursing care 269
second stage 272–3
third stage 273
uterus, rupture 271
in shoulder presentation 264
trial 266–7, 269
contraindications 266–7
management 267
in twin pregnancy 208–10
management 208–10
Laceration, causing haemorrhage 278
Lactation, inhibition 167
Lactogen, placental 322
Langhan's layer and cells 90
Language problems 403, 407
Lanugo 311
pre-term 353
Largactil (chlorpromazine) 304
Lead toxicity 405–6
Leboyer method of delivery 55
Lecithin concentration 318
sphingomyelin ratio 318
Legs, in puerperium 164
Length, pre-term infant 351
Leucorrhoea during pregnancy 62
Levatores ani muscle 115–6
Ligaments, pelvic, anatomy 107–8
uterine 66–7
changes during pregnancy 70
Lightening 22
Light-for-dates infants 357–9
causes 358
characteristics 358
complications 359
management 359
sequelae 359
Lignocaine 154, 159
Limb, deformity or absence 384
Lithopaedion 174
Local Authority Social Services Act 1970 426–7
Local Government Act 1972 427
Local Supervising Authorities 491–3
Lochia in puerperium 171
Long curved forceps 287
Lovsett manoeuvre 257
Low birth weight infants 350–9
classification 351
light-for dates 357–9
causes 358
characteristics 358
complications 358

Low birth weight (*cont.*)
management 359
sequelae 359
pre-term infants 351–7
causes 351
characteristics 351–3
complications 353–4
management 354–7
Luteinising hormone 13, 14
releasing factor 13, 14

Malposition of the occiput 249–52
Malpresentations 252–65
cord prolapse 282
see also Fetus
Mammary glands
anatomy and physiology 129–32
blood supply 130
changes during pregnancy 131
changes during puerperium 131–2
involution 138
lymphatic drainage 131
nerve supply 131
structure 130
see also Breast
Manic-depressive psychosis, puerperal 304
Marcain (Bupivocaine) 154
Mastitis 297–8
Maternal and Child Walfare Act, 1918 32
Maternal distress 268
Maternal mortality, *see* Mortality, maternal
Maternity
benefits 42, 438–9
allowance 42, 439
grant 42, 439
pay 439
leave 408–9
services, NHS 415
Mathews Duncan method of placental separation 77
Maturity of fetus 315–8
amniotic fluid studies 317–8
assessment 316–8
pulmonary surfactant 318
radiology 316–7
ultrasound 317
weight 315–6
Mauriceau-Smellie-Veit manoeuvre 257–8, 273
Mean corpuscular haemoglobin 29
in iron deficiency anaemia 217
Mean corpuscular volume 29
in iron deficiency anaemia 217
Meconium
after birth 337
in breech presentation 255
formation 333
ileus 387
passage into amniotic fluid 328
physiology 311
Meiosis 86, 468, 477
Membranes
artificial rupture, *see* Amniotomy
delivery methods 160–1
inspection 162
during first stage of labour 148
separation 77
Mendelson's syndrome 292–3
Meningitis, neonatal 378
Meningocele, neonatal 389
Menstrual
cycle 13–14
history 34–5
phase 13
period, last (LMP) 34–5
and calculation of estimated date of delivery 35
regulation 435
resumption after birth 79, 85, 168
Mental state in puerperium 165
Mestranol 417
Metabolic rate in pregnancy 30
Methoxyflurane (Penthrane) and air 153
Metronidazole (Flagyl) 232
Microcephaly, neonatal 389
Micturition
frequency, in pregnancy 18, 22, 24
physiology 141–2
in puerperium 164
Midwife (midwifery) 502–4
administration of analgesia 496
code of practice 442–4, 489, 498–501
Committee 491
definition 502
history 487–94
management of stillborn infant 447
notification of intention to practice 495

Midwife (*cont.*)
practice 495–501
records 497
responsibilities 495–501
Rules 495–8, 488–9
sphere of practice 502–4
supervision 491–3
supervisor 493–4
treatment outside province 495–6
Midwifery Care Plan 38, 144
Midwives Acts 1902, 1951 487, 488
Milk
breast, *see* Breast milk
free 441
Mineralocorticoids in pregnancy 29
Misuse of Drugs Act 1971 152
Regulations 1973, 1974 499
Mitosis 86, 468, 477
Mitral stenosis 222
Mogadon (Nitrazepam) 152
Mole
blood 174
carneous 174
hydatidiform, *see* Hydatidiform mole
stony 174
Mongolian blue spot 336
Mons veneris, anatomy 57
Moro reflex 336, 349
Mortality
maternal 453–7
abortion 176, 454
amniotic fluid embolism 286, 454
anaesthetic complications 291–2, 293
asthma 229, 456
cardiac disease 226, 227
causes 453–4
decline 454, 455, 457
diabetes mellitus 215, 456
eclampsia and pre-eclampsia 198
ectopic pregnancy 179, 454
enquiries into 455
epilepsy 231, 456
haemorrhage 187, 280, 454
hypertension 198, 454
labour, complications 273
notification, certification and registration 455
postpartum haemorrhage 280
puerperal sepsis (genital tract infection) 296, 454
pulmonary embolism 302, 454
suicide 304–5, 456
uterus, rupture 271, 454
perinatal cord presentation and prolapse 282
rate, infant 450–1
neonatal 449–50
perinatal 448
causes 448–9
predisposing 449
Moulding, fetal skull 124–5
Multiple pregnancy 205–10
aetiology 206
diagnosis 206
HCG levels 321
labour 208–10
complications 209–10
malpresentations 207
management 207
labour 208–9
pre-eclampsia 192
and preterm infant 210, 351
prognosis 207
puerperium 210
twins 205–6
types 205–6
Muscle(s) injury, birth trauma 350
tone, pre-term infant 353
Musculoskeletal system, abnormalities 382–4
Myelomeningocele, neonatal 389
Myometrium
anatomy 65
changes during pregnancy 69

Naevi 384
Narcan(naloxone) 153, 345
National Boards for Nursing midwives, and Health Visiting 490
National Health Service
cervical cytology 423–4
child health services 424–6
family planning services 416–23
health education 426
health visiting services 416
historical 410–2
maternity services 415
reorganisation 412–5
school health and dental services 425
vaccination and immunisation 426
National Health Service Act, 1946, 1980 32, 411

National Health Act (*cont.*)
Reorganisation Act 1973 32, 412, 427
Natural childbirth 54
Nausea and vomiting in pregnancy 17, 20, 24
Necrotising enterocolitis 376–7
Neonate, neonatal
complications 343–98
asphyxia neonatorum 343–6
'at risk' 397–8
birth trauma 346–50
cold injury 392–3
congenital abnormalities 381–92
diabetes mellitus 394
diabetic mother 393–4
general problems 394–7
inborn errors of metabolism 379–81
infections 371–9
postnatal 374–9
prenatal 371–4
jaundice, *see also* Jaundice 363–70
low birthweight infants 350–9
mortality rate 449–50
normal 331–42
Apgar score 334, 344
artificial feeding 337, 340–2
breast feeding 337, 338–40
care at birth 334–7
first ten days 337–42
eleventh to twenty-eighth day 342
examination 335–6
first feed 337
observations and recordings 337–8
physiological changes at birth 331–3
screening tests 338
Nephritis, chronic glomerular in pregnancy 200
Nephron, structure 136
Nerve injury, birth trauma 349
Neuralgia, brachial, in pregnancy 26
Neurohormonal reflex 132
Neurotic states, puerperal 303
Nidation, controlling 423
Nipple, anatomy 129
cracked 297–8
during pregnancy 131
in puerperium 166
Nitrazepam (Mogadon) 152
Nitrous oxide and oxygen 153
Nursery school 430
Nurses, Midwives, and Health Visitors Act 1979 489, 491, 492
Nutrition, pre-term infant 356–7
see also Diet
Nutritive function of placenta 99
Nystatin 232

Obesity in pre-eclampsia 192
Obstetric history 35–37
Occiput, malposition 249–52
definition 249
diagnosis 250
labour, outcome 250–2
persistent 251
prognosis 250
Oedema
during first stage 145
in pre-eclampsia 191, 194, 195,
during pregnancy 38, 45
pulmonary, in heart disease of pregnancy 224
Oesophageal atresia 386–7
Oestrogen
excretion 322–4
associated with pre-eclampsia 323
levels 323–4
measurement 322–3
production 100–1
Oligohydramnios 105
Oliguria
in eclampsia and epilepsy 230
in pre-eclampsia 192
One-parent families 427
benefit 440
Operative procedures 286–91
Operculum 68, 76
Ophthalmia neonatorum 376
Ortolanis's test 382
Barlow's modification 382
Os uteri
during first stage of labour 148
effacement and dilation 75–6
Osiander's sign 19, 23, 62
Osteomalacia 249
Ovaries
anatomy and physiology 82–5
attachments 82

Ovaries (*cont.*)
blood supply 83
changes during pregnancy 85
changes during puerperium 85
follicles 83–5
lymphatic drainage 83
nerve supply 83
relations 83
structure 83
Ovulation 15, 85
controlling 417–9
in puerperium 85
Ovum
fertilisation and implantation 85–8
fertilised, segmentation 87–8
maturation 15
Oxygen
administration, in resuscitation 345, 346
therapy in respiratory distress syndrome 362–3
Oxytocin 132, 160, 161, 173
infusion, in induction of labour 239–40
management 241
Oxytocinase, levels, indications 325

Pacemaker, uterus 72
Palpation during pregnancy 46–9
Palpitations in pregnancy 26
Palsy
Erb's 349
facial 349
Klumpke's 349
Paracentesis 104
Paraesthesia in late pregnancy 26
Parenthood preparation 43, 51–5
Partograms 145
Partographs 149, 244
Patau's syndrome 391
Patent ductus arteriosus 384
Pelves, pelvis, pelvic
abnormal 246–9
abnormalities of spine, hip joints, and lower limbs 249
android 247–8
anthropoid 248
contracted 247–8
developmental 249
disease or injury 249
fractured 249
justominor 247
Naegele's 249
platypelloid 248
Robert's 249
anatomy 105–14
angles 114
assessment in cephalopelvic disproportion 266
axis 113
bony, anatomy 105–8
cavity 110–2
diameters 111–2
diaphragm 115–6
in first stage of labour 149
floor 114–9
inlet 108–110
diameters 109–110
joints, anatomy 107
ligaments, anatomy 107–8
outlet 112–3
diameters 112–3
planes 113
Penicillin
in cardiac disease 224
in gonorrhoea treatment 235–6
in syphilis treatment 234
Penthrane (methoxyflurane) and air 153
Perimetrium anatomy 65
Perinatal mortality rate 448
causes 448–9
predisposing 449
Perineum, perineal
body 118
changes, in labour 118–9
in pregnancy 118
during puerperium 119, 164,
muscles 117–8
Perspiration during pregnancy 42
Petechiae, birth trauma 350
Pethidine 152–3, 155, 161
in labour, heart disease 224
Pethilorphan 153
Phaeochromocytoma in pregnancy 201
Phenobarbitone 230
Phenoxybenzamine (Dibenyline) 201
Phenylketonuria 379–80, 471
cause 379
diagnostic tests 379–80
diet 380
management 380
untreated, clinical features 380
Phlebothrombosis 300–1

Phototherapy in jaundice 368, 370
Phytomendadione (Konakion) 363, 390
Pigmentation, skin, in pregnancy 19
Pituitary gland in pregnancy 29
Pituitary necrosis 279–80
Placenta, placental
  abnormalities 96–8
  abruption
    abdominal examination 182–3
    aetiology 181
      bleeding 180
      combined 180
      complications 186–7
      concealed 180
      differential diagnosis 182–3
      management 183–6
      renal failure, acute 187
      revealed 180
      signs and symptoms 182–3
  accreta 96
    and postpartum haemorrhage 278
  battledore 98
  bipartita 96
  bleeding, after expulsion 276
    before expulsion 276
  calcification 97
  circumvallata 96
  delivery, methods 160–1
    controlled cord traction 160
    fundal pressure 161
    maternal effort 161
  development 90–3
  diseases 97
  in fetal distress 325
  functions 98–101
    assessment 320–5
    barrier 100
    endocrine 100–1
    excretory 100
    nutritive 99
    respiratory 99
    transfer 99
  hormonal excretion 100–1, 321–4
  increta 96
  infarctions 97
  inspection 162
  lactogen, human (somato-mammotrophin) 322
    functions 101, 322
  manual removal 278
  membranacea 96
  praevia 181–8
    abdominal examination 182–3
    bleeding 182
    causing post partum haemorrhage 275
    differential diagnosis 182–3
    management 183
    placental localisation 184
    signs and symptoms 182–3
  retained, and PPH 277–8
  separation 77–8
    and descent 77–8
    premature, in twin delivery 209
  signs of separation and descent 161
  site, bleeding from 274–7
    see also Postpartum haemorrhage
  succenturiata 96
  at term 94–5
  tissue changes 97
  transfer 99
  tripartita 96
Plasma fibrinogen concentration 29
  depletion 186
Playgroups 429
Pneumonia, neonatal 377
Polarity, uterine 74
Polydactyly 383
Polyhydramnios 103–5
  acute 104
  aetiology 103
  chronic 104
  clinical features 103
  complications 104–5
  contraindicating amniotomy 238
  and cord prolapse 282
  and diabetes mellitus 213
  indication for induction of labour 238
  pre-eclampsia 192
  and pre-term infant 351
  in twin pregnancy 207
Postnatal
  care 163–8
    preparation 52
  examination 168
  infections, *see* Infections, postnatal
  see also Neonate
Postpartum haemorrhage 274–9
  causes 274–5
  coagulation disorder 277
  definition 274

Postpartum haemorrhage (*cont.*)
diagnosis 275
following antepartum haemorrhage 187
from laceration 278
from placental site 274–5
management 275–7, 277, 278
manual removal of placenta 278
mortality 280
observations 276
obstetric shock 281
placental causes 275
primary 274–9
retained placenta 277–8
secondary 299
twin pregnancy 208
Preconception care 7
Pre-eclampsia 191–5
aetiology 191
clinical course 192
complications 192–3
and diabetes mellitus 213
hypertension 191
hypotensive drugs 194
indications for induction of labour 194, 237
management 193–5
observations 194
oedema 191
predisposing causes 192
proteinuria 191
severe 195
signs 191
symptoms 192
twin pregnancy 207
Prefixes used in obstetrics 2–3
Pregnancy 17–55, 171–210, 211–3
abnormal 171–210
advice 40–2
auscultation 48–9
care 32–50
first trimester 17–30
general examination 38–9, 45
high risk groups 43–4
investigations 39–40
late (third trimester) 22
midpregnancy (second trimester) 20–22
medical disorders 211–36
minor disorders 24–7
multiple, *see* Multiple pregnancy
normal 17–55
signs and symptoms 17–24
obstetrical examination 39
history 32–7
palpation 46–8
physiology, general 27–31
place of confinement 43
preparation for parenthood 51–5
prolonged 237
psychological aspects 458–60
Rhesus incompatibility 367
see also Rhesus
signs and symptoms 17–24
sociological aspects 401–7
tests 20
hormonal 20, 321
immunological 20
thirty-fourth week 49
thirty-sixth to thirty-eighth week 45
twenty-eighth week 49
visits, frequency 45
Prenatal screening and diagnosis 473–6
Pre-school child, community services 424–5
Prepuerin test 20
Prescriptions, free 43, 441–2
Presentation 47
breech, *see* Breech presentation
brow, *see* Brow presentation
face, *see* Face presentation
first stage 147, 148
secondary brow or face 251–2
Pre-term infant 351–7
causes 351
characteristics 351–3
complications 353–4
management 354–7
nutrition 356–7
observations and recordings 354–5
prevention of infection 355–6
respiration 354
temperature, regulation 355
mother-infant relationship 357
Primary Health Care Teams 414
Primitive mesenchyme 90
Primolut Depot (hydroxyprogesterone caproate) 172–3
Progesterone 101
serum levels 324
urinary levels 324
uterine therapeutic system 418
Progestogen 417
Prognosticon test 20

Prolactin 131, 167
Promazine (Sparine) 155
Prostaglandin
  infusion in induction of labour 240
  method 240–1
  natural, in late pregnancy 68, 71, 240, 243
  oral 241
  vaginal 240
Proteinuria
  in diagnosis of epilepsy and eclampsia 242
  in pre-eclampsia 200
'Prune belly' syndrome 389
Pruritus vulvae in pregnancy 26
Pseudo hermaphroditism 388
Psychological aspects of
  labour 459
  postnatal period 459–60
  pregnancy 458–9
Psychophysical preparation for childbirth 55
Psychoprophylaxis 55–6
Psychosis, puerperal 302–5
  care of baby 305
  conditions 302
  indications and influences 302
  mortality, maternal 304–5
  psychoses 303–4
  types, neurotic states 303
Ptyalism in pregnancy 26–7
Pubis 106
Puerperium (puerperal)
  abnormal 295–305
  and heart disease 225
  infection 295–98
    breast infections 297–8
    general management and signs 295
    genital tract infection (puerperal sepsis) 295–6
    respiratory infections 298
    thrombophlebitis 298, 299–300
    urinary tract infections 296–7
  management 163–8
    discharge 168
    education, supervision and advice 167
      general care 165–7
    mental state 165
    observations and recordings 163–5
    postnatal examination 168
  sepsis, following antepartum haemorrhage 187
    see also Genital tract infection
  following twin pregnancy 210
Pulmonary embolism 301–2, 454
Pulmonary oedema, in heart disease of pregnancy 224
Pulmonary sarcoidosis 228
Pulmonary surfactant 71, 318, 353, 360
Pulmonary tuberculosis, *see* Tuberculosis, pulmonary
Pulse
  in antepartum haemorrhage 183, 185
  during first stage 145
  in puerperium 163
Pyelonephritis in pregnancy 202–4
Pyelonephritis, chronic, in pregnancy 199–200
Pyloric stenosis 387

Quadruplets 205, 206
Quickening 21
Quinestrol (Estrovis) 167
Quintuplets 205, 206

Rachitic pelvis 249
Reflexes
  in pre-term infant 353
  in light-for-dates infant 358
  in normal neonate 336
Regional Health Authorities 413
Regional Team of Officers 413
Renal
  agenesis 388
  diseases in pregnancy 201–4
    bacteriuria 202
      asymptomatic 202
    causative organism 203
    chronic 199–200, 229
    clinical features 203
    fetal prognosis 204
    follow-up care 204
    management 203–4
    maternal prognosis 204
    predisposing factors 202–3
    pyelonephritis 202
  failure, acute 187
  tract, changes at birth 333
    in pregnancy 30
Reporting Officer 432
Respirations, maintenance, pre-term infants 354

Respiratory
centre, dysfunction 343–4
difficulties, neonatal, dyspnoea 396
diseases in pregnancy 227–9
asthma 229
chronic bronchitis and emphysema 229
pulmonary sarcoidosis 228
pulmonary tuberculosis 227–8
distress syndrome 353, 360–3, 396
acidosis, correction 362
cause 360
diagnosis 360
general care 361
incidence 361
management 361
oxygen therapy 362–3
in pre-term infant 353
prognosis 360–1
temperature control 361
ventilation 362–3
function of placenta 99
infections 298
rate at birth 331–2, 337
system, abnormality, neonatal 404
changes at birth 331–2
postnatal infections 377
in pregnancy 30
Rest during pregnancy 41
Resuscitation of newborn 345–6
Retained placenta, and PPH 277–8
Retraction, uterine 74
ring 74–5
Retrolental fibroplasia in pre-term infants 354
Rhesus
factor investigation 39, 49
(incompatibility) haemolytic disease of the newborn 365–9
causing jaundice 364–5
exchange transfusion 369
indication for induction of labour 237
isoimmunisation 366–7
management 367–9
at delivery 367, 368
of pregnancy 367–8
Rhythm method 419
Ritodrine hydrochloride 242–3
Rotation, in occipitoposterior position
long anterior 250
short posterior 250
Rubella
antibodies 40
effects 372, 467
risk to fetus 372
screening 9, 40
vaccination 9, 426

Sacrum, anatomy 106–7
'Safe' period 419
Salbutomol 242
Salivation, excessive, in pregnancy 26–7
Sarcoidosis, pulmonary, in pregnancy 228
Scalp, fetal 125–6
during labour 125–6
Schizophrenia, puerperal 303–4
School Health Services 425
Schultze method of placental separation 77
Septicaemia, postnatal 377–8
Serology 40
Sex
determination 87, 468
Sexually transmitted diseases 232–6
candidiasis 232
group B streptococci 233
herpes genitalis 233
trichomoniasis 232
Shaving, necessity 146
Sheath 419
Sheehan's syndrome (anterior pituitary necrosis) 187, 278–9
Shock, obstetric, causes 280, 281
Short curved forceps 287
Shoulder
dystocia in prolonged second stage of labour 273
presentation 263–4
cause 263
diagnosis 263
labour 264
management 264
'Show' 76
Sickle cell disease (HbSS) 471
management 220
Sickle cell trait (HbAS) 220
management 220
Sickle cell HbC disease (HbSC) 220
management 220
Singer test 330
Skeletal injury, birth trauma 349
Skin
abnormalities 384
care, at birth 334, 338
infection, postnatal 376

Skin (*cont.*)
injury at birth 350
pigmentation in pregnancy 19
in pregnancy 31
Sleep
during pregnancy 41
in puerperium 165
Smoking
during pregnancy 37, 40
preconception 9
Social
class, classification 409
security 438–42
services 426–38
structure 401–2
Somatomammotrophin, *see* Placental lactogen, human
Souffle, uterine 21
Sparine (promazine) 155
Special Care Baby Unit 243, 346, 355, 359
Spermatozoon, anatomy and physiology 86
Sphingomyelin 318
Spina bifida neonatal 389–90
occulta 389
varieties 389
Staphylococcus albus causing pyelonephritis 203
Statistics, vital 444–57
Status epilepticus in pregnancy 230–1
Stelazine (trifluoperazine) 304
Sterilisation 420
female 420
male 420
Sternomastoid 'tumour', birth trauma 350
Steroid inhibitors causing jaundice 365
Stilboestrol 167
Stillbirth
causes 447
predisposing 447
certification 447
midwife's duties 447
notification 447
rate 446
registration 447
Stony mole 174
Stools, following birth 338
Streptococcus faecalis, causing pyelonephritis 203
Striae gravidarum 31
Suicide, maternal 304–5, 456
Sulphadimidine in pyelonephritis 203–4
Supervisor of Midwives 493–4
Supine hypotension 26, 28
Supplementary benefits 441
Supplements, pre-term infant 357
Surfactant 71, 318, 353, 360
Sutures, fetal skull 119–24
Syncitiotrophoblast 90, 101
Syndactyly 384
Syntocinon (Oxytocin) 160
in labour induction 239–40
management 241
Syntometrine 157, 160
Syphilis and pregnancy 233–4
diagnosis 234
effect on fetus 234, 373
effect on pregnancy 234
Reiter Protein Complement Fixation Test 40, 234
stages 233–4
treatment 234
Venereal Disease Reference Laboratory (VDRL) Slide Test 40, 234
serological test 40
Syphilitic placenta 97
Syringomyelocele, neonatal 389

Tachycardia, fetal 326
Talipes 383
management 383
Temperature
body
control in respiratory distress syndrome 361
during first stage 145
intrauterine 311
maintenance at birth 334, 345
in puerperium 163
recording at birth 334, 353
regulation at birth 333
in pre-term infant 355
room, pre-term infant 355
Tentorial tear 347
Tentorium cerebelli 126
Terminology, basic 1–2
Tetrology of Fallot 385
Thalassaemia 220–1
management 221
Thromboembolic disease 299–302
Thrombophlebitis 299–300

Thrombosis, deep vein 300–1
Thrush 232
Thyroid gland in pregnancy 29
Thyroid stimulating hormone 101
Total parental feeding 357
Toxoplasmosis 374, 467
Transfusion, exchange 369
  complications 369
  infection 369
  ischaemic lesions 369
  procedure 369
  sequelae 369
Transposition of great vessels 385
Transverse arrest, deep 251
Trauma, birth *see* Birth trauma
Trial of labour 266–7, 269
  contraindications 266–7
  management 267, 269–70
Tricloryl (Triclofos) 152
Trichomoniasis 232
Triclofos (Tricloryl) 152
Trifluoperazine (Stelazine) 304
Triplets 205, 206
Trisomy syndromes 390–1
Trophoblast 88, 89–93
Tubal abortion 178
Tube feeding, pre-term infant 356–7
Tuberculosis, intrauterine infection 373
  pulmonary
    complicating pregnancy 227–8
    infant 228
    management
      labour 228
      pregnancy 228
      puerperium 228
Turner's syndrome 391
Twins
  aetiology 206
  binovular 205, 206
  diagnosis 206
  effects of pregnancy 207
  labour 208
    management 208–10
      complications 209–10
        first stage 209
        second stage 209–10
  locked 209–10
  monoamniotic 206
  puerperium 209
  types 205–6, 206
  uniovular 205–6
Type I dips (early decelerations) 327
Type II dips (late decelerations) 327

Ultrasonography 19
Ultrasound
  fetal
    breathing monitoring 321
    growth 316, 317
    heart monitoring 321, 327
Umbilical cord
  anatomy and physiology 95
  battledore insertion 98
  care at birth 334
  care after birth 338
  and fetal distress 326
  presentation and prolapse 280–3
    causes 281–2
    conditions involving 280–1
    diagnosis 282
    management 283
    mortality rate 282
    prognosis 282
  velamentous insertion 98
Umbilical hernia 388
United Kingdom Central Council for Nurses, Midwives and Health Visitors 153, 155, 489, 490, 491, 495
Ureter, anatomy and physiology 138–9
Urethra, anatomy and physiology 142–3
  effects of labour 143
  effects of pregnancy 144
  effects of puerperium 144
Urinalysis 39, 45
  during first stage 146
  in pre-eclampsia 194
  in pyelonephritis 203
Urinary tract
  anatomy and physiology 133–43
    development 133
    effects of labour 143
    effects of pregnancy 143
    effects of puerperium 143
    see also Kidney, Ureters, Urethra
  infection 296–7
  neonatal 377
Urine
  after birth 337
  formation 136–7
  incontinence 297
  retention in puerperium 297

Uterus (uterine)
  action, abnormal 243–6
    Bandl's ring 245
    constriction ring 246
    hypertonic 245
    hypotonic 244
    incoordinate 245
    precipitate labour 245
    tonic 245
  anatomy and physiology 63–79
  bimanual compression 276
  blood supply 66
    changes during pregnancy 69
  changes, during normal labour 70–8
    during pregnancy 67–70
    during puerperium 79
  contractions, *see* Contractions
    Couvelaire 180
    in primary postpartum haemorrhage 275
  growth in pregnancy 20, 22, 46, 67
  inversion 284–5
    causes 284
    degrees 284
    diagnosis 284–5
    management 285
    prognosis 285
    signs and symptoms 284
  involution 79
    in puerperium 164
  ligaments 66–7
    changes during pregnancy 70
  lymphatics 66
  nerve supply 66
  relation 67
  rupture 271
    maternal mortality 271, 454
  second trimester 20
  segments, upper and lower 74
    polarity 74
    retraction ring 74–5
  souffle 21
  tubes, *see* Fallopian tubes

Vaccinations 426
  programme 426
Vacuum extractor 288–9
  'chignon' 347
  indications for use 289
  in fetal distress 330
Vagina, vaginal
  anatomy and physiology 60–2
  blood supply 62
  changes
    in pregnancy 62
    in puerperium 63
  discharges physiological and pathological 231–3
  examination 39, 49–50
    in antepartum haemorrhage 183, 184, 185
    in breech presentation 255
    in brow presentation 262
    in face presentation 260
    indications 63
    labour, first stage 147–49
      technique 147–9
    in occipitoposterior position 250
    postnatal 168
    in prolonged labour 270
  introitus (orifice) anatomy 58
  lymphatics 62
  nerve supply 62
  pH 62
  in pregnancy 18
    changes 62
  relations 62
  secretions 61
Valium (Diazepam) in eclampsia 196
Varicella, neonatal 373
Varicose veins in pregnancy 25, 45
Vanillylmandelic acid (VMA) 201
Vasectomy 420
Venereal disease 233–6
  gonorrhoea 234–6
  syphilis 233–4
Ventilation in respiratory distress syndrome 362–3
Ventouse extractor 288–9
  causing 'chignon' 347
  in fetal distress 330
Venticular septal defect 384
Vernix caseosa 311
  pre-term 353
Vertex, positions 150
Vestibular bulbs, anatomy 59
Vestibule, anatomy 58
Villi
  anchoring 93
  chorionic 91
  nutritive 93
  primitive 91
Viruses, neonatal infections 372–3
Vital statistics 444–57
Vitamin K synthesis 332, 371

Vitamin supplements, pre-term infant 357
  welfare 441
Voluntary organisations 442
Vomit, inhalation 292–3
Vomiting
  neonatal 394–5
  observations 394–5
  types and causes 395
  in pregnancy 17, 20, 24, 188–9
Vulva
  anatomy and physiology 57–60
  and perineum in puerperium 165
  shave 146
Vulvovaginitis, and diabetes mellitus 213

Weight
  at birth 334, 338
  gain, excessive 191, 194, 223
  in pregnancy 30–1, 38, 45
  pre-term infant 351, 352
  see also Low birth weight infants
Welfare milk and vitamins 441
Welldorm (dichloralphenazone) 152
Winding the baby 342
Women
  employment 407–9
  role 401–2
    in society 401–2
    in ethnic groups 404, 406–7
Work during pregnancy 41, 408
Wrigley's forceps 287

X-ray examination 22
X-ray pelvimetry 270

Heasitate
Hesitate